Psychology Revivals

Psychology and Mental Health

First published in 1950, *Psychology and Mental Health* describes the origin of behaviour disorders and the psychoneuroses especially as regards their causes in early childhood. Most psychologists agree that such disorders as hysteria, sex perversion, the obsessions and anxiety states, as well as many behaviour disorders and delinquencies, find their roots in childhood experiences. If this is the case it should be possible to prevent them from developing into full-blown neurotic disorders which may take years to cure.

The purpose of this book is to describe the early causes of these disorders with a view to their treatment, but more particularly with a view to their prevention. As mental health is the concern not only of the doctor but of the parson and the priest, of the teacher and the parent, this book is written in non-technical language as far as the demands of accuracy will allow. It embodies the result of over thirty years' experience in the treatment of patients suffering from these disorders, and the views here maintained, which differ somewhat from the other analytic schools, are illustrated with clinical examples throughout. This book is a reissue originally published in 1950. The language used reflects its era and no offence is meant by the Publishers to any reader by this republication.

W0113274

Psychology and Mental Health

A Contribution to Developmental Psychology

J. A. Hadfield

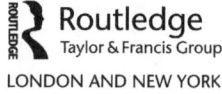
Routledge
Taylor & Francis Group

LONDON AND NEW YORK

First published in 1950
by George Allen and Unwin

This edition first published in 2022 by Routledge
2 Park Square, Milton Park, Abingdon, Oxon, OX14 4RN
and by Routledge
605 Third Avenue, New York, NY 10017

Routledge is an imprint of the Taylor & Francis Group, an informa business

© George Allen and Unwin, 1950

Publisher's Note
The publisher has gone to great lengths to ensure the quality of this reprint but points out that some imperfections in the original copies may be apparent.

Disclaimer
The publisher has made every effort to trace copyright holders and welcomes correspondence from those they have been unable to contact.

A Library of Congress record exists under LCCN: 50014388

ISBN: 978-1-032-19568-1 (hbk)
ISBN: 978-1-003-25985-5 (ebk)
ISBN: 978-1-032-19578-0 (pbk)

Book DOI 10.4324/9781003259855

PSYCHOLOGY
AND
MENTAL HEALTH

A Contribution to Developmental Psychology

by

J. A. HADFIELD
M.A.(Oxon), M.B.Ch.B.(Edin)

Lecturer in Psychopathology and Mental Hygiene
University of London
Late Director of Studies,
Tavistock Clinic, London (1935–46)

LONDON
GEORGE ALLEN AND UNWIN LTD

FIRST PUBLISHED IN 1950
SECOND IMPRESSION 1952
THIRD IMPRESSION 1960

THE ITALIAN EDITION
is published by Cherardo Casini Editore, Rome

THE SWEDISH EDITION
is published by Albert Bonnier Forlag, Stockholm

THE SPANISH EDITION
is published by Ediciones Morosta, Madrid

PRINTED IN GREAT BRITAIN
in 11 point Plantin type
BY BRADFORD AND DICKENS
LONDON, W.C.1

CONTENTS

PART I
GENERAL

CHAPTER I

INTRODUCTORY:

THE SCOPE OF MENTAL HEALTH

IT is generally agreed by psychopathologists that the psycho-neuroses such as Hysteria, Sex Perversions, Anxiety States, Obsessions, Depression, and many Behaviour disorders are traceable in their origin to abnormal conditions in the early years of life.

If this is so, it should be possible by providing the right conditions in childhood to prevent the occurrence of these disorders.

It is the function of psychological medicine to cure these disorders; it is the function of mental hygiene to prevent them.

Mental Hygiene is concerned with *the maintenance of mental health and the prevention of mental disorder*. Its main function is to maintain mental health; but to do so it sets out to discover the causes of mental disorders, so as the more effectively to prevent them. In practice mental hygiene is also made to include the early *treatment* of mental disorders, that is to say, to prevent their further development.

The prevention and early treatment of these psychoneurotic disorders is a matter of the greatest urgency; first, because of their wide prevalence in the population (there are few people who have not some form or another of psychoneurotic disorder); also because they cause the greatest incapacity, suffering and distress. But chiefly because once developed the psychoneuroses are difficult to cure by our present methods of treatment, and require a great expenditure of time and money. There are certainly not enough doctors the whole country over to treat all those requiring treatment. To cure these conditions in later life is extremely difficult; to prevent the formation of these complexes in childhood is comparatively easy. The only adequate way, therefore, of dealing with the psychoneuroses is to prevent them.

Mental hygiene is a *positive* science in that it sets out to establish a condition of healthy-mindedness: it is a *normative* and not a pure science, because it has a norm or standard at which it aims, namely that of mental health: it is an *applied* science in that it seeks to discover and apply the principles for the establishment of mental health and happiness in the individual and in the community.

But if the aim of mental hygiene is the establishment of mental health we must ask ourselves, what *is* mental health? What do we mean by healthy-mindedness?

We cannot define it as the absence of mental disease, or freedom from symptoms, for we cannot tell what is abnormal till we have a standard of the normal by which it can be judged. Is it abnormal to be angry? Is jealousy always to be regarded as pathological? Nor can we define mental health, as some do, as "freedom from anxiety." For some people are depressed without being in any way anxious, and some have a hysterical paralysis and are quite cheerful, for they have temporarily solved their problem. If there was an original anxiety it is no longer operative. On the other hand it is very natural to be anxious in a blitz.

In general terms, then, we may say that *Mental Health is the full and harmonious functioning of the whole personality.*

Let us take the analogy of the body: what do we mean by physical health? By physical health we surely mean that all the organs of the body are functioning fully and completely, and in harmony with one another.[1]

So it is with the personality as a whole. We have at birth a number of innate potentialities (often called instincts) each of which has its functions to perform, rage to overcome a foe, sex to procreate the species, and maternal love to care for the off-spring. We then *acquire* an infinitely larger number of potentialities and dispositions for the performance of new functions of service to the personality. The full expression and co-ordination of all these functions are necessary to a healthy life. But this co-ordination can come about only by directing them towards a common end or aim of the personality as a whole. These then are the three requirements of mental health: full expression, harmonization, and the direction to a common end of our native and acquired potentialities.

Full expression is necessary, for these potentialities are the "material" of our personality, necessary to our biological adaptation in life and necessary to a strong will and character. If they are *suppressed*, the personality suffers, and we become inefficient, weak of will, and feeble in character; we are good but sapless. If they are completely repressed they may later emerge in abnormal forms as the psychoneuroses.

---

[1] Socrates, in Plato's *Republic*, Book IV, defines health thus—"Now to produce health is to put the various parts of the body in their natural relations of authority or subservience to one another, whilst to produce disease is to disturb this natural relation."

Harmonization is also necessary; for each of these potentialities has its own aims and functions to perform, and these often conflict within one another, rage conflicting with sex and fear with both. More important, they may conflict with the aims and ends of the personality as a whole, leading to dispeace and disharmony. The harmonization and co-ordination of all these tendencies is therefore necessary to peace and health of mind.

We may again take the analogy of physical health: we should not call that man healthy in whose body all the organs are working completely and fully, but each on its own—the heart pumping away, the lungs breathing hard, the skin perspiring, the muscles tense—irrespective of the other organs. Every organism, whether plant, animal or man, functions as a whole, as well as in its individual parts. The body is an organism, and should work as a functional unity; and if any organ of the body works out of harmony with the rest, the result is not health but physical disorder. Indeed, there is in the body a system, the nervous system, whose specific function it is to integrate the whole so that all the various functions of the body work harmoniously together; the central nervous system bringing it into right relations with the outside world, the autonomic nervous system bringing it into right relations with itself, so that all parts of the body work as a unity towards the common end. As with the body, so with the personality as a whole. The personality is an organism, that is to say a group of units functioning towards a common end. It is therefore necessary for mental health that all our dispositions, native and acquired, should, like the organs of the body, work not only completely and fully, but harmoniously together. If those potentialities, whether rage, sex or ambition, function completely, but independently of the rest of the personality and its ends, they would produce not mental health but mental chaos and unhappiness, and ultimately the breakdown of the personality, as in the psychoneuroses.

The common end. Since ,these potentialities are dynamic tendencies, they can be harmonized and unified only by being directed towards a common end or aim. But there is in the personality as a whole, as there is in the body, a unifying principle for the direction of all these potentialities. In every individual there is a natural tendency to *identification*, corresponding to imitation in the lower animals but far more potent, by means of which the child takes over the moods, ideas and standards of life from those on whom it depends, and so, irrespective of any teaching or training, establishes within itself a standard of behaviour which acts as a co-ordinating principle towards which its whole life and potentialities may be directed. Ideals, aims and purposes in life are necessary to mental health.

But obviously some aims are more capable of directing the potentialities of the personality than others: personal ambition, libertinism or strict ascetism, for instance, are capable of engaging some of our energies but not others, and are therefore unsatisfactory from the point of view of mental health and indeed are often found to lead to psychoneurotic disorders. The problem of what are the right ends is the concern of ethics. But we naturally ask "right for what"? It would be an interesting subject of ethical study to investigate what are the right ends, not from the metaphysical point of view, nor that of the greatest good of the greatest number, but right ends judged from the point of view of mental health, namely those most capable of directing and co-ordinating the functions of the whole personality to health and happiness.

We may therefore define *mental health* more fully as *the full and free expression of all our native and acquired potentialities, in harmony with one another by being directed towards a common end or aim of the personality as a whole.*

Mental health as thus defined is *dynamic* not static, it is the *functioning* of the whole organism towards an end, not the attainment of a certain state: it is not stagnation but a harmony of movement, living and active.

This standard of mental health in principle *applies to everyone,* but in so far as we are all born with different potentialities, not to speak of those we acquire from our varied experiences in life, it *differs in practice for each individual.* Thus what is conducive to the health and happiness of a man of a placid temperament may be quite unsuited to the happiness of another: the potentialities of a man brought up in one set of circumstances, may best be directed towards business achievement, the interest of another is in a quiet and studious life; one woman finds her health and happiness in her domestic and family life, another in a career, whereas a third is more content with social service. The purpose of vocational guidance is to discover for what work each individual is most fitted, not merely for efficiency, but for individual health and happiness.

Whilst therefore the principle of mental health is the same for all, it works out differently for each person, and gives scope for the play of individuality; it does not turn out everyone to a pattern, but allows of infinite variety in our personalities.

The acceptance of such a standard of mental health with its

recognition of the varieties of human personality should also make for the greater toleration of our fellows, for we are not all alike, nor must we expect others who are temperamentally different to find their line of life in what may seem right for us, nor even to have the same moral standards.

This standard of mental health is also our *aim in treatment* which is not merely the abolition of a symptom, but the restoration of the whole personality to full functioning and happiness. In the psychoneuroses, this is best done by analytic treatment, the purpose of which is to release the repressed emotions causing the neuroses, and redirect them to the service of the personality as a whole.

This conception of mental health also applies to the *mental hygiene of childhood* the aim of which should be to give to the child the opportunities for the fullest development of his personality, by the full expression of his dynamic tendencies and their direction to healthy and voluntarily chosen ends.

Other standards. This standard of mental health differs from other standards which are, however, all legitimate in their way and for the purposes for which they are designed, such as the standards of biological efficiency, social adaptation and ethical ideals.

The standard of *biological adaptation* is a very common and useful one: it is a standard of fitness. If a man is fit for work, if he is a success in life, if he makes good, then that is all that can be asked of him. It is the standard adopted by those industrialists whose only concern is the maintenance of their workpeople in a state of efficiency; it is the standard of the medical officer in the Services whose main concern is the return of the men as fit for duty; it is the standard of the type of schoolmaster who thinks of little else than that his pupils should win scholarships, and distinguish themselves at the University, irrespective of their mental health.

This biological standard is a very practicable one; for it is the first business of man to live, and since, as in all the higher organisms, it is by his mind and wits that he adapts himself to his environment, success is a good test at least of his ability.

But obviously we cannot take biological efficiency as a standard of mental health, for there are thousands of men and women who are most efficient but who are most unhappy; they are very successful, but full of anxiety; indeed, it is often their very anxiety which drives them on to their success. They break down in the end, which proves that they never were really mentally healthy.

Another popular standard is that of *social adaptation*. This also is a useful standard, for we live in communities, and to live effectively should be socially well adapted to our fellows. It is also a fairly correct criterion of abnormality, for we found in the military Neuropathic Hospital that the psychoneurotic individual is one who is more commonly ill-adapted to his social environment than he is to his work.[1] But social adaptation is not an adequate standard of mental health, for on the one hand there are many people who by temperament and constitution are reserved and yet within the bounds of normality, whilst there are others who appear well adapted to their social environment and get on well with their fellows, but this may itself be due to an inferiority complex leading to ingratiation as a compensation.

Indeed, as we shall have ample opportunitites to observe, the neurotic is often one who is too "social," and has become neurotic because he has been led to conform too rigidly to social standards to the detriment of his mental health. He is so anxious to win the approval of others that he suppresses his own individuality and thereby does violence to his personality, with the result that he ultimately develops a neurosis which is a rebellion of his natural self against these too rigid demands. Not only so, but obviously the medical psychologist cannot be content with a sociological standard, since what is wrong in one society such as polygamy and stealing is regarded as smart in a neighbouring community: what to one person is ordinary politeness, to another person is being hypocritical: in one girl's school it is considered *infra dig* to have a "crush" on another girl, in another school it is the fashion and those who have not such a passion are looked down upon. Mental health cannot be made to depend on changing social fashions.

Mental health also differs from *ethical standards* in so far as they are conceived as objective standards of right and wrong, for there are unfortunately many men who are very moral but suffer from nervous indigestion, very religious but suffer from phobias or sex perversions. Goodness does not appear to be a protection against neurosis. In any case, moral standards change as a child progresses from one phase of development to another, so that the standards say of a boy of 14 whose main concern is loyalty to the gang are very different from those of the same individual at the age of 16 with his abstract idealisms, or of 24 whose main

---

[1] See *British Medical Journal*, February 28 and March 7, 1942. "War Neuroses." We found that 60 per cent were previously well adapted to school life and work, whereas there were only 40 per cent socially well adapted.

devotion is to his family. Standards differ not only for each individual but at his different stages of development.

But these standards of behaviour, though different from the standard of mental health, are not incompatible with it; indeed, mental health embraces them. The efficient man is not necessarily mentally healthy, but the mentally healthy man will be efficient, since mental health implies the utilization of all his potentialities under the direction of the will, and such efficiency will be devoid of anxiety. The mentally healthy man will, generally speaking, be socially well adapted because social propensities are part of the ordinary man's make up: he will desire to conform to the demands of the community in which he lives and on which he depends, but without being a slave to them. He is prepared to go against them if in his judgment these standards are opposed to the higher good of the community. But he does so not in rebellion against society as such, but for the well-being of the society he loves. So too, the mentally healthy man will be "moral" in the broad sense of the term, not merely by virtue of conformity to social standards, but because ideals, aims and purposes of some sort are necessary to mental health, for by them alone can an individual direct and co-ordinate the impulses of his personality. The mentally healthy man will be moral, though the moral man is not necessarily mentally healthy.

Mental hygiene covers *all forms of mental disorder*, including Mental deficiency, the Psychoses (insanity), Psychoneuroses and behaviour disorders, all of which fall short of the standards of mental health as we have defined it. *The mentally deficient* is mentally unhealthy because he is *constitutionally deficient* in some of those potentialities possessed by the ordinary individual; he is lacking in social sense, in intelligence and even in the basic interests which make for self-preservation. The *psychotic* is mentally unhealthy, for although he may not be lacking in intelligence, his personality is constitutionally *unbalanced and disharmonized*, his emotions uncontrolled, his mental life disturbed, his cognitive life in his delusions, his affective life in depression or apathy. The *psychoneurotic* is mentally unhealthy because although unlike the mentally deficient he is naturally possessed of all the natural potentialities, some of these have been *repressed* owing to untoward experiences in early childhood, so that he not only loses the normal expression of assertiveness, sex or love, but these repressed tendencies, forbidden normal outlet, emerge in the abnormal forms of psychoneurotic symptoms. *Behaviour disorders*, such as delinquency, are abnormal from the

B

social and often from the mental health point of view, because the natural potentialities, though fully expressed, are directed towards *wrong ends*, not merely socially or morally wrong, but ends incapable of co-ordinating and directing the whole personality.

Although mental hygiene is concerned with all forms of mental disorder, we shall confine ourselves in this book to the psychoneuroses and behaviour disorders, not only because they are the only ones of which we have any adequate experience, but because these disorders, most of which are derived from environmental conditions in life, are far more accessible to prevention and to cure; whereas the psychoses and mental deficiency, being largely hereditary and constitutional, are far less accessible to prevention, and much less amenable to cure; and such treatments as there are, like electric shock for involutional melancholia, insulin coma for schizophrenia, and malaria for general paresis, valuable as they are, are largely empyrical, since the causes of most psychotic conditions are at present unknown.

Further, in this book *we shall lay particular emphasis upon the predisposing causes in early childhood*, since it is there, rather than in the precipitating factors in adult life, that the root causes of the psychoneuroses are to be found, and therefore prevented. In the first three or four years of life we may observe the earliest manifestations of hysteria, anxiety states, obsessions or sex perversions. If these are taken early enough they can fairly easily be rectified, so that perhaps in a few interviews we may prevent the development of a full-blown psychoneuroses, which in later life might take two or three years to cure.

Mental hygiene therefore consists of two main branches: (*a*) child psychology, which is concerned with the proper conditions in early childhood so as to maintain mental as well as physical health and avoid the *predisposing* causes of breakdown; (*b*) social, including industrial, psychology, the function of which is to provide the right conditions of work and living and so to avoid the *precipitating* causes of the psychoneuroses, social unrest and other disorders.

Both of these are necessary, for only by a thorough understanding of the causes of these behaviour and psychoneurotic disorders in childhood, can we build up sound principles of mental health; and only by providing the right conditions can we prevent the precipitation of many neurotic disorders, which, though they may be latently present, might never have developed were it not for the untoward conditions in present-day life and circumstances.

But obviously child psychology is the more radical and effective, for experience goes to prove that people do not break down with neurosis unless they are predisposed to do so, either because of an unstable constitution, or because of a neurotic disposition developed by abnormal experiences in early childhood. It is in childhood therefore that these conditions are effectively to be prevented.

These early experiences tend to form themselves into complexes by the process of repression, and when once formed these complexes become a constant source of abnormal behaviour, whatever the environment and however perfect. Complexes will compel a man to be depressed irrespective of circumstances, discontented with whatever work he takes up, to be self-conscious in any society of people, to be irrationally jealous even of his own children, to be afraid of the dark and terrified of travelling in a train, though he knows these reactions to be stupid and irrational. Social psychiatry in adult life may remove him from bad conditions and so prevent an actual breakdown; it cannot rid him of such deep-seated complexes, for when the complex is once formed it is virtually impossible to eradicate it by change of environment. Even if we succeed in removing overt symptoms like fear or depression by change of work the neurotic disposition remains and is apt to emerge at the slightest provocation. Indeed, as we shall see, complexes have this quality, that they make trouble even where there is none; and the best environmental condition in the world may be inadequate to cure the grumbling man or suspicious woman. For this they require treatment of the predisposing causes which produce the complexes, as well as the precipitating causes which produce the actual breakdown.

Such deep investigation into the predisposing causes in early childhood is of the greatest value, and not only for treatment. For it provides us with a complete picture of all the more important factors which produce a neurosis, and explains as nothing else can, the present-day morbid attitudes of the patient. Not only so, but by throwing light upon the early causes of neuroses and behaviour disorders it provides us with a clue as to their prevention, and thereby points the way to mental health.

For these reasons also we shall confine ourselves to the *psychology of the individual* rather than the influence of culture patterns. In these days of social psychiatry it is almost necessary to apologize for writing on individual psychology, but the latter still has a most important contribution to make to the solution of these problems.

There is no doubt that the social environment and culture patterns have an important influence upon the life and character of the individual, and also in the production of the psychoneuroses, as Karen Horney[1] and others have ably demonstrated. Psychopathology, it has been stated, is a failure in human relationships.

The culture patterns are particularly important in early life, since the child is dependent upon its parents for comfort, happiness and for life itself, and therefore must conform to their demands and modify its own behaviour in accordance with what society approves or disapproves. In particular it is these influences which determine the standards, aims, and ideals which as we have seen are necessary to mental health. If these demands are too lax it may lead to behaviour disorders, if too severe it often leads to psychoneuroses.

It is said, for instance, that the arrogance of the Japanese soldier is to be traced to the fact that as a little boy he is considered superior to his mother. He therefore becomes aggressive towards her, but at the same time is submissive to other males. He therefore grows up to be sadistic towards the conquered, but cringing to his conquerors and superiors. That may be true, and no one denies that such character traits (which incidentally are not true neuroses) arise from culture patterns.

But such observations are too simple an explanation of the psychoneuroses. (a) In the first place, we may find *the same reactions in many cultures*. There are many other than Japanese children who are permitted to be aggressive by their parents, quite apart from cultural patterns, and a Jew may be as arrogant as a Nazi. The difference between the way in which a Japanese or Canadian mother brings up her children may be no greater than the difference between that of the Canadian mother and her next-door neighbour. There is cruelty, strictness, kindness, tenderness and spoiling with their varying effects in different homes in every land. Indeed, there is no culture which cannot be paralleled in other cultures: so that whereas there may be *more* of such children becoming arrogant in Japan than in Canada or Scotland, it is only a matter of quantity and less of the quality of such behaviour. The number of such people in a community is most important for the sociologist and the politician since it determines that Japan goes to war. But for the psychopathologist who is concerned with the nature and causes of psychoneurotic disorders it is less important. (b) Again, when we come to study the deep-rooted causes of the neuroses, we find *the basic symptoms*

[1] The neurotic personality of our time.

and causes of the psychoneuroses to be the same whatever the culture.
We have under treatment·at the time of writing an American,
an Arab, an Egyptian, a Russian, an Australian and a Swiss, as
well as various brands of British. But what surprises us is not
the difference that the cultural patterns have made, but the fact
that when one gets down to the root of the trouble, the fundamental
causes are ridiculously the same. Indeed, one soon forgets that
one is analysing someone who belongs to a different culture from
one's own. Every child of whatever race fundamentally needs love,
protection and security, and the denial of these produces anxiety
and insecurity the world over. The *symptoms* arising from these
cases are also the same, the claustrophobia of the American being
identical with that of the Egyptian, and the depression of the
Englishman not very different from that of the Russian. Guilt is
the same in individuals of all races, although the moral standards
concerning which they feel guilty may vary in different cultures,
as they do indeed from one Englishman to another. Aggressiveness
and hate can be repressed and its consequences feared in the
aboriginal as in the Swiss. There seems to have been as much
neurosis in the gay city of Vienna as in Cheltenham (Eng.) or
Boston (U.S.A.). (c) Not only do we find the same reactions in
different cultures but we find *varying reactions in the same culture.*
It is the *individual* differences in upbringing which determines
why it is that even in the same culture one child reacts by being
arrogant, another by being affectionate, one becomes mentally
healthy, one neurotic.

Thus individual psychology and social psychology are inextric-
ably related, and social culture is no more important in fashioning
the individual, than is the individual in the creation of the social
pattern.

Social psychology is after all the psychology of individuals; it is
the reaction of the individual to a particular environment, the
environment of a group. The individual behaves very differently
when in a group than when alone, and the study of such reactions
constitutes crowd psychology: but it remains the psychology of
the individual nevertheless—unless we believe in a group mind.
No society has yet been known to exist which did not consist of
individuals.

Not only so, but when the social psychologist makes his survey
of social trends he has to apply to individuals for his information
and data. Even the conclusion drawn about the Japanese had to
be discovered from the study of individual Japanese children and
the way they were brought up. So in this book we study the

individual to discover the deep-seated causes of disorders not only in the hope of curing that individual of his disorder, and of learning how to prevent such disorders, but for the light that they throw on the social problems of our time. But it must be left to those more competent in sociology than ourselves to apply these discoveries to social problems.

But there is a still closer link between the individual's problems and those of society, for by the process of identification already referred to, the individual incorporates into himself the standards of society, so that he becomes a *duality* consisting of his *ego* or natural self (developed as the result of the reaction of his native potentialities with environmental experiences) and his *super-ego*, which is the incorporation of society within his personality.

The relation between the individual's ego and his super-ego is therefore a replica and reduplication of the relation between the individual and society; and the problems arising from the conflict of the individual with society are precisely of the same nature as the problems arising from the conflict between the individual and himself, between his natural self or ego and his moral self or super-ego. If therefore we can work out in the individual the causes of disorder and breakdown, which are in fact found to be the result of the conflict between the ego and the super-ego, we might find some clue to the causes of neurosis and unrest in the community; and if we can discover in the individual a solution to this problem, it may throw some light on the solution of these problems in the community.[1]

No apology is therefore needed for studying these problems in the crucible of the individual personality. The atom which now dominates world politics was first split in a Cambridge laboratory; in a wind tunnel of a factory are learned the secrets of airplanes that now span the globe: so in the individual soul are to be found all the conflicts that rage humanity, and there also can be found their solution.

But before we can discover the principles for the maintenance of mental health and the prevention of mental disorder, we must understand as clearly as possible the basic causes of these disorders. This is the function of *psychopathology, which is the scientific study*

---

[1] For instance: just as the personality who has no aim and purpose in life disintegrates, so the nation devoid of leadership lands in chaos and disorder. On the other hand, just as a moral super-ego which is too rigid represses the natural tendencies instead of directing and controlling them, and produces psychoneurotic disorders, so restrictive laws that go beyond public opinion lead to open defiance of the law, as in racketeering in America during prohibition, and black-marketing in the post-war world in Europe.

of morbid states and processes. As we cannot forecast correctly the weather on the earth's surface without knowing conditions in the stratosphere, so we cannot diagnose or adequately treat problems on the surface of behaviour without knowing what is going on beneath the threshold of consciousness.

In this book, therefore, we deal primarily with psychopathology, and investigate the causes of mental disorder; but we do so with a view to mental health, which is our aim and purpose. That is why we have retained the term "Mental Health" rather than "psychopathology" in our title, which is intended to express the aim rather than the subject matter of the book. Moreover the use of terms of normality in our title is intended to convey that we regard the abnormal not as a separate entity, but as aberrations from the normal, which can only be understood by an understanding of the normal. It is with that in mind also, that we open our discussion with a chapter on the "Sources of Behaviour," as at least a brief gesture towards the normal.

This book contains the substance of some of the lectures given by the author as Lecturer in Psychopathology and Mental Hygiene in the University of London for more than twenty years. Its publication is at the request of a number of students and a few friends who have expressed a wish to have a more permanent record of the lectures. The delay in publication has been due not only to the fact that he finds writing a very laborious task, but mainly to a desire to subject the views here contained to further clinical investigation which has now extended to more than thirty years in the treatment of these disorders.

Brought up in the Schools of Academic Psychology,[1] the author belongs to no specific school of psychopathology, though profiting by all. In philosophic outlook, and in personal regard, he is most attached to Professor Jung, by whose method (though not by Jung himself) he was analysed. But as a mode of treatment he has found the analytical psychology of Jung less effective than more radical methods to be later described. Each psycho-physician must employ the methods and instruments most suited to his personality.

It will be obvious that he owes much to Freud, the originator

[1] Under Professor Smith in Edinburgh, for what experimental psychology was then taught, and Professor William McDougall at Oxford, with whom he did some research work in the relations of anthropology to psychology, soon to be abandoned for the more alluring and fruitful field of psychopathology. Six years Arts and Theology at Oxford before studying Medicine, gave him also some appreciation of ultimate values.

of the modern approach to psychological medicine, as indeed do all psychopathologists, however much they may disagree with him. He uses Freud's method of *free association* for the discovery of unconscious experiences, and he finds Freud's *mechanisms*, of conflict, repression, projection, symptom formation and the rest, of the greatest value in the explanation of human behaviour and of the psychoneuroses.

But in *psychopathology* he differs from Freud (as indeed he differs from Jung and Adler) in many fundamental respects, and as these differences have an important bearing on the prevention of these disorders, that is his excuse for inflicting yet another book on a long-suffering public.

CHAPTER II

THE SOURCES OF BEHAVIOUR

HUMAN nature is very complex; and this complexity of human behaviour is largely determined by the fact that we are the products of evolution, and carry within ourselves ancestral traits and forms of motivation from the lowest forms of animal life to the highest stages of human development.

Biologically every individual "climbs up his own geneological tree" and goes through the main phases of evolutionary process, starting from the single-celled organism at fertilization, through countless stages to the aquatic phase before birth when we have gills (which in some persons persist as such after birth, and in all of us persist in the Eustachian tube now serving as a passage from the mouth to the middle ear). We then reach the simian stage about the time of birth (some people are born with tails), when we ape the monkey and have abnormal powers of clinging, which tend to pass away after the third week of life. We finally reach the distinctively human phase, after which we pass through various stages of maturation, through childhood and adolescence, until we reach adult life.

At every stage of evolution the organism is motivated by a specific form of behaviour, at one time by purely physio-chemical mechanism, at another by tropism, reflex action and then instinct; and as it advances, new and more complicated modes of behaviour are developed adapting it more adequately to the emergencies of life, such as intelligence, reason and purpose.

This process is at first exceedingly rapid so that we go through aeons of evolution in the nine months before birth, through thousands of hazardous years of development in the first two or three years of life, and then progress far more slowly through adult life, after which the forces of evolution begin to spend themselves, till we decline into old age.

But as the organism progresses through these phases of evolution, it not only develops new forms of motivation but retains within itself the modes of behaviour and ancestral traits through which it has passed; so that when we reach the final stage in man we find his behaviour motivated not only by forms of behaviour characteristic of the highest stages, like reason or purpose, but by

residues of all the earlier stages of evolution through which he has
passed in his upward progress.[1] This accounts for the extreme
complexity with which we are confronted in human nature. At
one time his behaviour is determined by his *physiological* state,
and he is depressed because of his low blood pressure, or ready
to take on anything because he is in good health. At other times
his actions are determined by his *biological urges* like his sex
impulses, or aggressiveness. At another time these same impulses
are guided by the *conscious pursuit of ends*, such as the determination to achieve an ambition or to educate his family, or by
reason in the choice of ends.

Not only so but in one and the same act he may be *motivated
by several of these at once*. Activities such as that of sex which have
operated through most stages of evolution run the whole gamut
of motivations at once, from the purely tropistic tendency which
draws together the two human beings, so that they feel that they
are "fated" to meet one another; through physiological tension
which demands sexual relief; reflex action which comes from
physical contact; the pursuit of ends such as the begetting of
children, to the highest sublimation in a love which is prepared
to make the supreme sacrifice for the one loved. The various
phases of evolutionary development are so mingled in the same
act that it is often difficult in any particular case to discern what
is the real motive of any act without taking all these into consideration. The result is that we tend to choose out the motives
most likely to be approved by others, and therefore ascribe to our
actions "reasons" more plausible than the real ones. This is the
process of *rationalization*, a process met with in the neuroses, the
paralysed hysteric saying he cannot fight because he is paralysed,
whereas he is paralysed because he is afraid to fight. He not only
bluffs others but fools himself.

Our behaviour is still further complicated by the fact that as
often as not our acts are determined by motives of which we are
entirely *unconscious*, this being partly due to the fact that the earlier
modes of behaviour, like the tropistic or reflex action, are themselves unconscious and automatic; but also to the fact that a
higher phase, in order to establish itself, often refuses to admit
the operation of a lower, and represses it out of consciousness.
There are a thousand things we do every day, but do not know
why we do them. It is not surprising that man's ordinary conduct

[1] I am indebted to my chief, Professor Mace, for pointing out that Aristotle
held that whilst the lower function can operate independently of the higher, the
higher presupposes and incorporates the lower.

often appears irrational and contradictory, his motives often incomprehensible and his reactions to any particular situation uncertain and incalculable. The "inconsistency of human nature" which has so often been remarked upon, is often due to the fact that our actions are at various times determined by these different levels of behaviour, of which we may be entirely unaware. The saint and the glutton live in us all.

It is inevitable that there should be *clashes between these various phases* of development, so that a tropistic urge to wander or travel may be inconsistent with our duties to our family; emotion may urge us to act contrary to the demands of reason; and the natural urge to grow up and accept the responsibilities of life may be strongly resisted by the infantile desire to cling to dependence and security. Such conflicts are inevitable, and are of little consequence as long as they are conscious; they are necessary to progress. But where there are clashes between various motivations which are themselves unconscious, these subterranean eruptions may result in the gravest disturbances of human behaviour, and produce neurotic disorder.

A brief sketch of the more important of these sources of behaviour will therefore help us to understand human conduct better, and incidentally offer an explanation of some of the differences between the more important schools of psychology, such as the Behaviouristic, the Dynamic, or the Gestalt schools: for we shall come to realize that the differences between these schools are often based, not so much upon a radical disagreement, but upon the varied emphasis that each lays upon one or another of these forms of motivation. To the physiologically minded, behaviour is based on reflex action and can be entirely explained in terms of conditioned reflexes; or on the endocrine glands. Others emphasize the importance of "instincts" which may be defined as generalized responses of the whole organism as distinct from local reflexes: whilst the philosopher asserts the paramount importance of man as a reasoning animal. Each school naturally finds much to support its views since undoubtedly much of human behaviour is determined by each of these. But if we regard man from the point of view of evolutionary development, we shall realize that there is truth in all these schools of thought, *except in so far as they claim to be exclusive.* They err not so much in emphasizing the importance of these specific forms of behaviour, as in claiming them to be a complete explanation of man's complex behaviour and even cast reflexions on the honesty of those who differ from them. The philosopher who is impatient of acknowledging the irrational in man, thereby shows himself to be irrational; the physiologist who talks of "pain" is talking of something of which he has no physiological evidence; and the strict behaviourist who denies the existence of consciousness is denying the means by which he makes such an observation.

We cannot explain human conduct in terms of one formula, nor are we aiding the advancement of knowledge by emphasizing one aspect of human life to the exclusion of others. No man, however learned, can have the knowledge to be master of all forms of man's complex behaviour, but he may at least have the wisdom to recognize the value and importance of the contributions of others in this complex field.

TROPISM

As an illustration of the primitiveness of our mental attitudes and behaviour we may take the case of a Tropism. Tropism is defined as the tendency of an organism to move in a particular direction (Loeb). It is a form of behaviour so primitive that we find it in living organisms devoid of a nervous system; yet its influence survives in man. There is *phototropism*, the tendency of an organism, such as the shoots of a green plant, to grow towards the light, a tendency which may survive in man's attraction towards the sun, and perhaps in sun worship: and there is *geotropism*, the tendency of the roots of a tree to grow downwards towards the earth. There are biochemical causes for both these forms of movement, and in neither is a nervous system, as commonly understood, necessary. In the case of the eel the choice of a stream is said to depend on the amount of oxygen contained in its waters. Tropism is not to be regarded as the *cause* of these movements; it is merely the way in which the organism is observed to behave.

Tropism also operates in animals by means of reflex action, as in the case of the moth which flies towards the candle. This is neither a piece of sheer stupidity on its part, nor a masochistic desire to suffer pain, but a mechanical movement determined by stimulation from the rays of light entering the eye.[1]

[1] These rays, entering the eye on one side, reflexly increases the activity of the wing on the opposite side, and therefore turns the insect towards the side from which the light comes. If it overshoots the mark the light enters the other eye, and the opposite wing being stimulated the moth is again turned towards the light. These movements are purely mechanical in the sense that they are initiated by external stimuli acting upon the organism from without and determine its movements in a given direction.

Tropisms are of interest to the psychologist in throwing light on human behaviour. For instance, some of them represent primitive forms of *attraction* to particular objects, whereas others are negative tropisms which turn them away from certain objects, an instance of *repulsion*. So we have very early manifestations in behaviour of what appears later as *love* and *hate*. Indeed, Empedocles, of Sicily, writing about the year 450 B.C. maintained that the material universe was set in motion by two forces, love drawing the elements together, hate separating them. Probably many of our conscious likes and dislikes for which we can give no reason, such as our dislike for putrid smells, are determined by such tropistic influences of which we are as unaware as is the eel of the causes of its movements towards the source of a stream, into which reason does not enter, but which are nevertheless of biological importance. The significance of these tropisms in human behaviour may be illustrated in *Stereotropism*, the tendency of an organism to keep in *close contact* with another body. The starfish clings with its ventral surface to the rock; the worm burrows into the earth, not because of a geotropism, nor from a preference for the dark, but (as proved by experiment, for the worm prefers a narrow but light glass tube to a dark open one) from the tendency to have the whole of its body surface in close contact with something.

This stereotropic tendency may be observed in infants, who cling to their mothers, want to have the whole body in close contact with them, snuggle into them, almost burrow into them. To quote an example from a patient, reverting to infancy, "I am burrowing in till almost I want to be inside, enclosed in a great body on one side, and with a big arm on the other, and I want to remain there and not for anything else to happen: I want to lie and be my mother (primitive identity), and when I do not get it I hug the bed clothes." Mothers recognize this need in the infant and tuck the baby up close in its cot to make it sleep more securely. This tropistic tendency to get into closest contact with the mother has been interpreted as a desire to "return to the mother's womb." It may be this tendency which urges the sick or wounded animal, such as the domestic sheep and even man, to seek the thicket or the hole in which to hide itself and die. A boy of three getting scolded by his father said, "I crept back to a closed cupboard where I could get close and not be out in the open."

This primitive movement of the infant comes to be associated with sensuous pleasure so that the child comes to seek close contact with the mother in order to gratify this sensuous pleasure.

But that is secondary, and the tropistic tendency for such movement was present before the sensuous pleasure to which it gives rise.

This stereotropic tendency to be in close contact later subserves both protective and sexual ends. The *protective* value of this tropism is obvious in the cases illustrated, the attachment of the starfish to the rock, and the clinging movements of the infant to its mother when it is afraid. It is consciously experienced in the child as a *feeling of dependence* upon its mother, and later develops into *suggestibility*, or psychic dependence, which leads us to accept and submit to the opinions, ideas and moods of others with whom we are identified, and ultimately becomes the basis of social life.[1]

This tropistic tendency to be in close contact with others for protective purposes urges animals and men to herd themselves together into crowds and great cities, and may therefore be the basis of "gregariousness." It operates especially in the presence of a common danger, when men huddle together and are so bound emotionally that any feeling of apprehension spreads as a contagion through the whole herd, so that they act as one, whether by way of flight or attack. Even reasonable adults in a disaster like shipwreck, cling to one another for the feeling of protection it gives, although for actual protection it may be worse than useless.

This stereotropic tendency also serves *sexual functions*, as in the nuptial flight of insects, the clinging of the frog to his mate, and in the embrace of lovers. In the experience of "falling in love" the whole personality is involved, and both protective and sexual motives are combined, so that the desire to care for and protect the loved person may be as strong and even stronger than the sexual.

There are also *pathological states* associated with this stereotropic tendency. If the starfish is torn from its rock it waves its tentacles about with all the appearances of an anxiety state: if the infant in close contact with its mother is torn away from her, it gets into a similar state of distress and alarm.[2] This type of anxiety has been given the distinctive name of "separation anxiety."

The best illustration of a pathological state related to stereo-

[1] Trotter—*The Herd Instinct*.
[2] A patient reviving infantile feelings during analysis described it thus: "I felt separated, helpless and alone, like a leaf that has fallen off the tree, but hasn't yet got into the soil." Another, reviving a feeling of abandonment in infancy, waved her arms about for all the world like a starfish, searching for contact, something to cling to.

tropism is that of *agoraphobia*, the so-called fear of open spaces. This is not really, as the name implies, a fear of open spaces as such, but the dread of being isolated: the open space is feared because there is lack of contact with anyone or anything. The one thing the agoraphobic craves is to have something to hold on to: thus a patient who was terrified to cross a park or a bridge over a river alone, was given confidence and a sense of security if he held the hand of his little boy. The space remained the same; it was the contact which gave him the sense of security.[1]

We have dealt with the manifestations of stereotropism in some detail, because it suggests that a more careful study of human nature would reveal many other unsuspected evidences of such primitive tropistic tendencies operating even in adult human life, and would explain many modes of behaviour for which we have at present no adequate explanation. Man may be motivated by urges that are as unconscious and automatic in their purpose as the migration of birds or the turning of the leaf towards the light; and to follow such deep-seated feelings within ourselves (which we call our intuition), however irrational, may often be a surer guide than reason itself. We say that we go hiking at week-ends for our health, but it may be only, as with sheep, an urge to wander for pastures new.

PHYSIOLOGICAL SOURCES OF BEHAVIOUR

There can be no doubt that a great deal of our behaviour is determined by chemico-physiological processes. If there were any doubt upon that, one only has to observe the changing behaviour of an individual under increasing doses of alcohol. The loosening up of inhibitions, followed by excitement, then bad temper, then the comatose state. The allergic individual has not only a distinctive physical constitution but also a mental hyper-sensitivity. Varying amounts of thyroid produce varying degrees of dullness, brightness and fatigue. The "acidosis" child who is bright one day will be lethargic the next. The patient with latent jaundice will lose interest in life, and his interests returns when the jaundice is cured. All these constitute a person's temperament, which is the influence of the physiological constitution over the mental constitution. The shy, reserved, shut-in, sensitive, punctilious, schizothyme with the angular physical habitus is very different in temperament from the barrel-shaped extroverted cyclothyme

---

[1] See Chapter on Anxiety States.

(Kretschmer). We shall later deal with these under temperamental character traits.

A recognition of these temperamental differences as determined by biochemical influences is necessary for all those who have the care of children and who would understand the behaviour of adults, for many states of naughtiness and ill-manner are due to physiological causes. But to assume that because physiological changes can affect behaviour, *all* behaviour is due to physiological causes is to commit a logical fallacy of the crudest order.

REFLEX ACTION

While tropism may operate in the absence of a nervous system, reflex action, which we next consider, always works by means of a nervous mechanism, and has its *four* definite phases. The *afferent phase* is initiated by some stimulus from outside the body, such as heat, or the sight of prey; or from within the body, like hunger and pain. The *central changes* depend upon native dispositions already present in the organism, or such as are acquired in the course of experience, making possible specific forms of response. The *response* is of a dynamic nature and produces activities like flight, defence, attraction, seizing prey. The *end result* is an adjustment to the situation, either by changing the environment to meet the requirements of the organism, as in attack, or adjusting the organism to adapt itself to the environment, as in flight.

Various schools have emphasized each of these phases: the behaviourist and conditioned reflex school emphasizing the importance of the stimulus as determining behaviour; the association school and others, the central dispositions; the dynamic school emphasizes the responses, and the hormic school the end or aim.

The afferent phase. There is no doubt that the environment and the stimuli to which we are subjected from the outside world play an important part in deciding our behaviour, which is largely our response to those stimuli. A child, in the presence of something it fears, will become terrified; a child who is encouraged will become confident. Some schools of psychology, therefore, have based their theories of behaviour on this as the determining factor in behaviour. So extreme can be this emphasis that Watson (in the often quoted phrase) can say, "Give me a dozen healthy infants and my own specified world to bring them up in, and I will guarantee to train any one of them to become any type of specialist I might select—doctor, lawyer, artist, and even beggar-

man and thief, regardless of talents, abilities, or ancestry."
According to this theory all behaviour depends on stimulus.

Conditioned reflexes. Unacceptable as are these extreme views,
the Behaviourists have called our attention to the fact that the
number of reflexes present at birth are comparatively few in the
human child as compared with the animal, and much less fixed,
so that they can be modified in innumerable ways, as McDougall
has shown in his *Social Psychology*, and Pavlov in his work on
Conditioned Reflexes. They have proved experimentally that not
only can a response of the organism be produced by the original
stimulus, say fear from noise, but by any stimulus associated with
it in a particular way, such as darkness, so that a child *acquires* a
fear of the dark, which is not innate. By this means behaviour is
capable of infinite variation. Thus the dog instead of being made
to respond by defensive movements to a prick on the skin, can
be made to show signs of appetite; and instead of responding to
the sight of meat by a flow of saliva, can be made to respond by
defensive movements. Human as well as canine nature can be
modified indefinitely; and the old idea that you cannot change
human nature is an exploded myth. Conditioned reflexes determine
that many people take sexual pleasure in pain; whilst others acquire
a dread of innocuous things like a close space.

The obliteration of primitive and innate responses, and the
formation of entirely new responses and habits, is a fact of
importance for the social re-education of the individual.
It is scientifically used in the training of animals, and less
scientifically in the training of children. Indeed, conditioned
reflexes are, and always have been, used by mothers without
their understanding the principles governing them, as in the
establishment of "clean habits."[1] The infant in the first year is
almost a "reflex animal," and the best way of training him in
right habits is by the application of the principles of conditioned
reflexes. When however he gets to a later age of two, and develops
a "mind of his own," his aggressive impulses may break down this
nicely organized reflex system, so that the child refuses to react
in this mechanical way. Not only can physiological habits be thus
regularized without difficulty or distress, but times of sleeping
and times of waking can be thus established. Even *our desires and
pleasures can be conditioned* in this way: so the infant who is fed

---

[1] In an infant, a feed of milk produces movement of the bowels. If the child
is at the same time put on a pot, the sensation of being put on a pot will thereafter
act as a conditioned stimulus and produce a motion even in the absence of
feeding.

every two hours will get hungry every two hours; the child who is fed every four hours will become hungry every four hours and *at no other time*. We can condition ourselves to prefer classic literature to sensational, country life to town, cleanliness to dirt. Emotional reactions, say of pleasure at meeting foreigners, or generosity to those who wish us harm, may be cultivated by putting ourselves in their position, and by such means we may build up a new character.

So valuable has been this concept of conditioned reflex, that it is not surprising that some have attempted to explain the whole of human behaviour both normal and abnormal, and including the psychoneuroses, in terms of conditioned reflexes.

There is much to be said for this view. For the psychoneuroses are like conditioned reflexes in that they are not innate, though based on innate potentialities, but *originate in experiences during life*; they are *acquired* abnormal modes of response. Furthermore, like conditioned reflexes they are *disorders of function* and not of structure.

But there are objections to the use of conditioned reflexes as a wholesale explanation.

(i) It is no doubt possible to explain all human behaviour in terms of conditioned reflex: but it would also be possible to explain all human behaviour in terms of physics, of atoms, protons, and electrons, and it might be argued that there is therefore no justification for the science of physiology. But the physiologist claims that there are certain *group* activities, like the functions of the heart or the lungs which work as a unitary whole, which cannot be adequately described in terms of physics. He therefore finds it more useful to express the functions he describes in a series of terms of his own. The physiologist therefore speaks of respiration, circulation, and even of "living" processes, "nerve impulse," and uses other terms savouring of mysticism to describe certain types of reaction which the physicist would explain in quite other terms.

It is precisely the same claim that the psychologist makes. He finds the terms of conditioned reflexes inadequate to explain the whole of human behaviour, just as the physiologist finds the terms of physics inadequate for the investigation of the phenomena he describes. So the psychologist introduces conceptions of consciousness such as feelings, emotions, pleasure and pain, intelligence, aims and purposes, to describe certain group functions of the whole personality which cannot be otherwise adequately explained. Indeed, it is a great physiologist who has said, "Mind proves refractory to descriptions by physics and chemistry."[1] The value of any scientific concept is that it helps us to understand the facts presented. The term "conditioned reflexes" explains too little because it attempts to explain too much: it is not that the explanation is untrue, it is merely that it is inadequate. It omits, for instance, any reference to purpose or aim which the psychopathologist as well as the psychologist requires to explain a neuroses like a hysteric paralysis.

(ii) Again it would no doubt be possible to explain all psychopathological conditions in terms of conditioned reflexes, but there comes the time when the chain of reflexes is so complicated that the conception of conditioned reflexes no longer serves any useful purpose. It may be easy to discover how a child can develop a conditioned fear of goldfish (to use Watson's case) and also to get rid of so simple a fear by reconditioning. It is easy to explain the ordinary fear of water produced in Pavlov's dogs subjected to the flood; but such simple anxieties are a very different problem from the complicated anxiety neuroses with which we are presented by our psychoneurotic patients. The neurotic phobias, anxiety states, obsessions and sex perversions, are of so complex a nature that neither the physiologist nor the behaviourist has the means of discovering the long chain of reflexes which has led to the final state of the patient nor of discovering all the factors which go to produce it; still less can he cure them.

It is, however, precisely this complex chain of reflexes that the psychologist is able to discover by analysis, so that the long since forgotten experiences which caused the disorder, and every step in the process of the development of the psychoneurosis, are brought back to consciousness. Having discovered all the main factors of the disorder, the analyst is in a position to bring about a readjustment, reconditioning and cure of the disorder. On the other hand, we have yet to meet a case, say of true obsession or a sexual perversion, which has been cured by reconditioning alone. It is indeed a significant and surprising fact that there is at present no school of psychotherapy which sets out to cure psychoneurotic disorders by these means. To hold to the theory may give us the satisfaction of intellectual simplicity, but it is barren of practical results.

(iii) There is a further difficulty. Pavlov has shown that conditioned reflexes tend to pass away *unless they are reinforced* from time to time by later similar experiences. Therefore simple experiences of fear, from which most children suffer, fortunately do not

[1] Sherrington, *Man on his Nature*, p. 339.

alone produce the neuroses of adult life, but tend to die out when the experiences are not repeated. Why then do these fears persist, when there is no danger to reinforce them? Reinforced the fear certainly is, but the reinforcement comes not from an objective danger, but from impulses within ourselves of which we are often unconscious: these perpetuate the fear.

The main facts of the conditioned reflexes have been observed and studied under the term *Association*, namely, that if two presentations occur together, the arousal of the one tends to revive the other; so that a child who was once burnt thereafter develops a fear every time he sees a fire. A past generation has explained both normal behaviour and neurotic conditions in these terms. The essential differences between the theory of conditioned reflexes and that of association is that whereas the latter describes the phenomena in terms of consciousness, that of conditioned reflexes strictly speaking describes them in physiological terms— and only uses consciousness in the process of studying and describing them. In the second place, physiology has the advantage of measuring the reaction *quantitatively*, for instance, by the amount of saliva which flows. Moreover it has taught us much as to the ways those laws operate and added greatly to our knowledge of the laws of association.

It is well to remember, since the idea of association is in disfavour at the present time, that all analytic treatment is based on its principles, for it is by virtue of links of association between events and experiences that we can analyse a neurosis by the use of "free association" and trace back a symptom to its causes.

Most of our adult habits, our tastes, our likes and dislikes, our desires, even our aims and purposes, have been formed in this way, often by accidental occurrences in early childhood, as we discover in the process of analysis; e.g. a man's linguistic interests were traced back to the fact that his mother, to whom he was devoted, used to sing him to sleep as an infant with German and French songs. Another developed her artistic talent because, denied her mother's affection, she found her only joy in the sights and sounds and colours about her. These, however, should not be regarded as the *only* causes.

The principles of association, like conditioned reflexes, have of course been largely used in *education*: the child who associates the washing-up of dishes with the receiving of a reward, will associate washing-up with pleasure, till it becomes a habit. Children given candy when vaccinated returned surreptitiously to get a second dose of vaccination!

Some psychologists regard any kind of training of children as disastrous to their freedom: but there is nothing abnormal in the formation of such habits by these means: indeed, it is unavoidable, since the child is bound to encounter conditions in life which inevitably produce such conditioned reactions. He may therefore as well be given such reactions as experience has proved to be of social and personal value, provided it is done, as it can be, without repression and without fear. Instead of regarding the child as "naughty," we now realize that his behaviour has often been conditioned by the circumstances under which he has been brought up, and instead of scolding him, we set about forming a new and healthier reaction. Better still, we should be able to prevent a child's developing bad habits, like bed-wetting, secretiveness or cruelty, and even morbid emotions like fear, by a better understanding of these laws, and, by discovering their causes, remove them when formed.

The principle of association, like that of conditioned reflexes, has also been used to explain pathological conditions. A child at birth is afraid only of a limited number of situations, but anything that becomes associated with them in a particular manner may become the object of fear. The child is not naturally afraid of the dark, and darkness is not a primitive stimulus of fear: but the child who is awakened by noise, such as a clap of thunder, which *is* a primitive stimulus, may thereafter develop a fear of the dark, which was associated with it. The fear of the evil eye which affects so many people in their dreams, is frequently found in analysis to be derived in infancy from the look of anger of the mother or nurse. A child who is nearly suffocated with the skim of milk will thereafter get sick with milk.

Many adult psychoneuroses may be explained as the result of association. A man always got a fit when he was on a road with a grass field on one side and a ploughed field on the other, and only on those occasions; which corresponded to the original situation when he was blown up in France. Another patient always had a suspicion of kindly people, which came from the fact that his mother used to be particularly nice to him when about to coax him into doing something particularly distasteful.

On the other hand, the principles of association has been utilized for the breaking up or abolition of abnormal reactions. A boy who is afraid of diving because of a previous experience, has a penny thrown into the water and is told he can have it if he dives for it: he does so under stimulus of this reward, finds there is nothing to fear, loses his dread, and thereafter dives for the pleasure of the diving.[1] Both *rewards* to encourage action, and *punishment* to inhibit action, are based on these principles.

The typical form of treatment which is based on association is that of *Suggestion*, which sets out to break morbid associations and to form healthy ones. The man who cannot think of the after-dinner speech he has to make without nervousness, is given suggestion which associates his after-dinner speaking with the feeling of confidence: and it is remarkable how effective can be the results of such treatment.

A youth got sick if ever he tasted milk, because as a child (as was later found in analysis) he was given some Gregory's Powder in milk and got sick. It was not, of course, the milk but the powder that made him sick, but thereafter milk alone made him vomit. The discovery and breaking of this association under hypnotic suggestion cured him. A man who had a craving for opium would buy laudanum in small quantities as he passed a chemist's shop. Under hypnosis the suggestion was implanted in his mind that whenever he saw a chemist's shop he would have the impulse to pass it. So strongly fixed was this suggestion and so effectively did it work that he returned later to have some of the injunction removed because when he wanted to go in to buy a toothbrush, he found he could not do so! Not all people are so suggestible.

Suggestion treatment is criticized on the grounds that it is superficial; but in some cases it breaks a vicious circle and can therefore produce a permanent cure. But as it does not reach the deep-rooted causes of the disorder, its cures are often transitory. In particular it has failed to cope with the *purposiveness* of the symptom.

Morton Prince has described a group of morbid conditions as "Association Neuroses," and gives as a typical instance the woman who had an attack of asthma whenever she came into a room with red flowers—even if those flowers were artificial. But further investigation of these cases suggests that there are other factors at work. Everybody who has had an attack of asthma does not thereafter get attacks whenever he sees something which was originally associated with it; nor does everybody who is shut up in a cupboard thereafter suffer from claustrophobia. These experiences may be an important factor in the case, and may determine the type of symptom; but would this association between

---

[1] This is taken by some to be bad treatment because it will induce the boy to dive only for rewards: in actual fact, twice was enough to abolish the fear, and restore the original habit.

the flowers and the attack of asthma have operated so effectively had the lady not already been predisposed by a desire for sympathy and attention, which she hoped to secure by her attack? Would the symptom have persisted had it not been reinforced by such a desire? The theory of association, like that of conditioned reflexes, is inadequate to explain all the facts, however valuable in practice it may be, and must give way to dynamic concepts such as the wish to get attention, and the purpose served by the symptom, which Freud has so convincingly brought to light. It is this persistent though unconscious wish which reinforces the reflex and perpetuates the original association.

CENTRAL ORGANIZATIONS

Conditioned reflexes depend on the nature of the stimulus. But to elicit a response there must already be present within the organism certain permanent and abiding nervous organizations or dispositions *capable of responding in these ways*. We cannot observe these dispositions directly any more than we can observe the structure of the atom; we can only presume them because of their extraordinary effects on behaviour.

Some of these are localized in their effects, like the sucking reflex; some are more generalized responses of the whole organism, such as fear or anger, which are often referred to as "instincts" or "propensities." But to avoid the controversy regarding the term "instincts," we shall simply refer to these dispositions as *potentialities of response*, since they are the conditions which make the response of the organism possible; they are potentialities which "dispose" us to act in this way or that, to be depressed, to be cheerful, to be suspicious. Dispositions, whether native or acquired, are the abiding conditions determining our behaviour. But when activated, these dispositions become the sources of dynamic forces expressing themselves in action, the nature of the behaviour, whether kindness or suspicion, depending on the nature of the disposition activated, as well as on the nature of the stimulus.

Some of these are innate like the instincts in the animals, and fear and rage in man. Others like honesty are acquired dispositions.

Innate dispositions. Instincts in animals, like the migration of birds, are innate dispositions, for though they may depend to some extent on climate or other conditions, there is obviously a native proneness of the organism to act in these ways. Some of these innate dispositions are operative even at birth—like fear of noise: others are potentially present at birth, but only become operative after further development of the organism, like nest building, the broodiness of the hen, the development of a bass voice in a male, or romance in a youth of 16 who suddenly finds himself in love with a girl to whom he was yesterday completely indifferent. This is the process of *maturation*, the changing phases of which it is most important for those to understand who deal with the education of the young, since mental health requires that all these naturally emerging tendencies at each phase of development should have full opportunity of expression in their own time. Only by the full expression of one phase can the youth satisfactorily pass on to the next.

Some of these innate potentialities are more primitive and necessary, like fear, aggressiveness and sex, and therefore are more firmly established, whereas others like curiosity and the maternal are a later development in evolution, and therefore more variable and unstable. The former can only be obliterated with the greatest difficulty, if at all. The others like the maternal which emerge in the later phases of evolution, are less well established and therefore more variable from individual to individual and more easily obliterated. There are many women who have no love for children, and even hate their own, as in two cases being treated by the author at the moment of writing.

From these conjectures we may draw some conclusions.

First, that the non-appearance of a propensity in an individual is no proof that it is not innate. Not only are some people constitutionally deficient in certain propensities because of their individual glandular make-up, but in others they are innately present but obliterated, as sex functions may be by an attack of mumps, or repressed by experiences in early childhood, such as affection by the jealous hatred of a baby brother, this being the case in one of the women above mentioned.

Secondly, the strength of these tendencies vary enormously from individual to individual, which determines to a large extent the difference in our character traits, as we shall see later. One person is by nature aggressive, another meek. The sex instinct is far stronger in some individuals than in others who take little interest in it, owing to their glandular development.

Thirdly, because the more established propensities like fear, sex and aggressiveness cannot easily be obliterated but only repressed, it is they which so commonly appear as the cause of the psychoneuroses, whereas other tendencies, like the maternal, acquisitiveness and curiosity (all of which are found in the most primitive races), being less strongly established, are less likely, even if repressed, to emerge in abnormal forms. The more primitive the potentiality of response, the less easily will it be obliterated, and the more likely, if repressed, to produce psychoneurosis.

Acquired dispositions. As soon as any native disposition, such as fear or aggressiveness is called into activity, it is immediately modified by the circumstances of the environment to form an acquired disposition, such as courage, generosity, stinginess, suspicion, kindness, cruelty, determination or ambition. Thus by the interaction of environmental conditions with native dispositions, new dispositions are formed within the organism, which may be infinite in number and give rise to an infinite variety of responses.

There seems little doubt, as American psychologists particularly have emphasized, that by far the majority of our behaviour reactions are determined by these acquired dispositions, which are also the prolific source, though not the only cause, of individual differences of behaviour and character. Acquired dispositions or potentialities of response are variously described as sentiments, complexes, drives, interests, habits, and attitudes, all of which are primarily developed as the result of the interaction between the innate dispositions, and the environment.

Once formed, these acquired dispositions become permanent qualities of mind, and thereafter determine a man's response to the outside world; so that because of environmental experiences, some people are optimistic, others sullen, suspicious, timid, kindly or harsh: whilst others still are more sensitive to rebuff or disposed to jealousy or hate owing to such acquired dispositions. At this stage of development, therefore, *the nature of the response depends not so much on the nature of the stimulus but on the nature of the disposition,* a fact of the most profound importance in human behaviour. Ordinarily an individual will respond to pleasant conditions by happiness, and by depression to adverse conditions, the nature of the response depending on the stimulus. But the man who develops a cheerful disposition will be cheerful in almost any situation in life, even the most adverse. The person with a depressed disposition, on the other hand, will react to everything by gloom, even the most pleasant things in life: the person with a suspicious nature will respond with suspicion to the most kindly approach; while the man with the inferiority complex will react to everyone, however amiable, by shyness and self-consciousness, or possibly by boasting. Everyone's personality, or pattern of behaviour, depends largely upon his individually acquired dispositions. Usually one or another of these acquired dispositions is dominant, in which case we regard it as his "Disposition"; so a man is said to be of a kindly disposition, a sullen disposition, not that he is necessarily always so, but that it is his prevailing response to life.

When once these dispositions are established, instead of the individual being affected by the outside world, *he himself affects and changes his environment*. The cheerful man will not only be cheerful under adverse circumstances, but will cheer everyone else up, and in doing so turn adversity into victory. So man becomes the creator and no longer the slave of his circumstances: he no longer has to wait on external stimuli, he acts spontaneously, that is to say from within, on account of the nature of the dispositions within him. He is no longer a blind spectator of forces which inevitably work their will upon him, but he becomes master of these forces by determining the conditions under which they are operative. The realization of this power over circumstances gives man the sense of freedom and belief in the freedom of his will, since circumstances no longer determine him, but circumstances are determined by him.

The importance of these central organizations has been recognized in education, the chief function of which should be the development of *right dispositions* in the child. It is better that a child should have the right dispositions, say of sociability, cheerfulness, determination or fair-mindedness, than that he should be conditioned merely to *behave* in a fair-minded way; for if he has such a disposition, the actions will naturally follow, whereas he may act in a kindly way for motives that are anything but kindly. Once he has developed a determined disposition, he can apply it with effect to anything he chooses to do, even to the distasteful. So it is better that a child should be *disposed* to act in certain ways rather than that he should be compelled to act so, or even merely have the habit of doing so: a generous disposition may be good, but the habit of giving to every beggar may be bad. The nature of an act is to be judged by the disposition which inspires it. "Out of the heart . . ."

Normal acquired dispositions we call "sentiments," like loyalty to one's family: *morbid* acquired dispositions we call "complexes." *Complexes are morbid acquired dispositions which compel the individual to behave in an abnormal manner*; as in the phobias, anxiety, depression, morbid sexual reactions and other forms of psychoneuroses: they are the abiding conditions of abnormal response.

Complexes, like sentiments, are a group of tendencies centred upon some particular object or person. We may then call a complex by the name of the dominant emotion or tendency itself, such as in inferiority complex, or a guilt complex; or we may call it by the name of the object idea or person upon which it is centred, such as a castration complex. The term "mother complex" may refer to a personal attachment to the mother, or it may refer to a tendency to be dependent and to rely on others to do everything for one.

These complexes, once formed, affect not only the nature but the *extent* of our responses to the environment, so that trifling stimuli may precipitate a response out of all proportion to the stimulus. A slighting remark may put a man into a fury, a casual joke make him weep. We may become allergic to certain mental as well as physical stimuli because of our complexes. On the other hand, a violent occurrence like bombing which puts one man into a panic may leave another unmoved, pointing to the establishment of dispositions of courage and self-control. It is not only the strength of the stimulus, it is the nature and strength of the sentiment or complex within the personality which determines the violence or otherwise of the response, and which makes the bigot, the saint and the criminal.

The most persistent of these complexes are those developed in early childhood when the mind is plastic and dispositions are most readily formed. These complexes may give rise to phobias, sex perversions and other abnormal reactions which may persist all through life. Indeed their abnormality often consists in the fact that, however justified they may originally have been, they persist under later circumstances when they are no longer justified or called for. Most psychoneuroses are found to be the persistence of such infantile complexes, whether childish fears as in the phobias, craving for sympathy and shrinking from responsibility as in the hysteric, resentment in the obsessional, or sensuous pleasure in the sex pervert. But they may lie dormant and produce no very marked reactions unless they are precipitated by later untoward circumstances which are then considered to be the cause of the breakdown. We all have complexes, but only some suffer a breakdown.

These complexes have their biological value, for once we have experienced a danger, it is in our interest that the anticipation of coming dangers should fill us with alarm, so as to warn us of them. But what is of value biologically can be most distressing psychologically and produce exaggerated reactions of fear, depression or anger which are now quite uncalled for.

Because these complexes are alien to present-day life, because they are painful, because they are incompatible with the rest of our personality, they tend to be excluded from conscious participation in life. They are in brief repressed. The term "complexes" is therefore used, not only of dispositions which are morbid, but more particularly of those which, being morbid, are repressed and have become unconscious.

Complexes then are the springs of morbid actions, for which the individual may no longer be, if he ever was, responsible. His complex compels him to do things and have feelings contrary to his will: he is compelled to be afraid when reason tells him that there is nothing to fear; he is suspicious and jealous when he knows that the grounds for these feelings are ridiculous, but he cannot help himself. He then becomes aware of the fact that his will is not free, and that he is no longer master of his fate. He has in fact become a neurotic, a slave to his complexes.

Most medical psychologists recognize *the importance of these central organizations in the treatment of the psychoneuroses*. Just as in education there are those who concentrate their attention upon forming right dispositions in the child, and let behaviour take care of itself, so in treatment the psychotherapist directs his treatment towards morbid complexes and lets the symptom take care of itself. When the complexes are discovered and broken up, the energies contained in them are released and directed to more useful ends. Where the causes of morbid states of mind such as anxiety and depression are known, or primarily due to present circumstances, a change in environmental conditions may change the morbid disposition: and everyone knows that a person made gloomy by ill luck may be cheered by encouragement. The same applies to the treating of children, in whom the complexes have been so recently formed that they may often be cured by changing the mother's treatment of the child. But where the complex is more deeply fixed this is inadequate. The child with night terrors or enuresis, may get over them by reassurance, but if they are due to a secret sense of guilt, the reassurance will have little effect. We may submit a sex perversion to every kind of environmental treatment without result: and the man who is depressed and is told to go out to the theatre more, will groan at the jokes of the comedian, because his depression is due, not to environmental stimuli, but to his own complex, and nothing short of eradicating this will cure him.

THE DYNAMIC APPROACH

Dynamic psychology concentrates its attention particularly upon the third phase of the reflex, namely the efferent phase or response. These responses (except the morbidly acquired ones) correspond to biological needs of the individual, and serve some function. The behaviour of animals and men cannot be satisfactorily explained without reference to the function it serves; even the reaction of the lachrymal gland to dust in the eye is understandable only in relation to its biological utility.

Most modern schools of psychopathology are dynamic in their conceptions, finding this the most adequate way of explaining the psychoneuroses. Freud's theory of the libido is dynamic; the mechanisms of conflict and repression, resistance and displacement of affect are all dynamic in nature, and symptoms are regarded as repressed urges forcing their way into conscious life and activity. Jung's theory is dynamic, though his conception of the libido differs in that it includes hunger and other instincts as well as sex. His conception of the collective unconscious is concerned with primitive dynamic forces. Adler is no less dynamic when he bases his psychopathology on the masculine urge for power, the desire to be supreme, to achieve the fictitious goal. Janet is the least dynamic of modern psychopathologists, regarding the personality as a synthesis of experiences: but even he postulates "psychic energy" or tension, to keep together the synthesis which constitutes the personality. It is the lowering of this psychological tension which gives rise to the splitting of the personality in hysteria, and to the weakening of the personality in psychasthenia. McDougall's system of psychopathology is also dynamic in the insistence upon the instincts or propensities; the modifications of these instincts being the source both of normal social behaviour and of psychoneurotic disorders.

The dynamic concept has been a great stimulus to the study and understanding of human nature. But a too exclusive emphasis upon this aspect may lead to a lack of balanced judgment; there is nothing sacrosanct about it, though it appeals to the western mind, which is characterized by energy as distinct from the apathy of the eastern mind; it appeals to those who like to "get things done." Moreover it has the advantage of being manifest in behaviour, and therefore it appeals to those who are reluctant to presume any processes in the mind which they cannot observe. But these dynamic processes obviously need to be stimulated by something, and also require some central organization which makes the response possible, and determines the type of response. The abnormal response of an individual is often based purely and simply on a false *idea*, say that someone intends him harm, that his mother did not love him, that masturbation led to insanity, or that he was the most important person in the world. In such cases there was nothing wrong in the dynamic reaction, granting the truth of these ideas; it is the falseness of the ideas which produced the abnormality in the response. Again, the dynamic response depends both in its nature and force upon the dispositions and complexes already formed; and most important in human nature, upon the aims, ends and purposes towards which the dynamic processes are directed.

PURPOSIVE ACTION

Purposive action depends on the conscious pursuit of ends. It is of all forms of behaviour the most significant in human life. In this pursuit of aims there are three stages relating to consciousness.

In the first, movements and responses take place in the absence of any consciousness. The amoeba absorbs food, our pupils dilate, our endocrine glands function, our stomach's digest without the organism being aware of it. We may speak of these as the *results* of these activities.

Secondly, there comes the stage when we become *aware of our actions and their results*, but without that awareness having any effect upon the action. We swallow if something is put on the back of the tongue, but the consciousness of the process and its result has no influence upon the reflex action; the swallowing occurs anyway. The seasick person experiences great nausea, "he is afraid he is going to be sick, then he is afraid he is not; then he is afraid he is going to die, then he is afraid he is not"—but all to no purpose.[1] The man who gets into a blind rage may know that the results of his fury will be disastrous, but he must strike. At this stage we are like spectators in a drama in which we ourselves are urged by our impulses to do things, the consequences of which we know and fear, but cannot avoid. As Nietzsche says, we not so much live, as are lived by great impersonal forces over which we have no control, and in the power of which we are helpless spectators.

Thirdly, there comes the stage when we are not only conscious of the result of our impulses, but *the consciousness of this end has a*

[1] This fact was appreciated by the ship's steward who was asked by the lady passenger, "What do I do when I feel sick?" He rightly replied, "You don't do anything; it does itself!"

determining effect upon our actions. This is *purposive action.*[1] Sneezing is a reflex: we may be aware that we are going to sneeze, but that awareness has no effect upon our action; we sneeze all the same. But later on, conscious that we are *going to sneeze* and of its inconvenient consequences, we may press upon the upper lip, and so by sidetracking the impulse avoid the inconvenience of sneezing. The man who realizes that if things go on he will lose his temper, puts a check on it in time.

Thus it comes about that what was at first merely reflex response, producing a *result*, gradually acquires consciousness of the *end*, and finally becomes a *purpose* when the consciousness of the end has a determining effect upon our conduct and directs our energies by intelligence to whatever appears desirable. The peacock spreads his feathers as a reflex action, and is presumably unaware that they are attractive; and the peahen is attracted by them, without knowing what she is letting herself in for; but it is a very different matter with the gay lady who knows very well what she is doing and what she is after.

The conscious pursuit of ends means that at this phase of the evolutionary process, no longer is behaviour determined by an objective stimulus, nor even altogether by our dispositions, but behaviour is determined by ends and *purposes*.

The most important actions in our lives have this consciousness as one of the determining factors. We do things because doing them will lead to certain ends, and we refrain from giving vent to impulses which we should otherwise have expressed because we are conscious of the undesirable results to which they will lead. It is the memory of our past experiences or their consequences which enables us to do this. Not only so, but because man is possessed not only of memory, but of *imagination*, he is capable of directing his actions to possible or probable results which he may never in fact have experienced. The same is true of our *beliefs*. The belief in the possibility of something such as victory of our cause, or the ultimate triumph of good, or the building up of a business, or the belief in a person, may bring about a result which would never have occurred were it not for the belief. Thus faith can remove mountains.

Consciousness. It will be observed that we have surreptitiously assumed consciousness, and this for the simple reason that there is not much else we can do about it but assume it. No one has ever adequately defined it; no one knows what it is. Some have therefore denied it, but in denying it, assume it. Consciousness is a fact

[1] McDougall, *Outline of Psychology*, p. 48.

of experience and a fact of observation like any other. The peculiar thing is, however, that we can only observe consciousness *by* consciousness itself; but we can only observe anything by consciousness, so the one is as valid as the other. The emergence of consciousness on to the stage of evolution is of the greatest biological significance, for those species have survived which have the capacity to visualize the result of their action so as to pursue or avoid them. Biologically speaking, the value of consciousness in the struggle for existence is that it can literally "jump to conclusions" and foresee possible consequences before the behaviour has taken place, and so can either check or encourage it. It is therefore the animals which have the greatest capacity for this revival of experiences as ideational processes and so can anticipate results by imagination, which have the greatest chance of survival. If consciousness were not of some value it would not have survived. "The most fundamental function of the mind," says McDougal, "is to guide bodily movements so as to change our relation to subjects around us." There are some men who see nothing but the immediate consequences before them; other people of wider experience, and with a capacity to make use of the experiences they have gained have more foresight to see ultimate ends, and are much better able to decide upon courses of action. But even the greatest philosophers and statesmen fall short of complete wisdom and foresight; hence the appalling mistakes in international politics which we have witnessed in our time. The talk about a possible war may prevent war or it may incite one. Who is wise enough to decide?

But the part played by consciousness in the determination of behaviour has always remained a puzzlement to physiologists and psychologists alike. How can we conceive of so ephemeral and immaterial a thing as an idea or state of consciousness having an effect on physiological activity? How can so evanescent an experience as a "thought" produce a physical result or affect material energy? In brief, how can an idea move a train? Surely it is at variance with the law of cause and effect, which insists that whatever is in the effect must have been in the cause.

The answer to this problem becomes simpler if we remember that consciousness of the end is not the complete "cause" but only the stimulus to the activity, the trigger which sets the activity in motion: like any other stimulus it does not create, but only releases energy, and directs the energy so released.

Conscious states may therefore be regarded as of the nature of a conditioned stimulus. To take the well-known case: the stimulus of meat on the tongue makes the saliva flow: if a dinner bell is rung at the same time, the ringing of the bell will make the saliva flow even in the absence of the meat. But the stimulus of meat on the tongue is also associated with the conscious pleasant sensations it produces, the experience of which is retained as a residual disposition in the mind. Thereafter, the revival of these conscious sensations as an image or memory can act as a conditioned stimulus, in exactly the same way as the ringing of the bell, so that the mere conscious imagination of meat will make the saliva flow, as we have all experienced. In such a case, the imagination of the meat is not the complete cause of the reaction any more than the sound of the bell, but it is the trigger stimulus which sets the movement in process. In this way consciousness can initiate action, even when it does not originate in some external experience but from ideas, desires or dispositions in the mind.[1]

Now this determination of behaviour by the anticipation of ends or results is made possible by virtue of the rapidity of consciousness, which makes it possible to foresee results and so determine behaviour. For when some past experience is revived in memory, *consciousness outstrips action, and reaches the end of the experience before the action has even begun to take place.*

The consciousness of the end now occurs at the beginning of the process and is therefore capable of determining the action either by encouraging the activity if the end is pleasurable, or inhibiting it if it is undesirable.

If we are walking in the mountains and see a hotel, the very sight of it urges us to go there for a meal; but before we begin to move towards it we recall a previous occasion when we went there and the food was bad and the beds damp. We are able to inhibit our action because in the revival of the previous experiences consciousness is more rapid than action and foresees the end of the proposed action even before the action gets started.

Consciousness of the end is then able to determine our behaviour by virtue of the fact that coming at the beginning of the action it *seizes the "final common path."* The principle of the "final common path" is that if two impulses try to gain entrance to a new path in

---

[1] This offers an explanation of the relation of body and mind. We may conceive that in the first place physiological processes such as reflex action gave rise to consciousness, but that then consciousness acting as a conditioned stimulus can initiate physiological action; so that body can affect the mind and mind affect the body. Thus we may have bodily disease like hyperthyroidism or syphilis producing mental disorders, or we may have mental and emotional disorders producing physical symptons such as hysterical paralysis or nervous indigestion. This shows the possibility of some disorders being psychogenetic.

the nervous system, the first arrival secures possession, and the impulse that gets in first inhibits, at any rate for a time, the other stimulus, and so determines the resultant action.[1]

The baby given a bottle sucks reflexly: and that gives it pleasure. Next time it sees a bottle the anticipation of the pleasure is revived and the child gets excited. Thus what was previously the result of the sucking, namely the conscious pleasurable sensation, now comes before the sucking, and encourages the activity. If the result of taking the bottle had been that the child got sick, the next sight of the bottle would revive the whole experience, including the consciousness of the sickness at the end, and this feeling of repulsion, getting in first, checks any impulse there may have been to take the bottle and the child refuses the bottle before even touching it. The image of the end determines the action, by siezing the final common path.

In other cases, however, consciousness of what happened before may be so vivid that it reproduces the whole experience, behaviour and all, so that the child gets sick at the very sight of the bottle before it has touched it. In such a case the consciousness of the end, instead of avoiding the sickness, has actually induced it, but that is an even more effective way of avoiding the bottle, the contents of which are presumably noxious.

This appears to be what happens when we stop ourselves sneezing by pressure on the lip: before the nasal irritation which makes for sneezing has a chance to capture the neural path and start the sneezing, we foresee the inconvenient result of sneezing, and thrust a new irritation by the slight pain of pressure, and that side-tracks consciousness, so that the sneezing is inhibited. By the rapidity of our thought we anticipate the result and produce the pain which seizes the final common path. The introduction of the "red herring" is a common illustration in politics, diverting the individual's attention and so inhibiting the real point at issue, before the latter can get a real hold. Thus, when in a rage and about to strike, a rapid vision of the consequences captivates our imagination and seizes the common path before we make the movement to strike, and inhibits it. In other cases we are too late to capture the "common path" and the original impulse captivates our behaviour; so we give way to impulses which are against our better judgment, and even though we know the consequences will

---

[1] The latter may however bide its time, and we have a delayed action, as in the case of people in a blitz whose immediate need was action; but who suffered later from trembling and anxiety which was at the time aroused but excluded because of the present need to act.

be disastrous. We cannot help ourselves; for we are driven on towards our fate by impulses which have got in first, and neither threats of disastrous consequences nor idealistc principles have now any effect over impulses which get the better of our true aims and purposes. The practical solution is a more speedy recognition of the ends of our action and prompt decision to avoid its consequences, before the other impulses get a hold.

The rapidity of conscious processes in anticipating the end, together with the law of the common path help to explain why it is that those animals, mainly human, who, by the production of images, are best capable of anticipating the end, can avoid dangers which those less gifted with imagery and foresight like the moth cannot avoid. This is also one of the main ways in which we "learn by experience." Intelligence, or the capacity to profit by experience, is largely foresight, and tests based on the *recognition of anticipated results* (like that of the man sitting on a branch and sawing it off on the tree-ward side) are of particular value in testing intelligence.

This principle of the final common path also explains why an idea once having taken root in the mind is very difficult to dislodge, such as our prejudices which any amount of reasoning will not move. Similarly, as we shall see, once a child has received a strong impression, that the world is a terrifying place, that people are cruel, that it is inferior, this idea may persist in spite of many later experiences to the contrary. It also explains post-hypnotic suggestion such as telling a man under hypnotism that in an hour's time when he is awake he will sing a certain song; and although he feels it foolish to do so, the idea once taken root in the mind and got possession, is so potent that he cannot help himself. This getting in first with a strong enough idea is one of the essential devices in propaganda. The lie must not only be a big one, as Hitler insisted, but must get in first.

To summarize: consciousness of the end which was at first only the result of a reflex and instinctive action, is capable on a revival of the experience in memory, of acting as a conditioned stimulus and releases energies which find expression in action. It is capable of doing this by virtue of the fact that in the revival of a previous experience consciousness outstrips action and rapidly reaches the end of the experience before action takes place; so that now, coming at the beginning, the idea of the end can seize the final common path and so determine action either to encourage or inhibit it. What determines the organism to choose this end as desirable or otherwise undesirable does not concern us for the moment, but in general it is that that end is desirable which is conceived as satisfying and completing the personality.

If we look at ideals and purposes in this way, there is less difficulty in accepting the idea of "purpose," for what we call purpose is merely motivation of our behaviour by the idea of ends, or possible ends, of our action, the consciousness of which may become the determining factor of our conduct.

Whether we regard such a process as *teleological* (*vis a fronte*), because our action is determined by ends, or *mechanistic* (*vis a tergo*), because the consciousness of such ends now comes before the action, is from the practical point of view of little importance; nor are we competent to discuss the philosophic implications of this problem. What is of importance is that *the idea of the end may make something happen which would never have occurred were it not for the idea of the end.* Thus the idea in the mind, the image of what has never happened but which might happen, becomes one of the most potent factors determining men's conduct, capable of releasing forces within the personality which are then directed towards those aims, and helps him to avoid disaster.

This purposive view though constantly denied by the mechanists is implicitly accepted even by those who deny any belief in purpose. The behaviourist proves himself an idealist when he says that a child "ought" to be brought up in certain ways, in order to achieve certain desirable ends. Pavlov is teleological when he aims at explaining human behaviour in terms of conditioned reflexes, and is an idealist when he describes the benefits likely to accrue to man by an understanding of man's behaviour in these terms. Freud claims to be dynamic but not teleological, yet it is difficult to see how he can avoid a teleological interpretation when he holds, for instance, that the symptom is the expression of a "wish to be ill." If that is not teleological, it is difficult to see in what sense we are to use the term. Thus many, even of those who deny purpose, are themselves in fact teleological and idealistic.[1] The

---

[1] Mapother, in a paper designed to condemn animism, conceptional thinking and purposiveness and to approve phenomenalism, twice quotes with approval the statement that "Science aims at the power of prevision based on quantitative knowledge." In this one sentence he manages to personalize science (which is animistic), and ascribes to it an aim (which is purposive and teleological). In approving phenominalism, he is approving something purely conceptual, and in spite of his disclaimer proclaims himself to be an idealist in holding this to the aim and ideal of scientific work. Nevertheless, Mapother's warning is a timely one in making us distinguish the phenomenal facts which are scientifically established from the conceptions and abstractions by which we try to explain them, a warning which he himself has unfortunately not heeded. (*Proc. of Royal Soc. of Medicine*, Vol. 27, 1934. "Tough and Tender.")

greatness of these men is beyond dispute in their contributions to science. They are only wrong in their too exclusive claims for one particular form of motivation, and in their failure to admit other equally relevant ones without which human behaviour cannot adequately be explained. Sherrington, on the other hand, as we have seen, has a large enough vision to appreciate the teleological functions of the nervous system in bringing about co-ordination. He has stated that the main factor which determines that a stimulus gets possession of the "final common path" is its strongly affective tone.[1] We may assume, therefore, that either the desirability of an end, or an anticipated pain, is one of the main determinants in our action. To quote him: "*Expressed teleologically*, the common path . . . is adapted to serve but one purpose at a time. Hence it is a co-ordinating mechanism and prevents confusion by restricting the use of the organ, its minister, to but one action at a time." We could not wish for a more convincing statement from a physiologist of the teleological point of view, nor better support of the ultimate aim of mental health as a co-ordination of the whole personality.

The introduction of purpose makes behaviour more variable and more unpredictable. Because of the process of conditioning, a number of different causes and stimuli may produce a similar response, say that of suspicion, or depression. On the other hand, because of purpose, a single stimulus, like a situation of danger, may evoke a variety of responses, such as flight, clinging, calling out or immobility, not only according to the situation involved but *according to the end we want to achieve*. In man, therefore, there is a "variability of response" which is in marked contrast to the relatively fixed behaviour in the lower animals. An impulse is no longer merely aroused as a response to a specific stimulus, but it may consciously be used to bring about a certain end. Both are dynamic, the latter alone is purposive. Impulses have now become the servants, not the masters of our will.

The neuroses may be understood in this light: paralysis may be originally a natural biological response to danger (we become paralysed with fear); but this reflex having now given rise to consciousness, we may use and even produce a paralysis to serve our ends of escaping from responsibility. The disorder which was originally a biological result is now purposive, and the paralysis psychogenetic, originating in mental processes.

[1] Sherrington, *Integrative Action*, p. 231.

ETHICS

But it is obvious that we must not only have ends, but the *right ends*, for some are capable of bringing about this co-ordination of our personality, and some are not, and everything will depend upon the nature of the end or aim. The practical task of ethics is to discover what are the right ends for man to pursue.

But right for what? On what criterion are we to determine which are the right ends and which are not? In mental health we have such a criterion, for *as far as mental health is concerned, those are the right ends the pursuit of which give the greatest fulfilment, completeness and happiness to the personality as a whole*. It is this which, consciously or unconsciously, determines our choice of ends. Regarded in this light, ethics, in its search for the right ends, plays a necessary part in mental hygiene.

In the main issue the *common end characterizing every organism is the urge to completeness*. This urge to completeness is a principle to which we called attention many years ago.[1] It is deep-rooted in all forms of organic life, physiological as well as psychological, unconscious as well as conscious. A tree lopped of a branch grows another branch; if we suffer a wound in the skin the whole resources of the body—the circulation, respiration, glandular secretions, production of white blood corpuscles, and the whole nervous system—are mobilized for the cure of that wound, however trifling, so that the body is restored to completeness. So it is with the personality as a whole which is ever striving towards its own fulfilment, whether we realize it or not. Indeed, this urge itself is so deep-rooted in all life that it may be conceived of as a tropism, based on deep unconscious processes. This applies equally to the worm, which seeks its completeness, as to man in spiritual aspirations. *If the struggle for existence is the primal necessity of the living organism, fulfilment is its final goal*. The urge to completeness is therefore the main motive of life; aims and ideals are the means whereby the personality seeks to gain such completeness.

Our ultimate aims in life are therefore chosen, consciously or unconsciously, according to their capacity to fulfil our personality, to make us whole. We seek for success or for pleasure because we believe that in it we shall find fullness of life: we live a life of service in peace, and self-sacrifice in war, because in them we find the greatest happiness and completeness of our lives. The mother finds the fulfilment of her life in giving her life for her child, and the soldier for the country and friends he loves. Indeed,

[1] *Psychology and Morals*, chap. viii.

such a sacrifice goes beyond happiness; it is a state of blessedness.

Amongst the schools of psychology, the Gestalt school has emphasized the "wholeness" of human experience; it has pointed out that intelligence and intuition are functions of the whole self, and our behaviour is determined not by this instinct or that, but must be considered as the personality acting as a whole. The ape who is faced with the problem of getting a banana which is out of reach solves this not by trial and error, nor by the operation of a specific instinct, but arrives at its solution by intuition, a function of the whole mind acting as a unity. It may be that in imagination the ape gets a picture of the completed action and the object achieved, and this suggests the means of attainment.

The study of the personality as a whole has received special attention from American writers, especially Allport in his standard book on *Personality*. By *personality* we mean "the individual as potentially active" (to add another to the hundreds of definitions!), that is to say that it possesses latent power capable of development into activity. This definition relates both to man's latent potentialities, and to his capacity of expressing it in action and behaviour. It refers both to personality in its external presentations (the *persona* or mask), but also to those latent qualities within the individual which determine the nature and strength of his character. The ordinary person has both of these in mind when he speaks of a person as having "personality." The particular quality characterizing such behaviour may vary, but when we speak of a charming personality, a forceful personality, or a niggardly personality, we refer not only to how he behaves but to what he is.

But unfortunately the personality does not always function as a whole since its functions, derived as they are from all stages of evolutionary development, often conflict with each other and with the aims of the personality as a whole. The sense of incompleteness is consciously experienced as discomfort, hunger, restlessness and fatigue and the conflict often leads to nervous breakdown, which is a failure of the personality to achieve this co-ordination, with the development of neurotic symptoms.

The symptom is an indication that the personality is wrong somewhere. Yet even a neurotic symptom, as we shall see, is an attempt to complete ourselves, for it represents an effort of the repressed and therefore unfulfilled part of our personality to find some form of expression which it is at present only permitted to do by way of the symptom; a hysteric pain for instance being an appeal of the personality for the sympathy he has been denied and has denied himself, the obsessional propitiation an expression of guilt he has ignored, but should recognize. Our aim in psychological treatment is therefore not simply to abolish the symptom, the headache or the phobia, but, by liberating the repressed parts of the personality which these symptoms represent, to restore the personality to function as a whole. That is why analytic treatment which is a process of release has proved more effective than more superficial forms of treatment, like suggestion or persuasion. Medical science should be satisfied with nothing less than the restoration of the whole personality to a state of complete mental health.

CHAPTER III

TYPES OF CHARACTER TRAITS AND DELINQUENCY

No one who studies human nature can fail to be struck by the extraordinary differences in individual character traits. Some people are jolly, some are sad; some humorous, others serious; some are vivacious, others reserved; some intelligent, others dull; some are cautious, others venturesome; some are sweet-natured, affectionate, tender, others rough, aggressive, masterful; one is vacillating, another determined; some shy, others self-assured; some are sensuous, others ascetic; some are sociable, others reserved; some materialistic, others idealistic. Such individual differences are almost infinite in their variety and make as many individuals as there are persons in the world. It is the particular quality and nature of these various characteristics in any person which we term *individuality*, and it is that which makes every person different from every other.

How are we to account for the extraordinary varieties of character traits in different individuals, which constitute the essential differences between them? Where do they originate? Why is it that in the same family, and in apparently the same environment, one child is imaginative and adventurous, the second studious and conscientious, the third has practical ability and intelligence, whilst the fourth is sociable and likes doing things for others? Some would say that it is a difference in physiological constitution and that it is hereditary factors which determine the character; others, that these traits depend upon environmental conditions and early training. To answer these questions we must of course investigate the *causes* of these various conditions.

The criterion of normality. Some of these characteristics we regard as normal and some as abnormal. We regard cruelty as a vice, kindness as a virtue, indolence as reprehensible, determination as desirable. One child is masterful, and his parents regard him as a boy of spirit; while other parents regard him as an objectionable nuisance. Homosexuality is regarded as a perversion by some people, natural by others, a mark of superiority by homosexuals themselves. To be conscientious is regarded as a virtue, yet it is possible to be overconscientious, morbidly

punctilious and over scrupulous. We may be kind to a fault, and
we may be cruel to be kind. But on what criterion are we to base
our judgment of which are normal and which are abnormal?
Obviously a character trait cannot of itself be regarded as normal
or abnormal without further reference.

To the question what is normal and what is abnormal, we cannot
give a categorical answer, until we have decided upon our standard
of judgment whether from the point of biological adaptation, by
social or moral or legal standards, or according to the standards
of mental health; for what is wrong by one standard may be right
by another. "Is jealousy normal or abnormal?" we ask. "It all
depends," we reply, "sometimes it is, and sometimes it is not."
"But depends on what?" It depends on circumstances, on motives,
and above all on our standards of judgment. Jealousy may be
regarded as the guardian of marital fidelity; but it has been known
to wreck homes and married happiness. It is obviously sometimes
normal, sometimes abnormal. It is therefore pertinent to ask for a
criterion of what is a normal and what an abnormal character trait.

*From the point of view of mental health those character traits are
normal which are in harmony with the remaining tendencies and
dispositions in the mind and with the aims and functions of the
personality as a whole.* They are abnormal when they are so
exaggerated or perverted as to be out of harmony with the rest
of the personality, in which case they conflict with and may
repress other tendencies which ought to have expression in a full
and complete life. This gives us a standard of normality and yet
allows for considerable scope for individuality within the bounds
of the normal. If jealousy therefore is in conformity with the
fulfilment of the aims of the personality, such as the guardian of
married fidelity, it is normal; if on the other hand it tends, as it
often does, to break up the marriage, it does violence to that aim,
and is abnormal.

Before discussing types of character trait some definitions are
necessary.

The Temperament is the mental constitution in so far as it
depends on the physiological constitution; as in the person who is
innately aggressive, cheerful by nature (like the cyclothymic), or
constitutionally unstable.

The Disposition is the mental constitution in so far as it depends
on environmental conditions: it is the result of nurture not of
nature. So a child may develop a kindly disposition or an arrogant
disposition according to the environment in which he has been
bred.

The Character is the quality of the personality as a whole in so far as it is determined by our aims, purposes and ideals in life. According to whether these ideals are or are not in accordance with accepted standards, a man is said to be a "good" character or a "bad" character.

The Will is the function or activity of the personality as a whole as directed towards its aim: the more completely the forces of the personality are mobilized towards a common end, good or bad, the stronger and the more effective is the will.

Our temperaments are mainly inherited; our dispositions are what our environment makes of us; our character is what we make of ourselves. A man may be temperamentally cruel, as in some psychopathic or epileptic personalities: he may have a cruel disposition if he becomes cruel because of example, encouragement or other environmental influences; he has a cruel character if he deliberately sets out to be cruel.

The Personality is, as we have said, the whole personality as potentially active, and is the sum total of the functions and potentialities of the whole individual, including his physiological make-up, his acquired dispositions and his character as determined by his ends, aims and purposes in life.

Character traits. By the term "character trait" we mean those behaviour patterns which, though not the dominant "character" of the individual, are nevertheless outstanding qualities in his personality determining his modes of behaviour. A man of cruel character may also be sentimental, vain, or even generous to his friends, and the man of religious character with ideals of tolerance to all men, may in fact be sometimes bigoted, bad tempered or unforgiving, which are his character traits.

Clinical classification of character traits. At first sight it might appear that the varieties of character traits, such as those we have enumerated, are so numerous that it would be impossible to classify them; and indeed many clinicians when confronted with a case of jealousy, suspicion, or depression, take each case separately and try to find out its specific causes. But a further consideration of such traits will help us to realize that there are not only individual differences, but different *types* of character trait, the recognition of which greatly simplifies the task of diagnosis and the problem of treatment.

A scientific classification of character traits, whether normal or abnormal, must have reference not merely to their manifestations in behaviour, but also to causation. This is necessary not only for a proper understanding of the character traits themselves, but also to their proper handling and treatment, and especially for their prevention.

We classify character traits, normal and abnormal, into four groups: (1) Temperamental, (2) Simple, (3) Reaction, and (4) Psychoneurotic character traits. These differ in their causation, in their manifestations as types of behaviour, and in their treatment.

Temperamental or physiological character traits, whether normal or abnormal, are those which are determined primarily by the physiological constitution. *Simple or ordinary character traits* are those which are determined by the direct influences of the environment. *Reaction character traits* are those which are a reaction to some other tendency in oneself which is repressed. *Psychoneurotic character traits* are those which are due to the emergence of these repressed tendencies.

There are of course combinations of these types, but that makes it the more necessary to distinguish them.

To make clear the distinction between these various types of character trait, we may take a specific case, say that of *stealing* in a boy of fourteen. From the point of law, stealing is stealing, and must be punished without respect of persons, and with very little consideration for the reasons and motives for the stealing. Extenuating circumstances are sometimes taken into consideration, and sometimes the previous character of the boy, but the first duty of the magistrate, even in the children's courts, is the protection of society and therefore only limited investigation is made into the type of delinquency or its psychological causes. But this boy may steal:

(*a*) Because he is constitutionally feeble-minded, and therefore weak-willed, a psychopathic personality with no moral sense nor power of self-control, or because he has been permanently affected by sleepy sickness: indeed, he may not even have the sense to cover up his misdeed, or know that he has done wrong. Such is a *temperamental or physiological character trait*.

(*b*) On the other hand, the boy may steal simply because he wants to; because he has been brought up in a bad home, with bad ideals by bad parents, or with bad companions. He may even have been taught to steal by his parents. He is lacking in moral character not because of any physiological defect, but because of low ideals. He knows the difference between right and wrong, and can do otherwise if he chooses to, but he does not want to: he has no qualms about stealing, except from the point of view of punishment, and takes skilled precautions against discovery.

Such is a *simple character trait*. It is psychologically uncomplicated, and involves no repression.

(*c*) In the third case, the stealing is from an entirely different motive: the boy has a good home and good parents, and has been well brought up morally, but when another child was born he felt deprived of affection, developed a feeling of inferiority and reacted in the opposite direction by jealousy. Craving for affection and attention he nevertheless represses it, and going to the opposite extreme says, "I don't want their love; I don't care about anybody," becomes rebellious, antagonistic, sullen, anti-social, and steals to get his own back. When he is discovered he is defiant, refuses sympathetic advances and takes his punishment sullenly. This is a *reaction character trait*, by which we mean not so much a reaction to environmental conditions (for simple traits are also that), but a reaction *against himself*—in this case against his latent need for affection, which he represses.

(*d*) Finally, there is the boy of quite different character from these others. Far from being a bad boy, or anti-social, he is of good character, hard-working, clever, the model pupil at school; and yet to everybody's surprise as well as his own, it is found that it is he who has been taking money from other boys' lockers, or stealing books from a shop. As likely as not he does not want these things, makes no use of them when he gets them, and cannot understand why he should steal them, and may take little precaution against discovery. When he is discovered he is not defiant, as the last type, but full of remorse for all the pain he has caused his parents, and the disgrace he has brought on himself. This is typical pathological stealing and his case baffles his schoolmaster, parents and himself alike. It is a *psychoneurotic character trait*, which is the emergence of a repressed tendency—in this case a repressed resentment and aggressiveness.

Now even on superficial observation it is obvious that these four types of stealing differ very much in nature and character the one from the other: in the first case the stealing is done quite openly and without any sense of wrong and therefore often clumsily; in the second it is done deliberately, surreptitiously and is well planned; in the third it is done defiantly, and in the fourth case (as may be in the third), the object stolen is not wanted, and of no use to the boy, but unlike the third case this boy may be of good character, and the stealing quite alien to his character. They are all acts of stealing, but the *type* of stealing is different, the *causes* are different, and the *type of treatment* must obviously be determined by these differences. To treat the post-encephalitic or mild mental defective as though he was of bad character and responsible for his actions would be unjust and futile: his deficiency makes it impossible for him to appreciate the difference between right and wrong, and impossible to control his impulses if he did. It would, on the other hand, be futile to psycho-analyse the *simple delinquent* with the bad upbringing since his stealing is not due to any repressed complex. What he requires is new ideals and standards of conduct. It is no use treating the boy with a *reaction* delinquency either by endocrine glands, for there is nothing physically wrong with him, nor by good advice, for his defiance would make him reject all advances, nor by punishment which would increase his resentment and make him a worse delinquent. What he and the *psychoneurotic* require is specific analytic treatment. As with stealing so with any other type of abnormal character trait: before we start to discover the individual causes in any particular case, we should determine the nature, and particularly the type, of character trait presented.

TEMPERAMENTAL CHARACTER TRAITS

Temperament we have defined as the mental constitution in so far as it depends on the physiological constitution: it is the influence of the body over mind.

Temperamental character traits are therefore physiologically determined potentialities of response.

There is no doubt that physiological changes in the individual can bring about changes in the mental attitudes and produce character traits of a specific nature. There are people of a cheerful optimistic type, but subject to ups and downs of emotion, who are of the "cyclothymic" temperament. Others are shy by nature, reserved and shut in, namely those of the "schizothymic" temperament. Those deficient in thyroid are dull and phlegmatic. These conditions are almost certainly constitutionally determined.

This definition of temperament agrees so far with the traditional view of temperamental as being due to the "tempers" or "humours" of the body. Also with that of McDougall, who defines temperament as the "sum of the effects upon mental life of the metabolic or chemical changes that are constantly going on in all the tissues of the body."[1] Others, however, define temperament as the affective constitution of the individual, as against the intellectual. This difference in definition is not so great as appears at first sight since the affective

[1] *Outline of Psychology*, p. 354.

life is so closely related to physiological functions, especially of the autonomic nervous system.

The physicians of old who regarded the sanguine, the choleric, the melancholic and the phlegmatic temperaments as due respectively to the influence of the physiological organism upon the mental life of the individual had a true conception of temperament. This old classification has found some support in the work of Pavlov, who finds such differences of temperament in his dogs. His opinions are, however, vitiated by the fact that he makes no attempt (as far as we know) to discover how far those "temperamental" differences may have been due not to constitutional causes, but to earlier experiences in the lives of his dogs, that is to say, due to the dog's previously formed conditioned reflexes. Kretschmer[1] has attempted to correlate four groups of phenomena, namely, physical habitus, temperament, psychopathic disorders and psychoses, and his classification into the schizothymic, shy, sensitive type, and the cyclothymic, cheerful and depressed type, correlating with certain types of physique is widely though not universally accepted. But it is important to recognize that a person may develop these characteristics of sensitivity or depression as a result of environmental conditions, so that even a cyclothymic may be made shy and shut in by the treatment he receives in early childhood, and therefore does not develop the characteristic social traits. A person who is shy and reserved is not necessarily schizoid. Possibly many of the "exceptions" to his correlations of the physical habitus and mental character are due to this fact. Hess and Erlinger have differentiated the tense "vagotonic" individual and the "sympatheticotonic" type, which correspond somewhat to the schizoid and cycloid, and to the introvert and extravert types as described by Jung.

All these are constitutional types.

We shall therefore use the term "temperamental" only of those mental characteristics which are physiologically determined and not of those traits of character like kindness, courtesy or spite which are purely psychologically determined, however deep-rooted they may be in the personality.

The term *constitutional* like the word temperament we use only of those conditions which are physiologically engendered and are usually hereditary and innate (the exception being cases in which glandular changes develop and produce constitutional disorders). We should no more say that a man is a "constitutionally" good tennis player (though he may have a good constitution for tennis playing) than that a woman has an "instinct" for arranging flowers, though her artistic temperament may conduce to it. But the term constitutional has a wider application than temperament, for temperament refers only to mental and emotional characteristics, as derived from the physical make-up, whereas constitution refers also to physical characteristics and disorders like the allergies and rheumatic constitutions. But since those suffering from the

[1] *Physique and Character.*

allergies are often subject to mental characteristics such as over-sensitivity, we may speak of the allergic "temperament" to call attention to the mental accompaniments of these constitutional disorders.

Further, the term temperament is usually used only of the *milder* types of character trait, and not of the more severe ones such as the psychoses, mental deficiency or psychopathic personality. So we may speak of an optimistic temperament, or a pessimistic temperament, but not when the optimism reaches the stage of mania or the pessimism the stage of deep melancholia.

Kretschmer, indeed, uses the term temperament not only of the *mild* types but only of the *normal* types, and there is much to be said for this use. But we always prefer to use a term as much in conformity with common usage as possible as long as it is within the bounds of scientific accuracy, and so feel justified in speaking of a melancholic or arrogant "temperament."

Again the word temperament is used of the more *persistent* though mild phases, whereas the word "mood" is more often applied to passing affective states such as being in a good mood or a bad mood, a generous mood or a sulky mood: indeed, a stingy man may for a moment be in a generous mood. Not only so, but a mood may arise from either physiological causes like a "hang-over" or psychological causes like disappointment, whereas temperament is best used only of the former.

Even *transitory* physiological conditions have their effects upon the mental life and character. Gout makes us irascible, jaundice makes us pessimistic, alcohol makes us cheerful, then sentimental, then irascible, then depressed, then comatose. We may for convenience refer to these transitory conditions as "physiological character traits" as distinct from the temperamental, reserving the latter term for the more abiding states.

But as these conditions are all physiologically determined, we shall in our discussion consider them all together as temperamental.

The fact that our mental make-up depends very largely upon our physiological constitution is a matter of common knowledge, some people being constitutionally and by nature more gentle, others more aggressive; some more sensitive, others coarse. We recognize this influence of the physiological factors in the determination of individual characteristics in everyday language. The "thick-skinned" person lacks sensitivity, and we speak of a person as dull and "heavy," recognizing that a certain type of heavy person, the sub-thyroidic, is also intellectually dull, the mental characteristic in these cases being named after its physiological counterpart. Another person we speak of as "fat and jolly," having recognized a connection between fatness and jollity even before psychiatrists described the cyclothymic temperament. The plump and petite woman is of a very different mental make-up from the tall, thin, angular, punctilious, intellectual type of woman. Again, the big-boned man of the policeman type with his slow deliberate movements is very different from the typical fireman, short, thick-set, alert, quick and active type. It is probably some physiological difference which gives the typical tenor singer his feminine characteristics, his high-pitched voice, feminine distribution of hair, and his tendency to be "temperamental," highly emotional and fond of self-display. Those who have to do with church choirs tell us that they have more trouble with their tenor singers than with all the rest of the choir put together, and after the opera you will see the tenor surrounded by a throng of adoring females, while the bass goes home to his wife! One finds women, on the other hand, of the short, strong, thick-set, hairy masculinoid type, of whom Leonard Williams says: "These women rarely get husbands, and when they do, their husbands are sorry! No doubt they have their place in the scheme of things; but they are not usually regarded as domestic treasures." Temperamental changes occur more particularly in women, because of the greater changes in their physiological make-up, after marriage, childbirth and the menopause, with the result that "the butterfly of our dreams turns into the scorpion, which like that of the Zodiac may be accompanied by twins." The bright-eyed, warm-hearted little bride turns into the cold-blooded, myxedematous heavy-weight; fair and fluffy at fifteen, she is fat and formidable at forty. The hierarchy amongst hens, which determines that each hen in a group pecks every hen beneath her social status, but respects the ones above, is probably due to endocrine glands producing grades of masculinity as measured by the comb. The same may be observed in women in society.[1]

Our temperament may change during the course of life, so that the energetic young idealist may turn into the flabby, indolent and self-indulgent man of middle age, on account of changes in his endocrine secretions. He follows the life history of the sea-squirt, which in its youth is lively and has an alert and active nervous system; but as it gets older and discovers that it can get all that it requires by sticking to a rock and letting water pass through its body, it loses its energy, its vitality, and even its nervous system, and in fact becomes a squirt! You can get nothing out of it except by squeezing. So with some humans.

These temperamental differences depend upon biochemical changes of which we know little, and therefore it is impossible for

[1] Nevertheless if two hens however socially remote are segregated they make friends like the Duchess and her maid on a lonely island. So circumstances can triumph over glands!

us at present to differentiate all the types of temperament. Yet it is important in judging people's character to consider such differences, for we cannot expect the same physical courage from the sensitive nervous type as from the robust thick-set type, though he may be possessed of much greater moral courage. Nor can we expect of the highly-sexed type of girl, whose interests are mainly physical, the same devotion to study as her cold intellectual classmate. Since the endocrine system of each individual is different so this may be a cause of individual difference.

The recognition of temperament is also important in *vocational guidance*. The son who inherits the physiological make-up of his father and is a "chip of the old block," having inherited his physiological make-up, may successfully follow in his father's footsteps. The father on the other hand with a masterful temperament who compels his only son to follow him in business irrespective of the fact that the son has the artistic temperament of his mother, is inviting failure. Yet if the son is sufficiently robust he may bring his artistic talents to bear upon his business, and become a theatrical producer, as in a case under our care.

Adolescence seems to be an age particularly prone to "temperamental instability" which may in fact be temperamental in the true sense. But it is sometimes difficult to diagnose to which type the instability belongs, whether it is constitutional, or due to environmental conditions such as frustration and thwarting of natural tendencies, or to the emergence of repressed psychological complexes, or to deficiency in discipline and character, all of which tend to be accentuated in adolescence. But every parent and teacher should recognize that the lethargy of the adolescent who "outgrows his strength" (due perhaps to the overactivity of the pituitary gland followed by its exhaustion) is a physiological characteristic in which scolding does no good. It merely adds an "inferiority complex" to his constitutional disability.

One of the most interesting clinical types of constitutional disorder, commanding some attention in recent years on account of the legal implications, is that of the *Psychopathic personality* which we may define as *a constitutional disorder manifesting itself especially in anti-social behaviour*. If the moral sense can be destroyed by injury to the brain in sleepy sickness, there seems no reason against the possibility of an individual being *congenitally* deficient, though this has not, as far as we know, been scientifically demonstrated. These people are not insane, nor certifiable; they are not mentally defective, and so cannot be classed with the old "moral defectives"; indeed, they are often intelligent and shrewd. But they are lacking in social and moral sense, and this defect appears to be due not to bad upbringing, but is an innate constitutional defect, which renders the individual incapable of appreciating social demands. He is therefore inconsiderate, breaks rules in the Services, is quarrelsome, egocentric, vain, and a nuisance to everybody. These same characteristics may of course be derived from other causes such as early training, which may make an individual a rebel although he knows quite well the difference between right and wrong. But the psychopathic personality is not an ordinary rebel, and the term is best applied only to those in whom these characteristics are deemed to be of a constitutional nature beyond the capacity of the individual to control. They are also beyond the capacity of the adjutant to discipline, of the magistrate to correct by punishment, and of the medical man to cure. There was little we could do with such men in the Services, except to discharge them for the civilian doctor to cope with! Mild instances of these "difficult" or cranky people are not uncommon in civil life, though they do not excite so much notice as in the Services with its stricter social demands. These people may be of specific psychotic types such as schizoid or paranoid, but not necessarily.[1]

Crimes are sometimes of this constitutional nature. As tested by the Electro-encephalograph (the measurement of brain waves) not only epileptics but 65 per cent of soldiers who had committed acts of violence of a senseless and unpremeditated kind, and were generally of an aggressive turn, were found to have a disturbed rhythm of the brain wave.[2] Probably a still larger proportion as yet undetected by physical measurements can be ascribed to physical disorders of the brain. But senseless and apparently unpremeditated attacks can also be produced by men who have been nursing a grievance, without any corresponding physiological defect, and the question arises whether it may not be that such emotional disturbances themselves cause the disturbed physiological rhythm.

The characteristics, then, of temperamental character traits are (a) that they are always determined by *physiological factors*, whether hereditary, constitutional or acquired: (b) they are usually *accepted* by the individual, who may not recognize them as abnormal since they are so part of his nature. But there are some more sensitive to social opinion and criticism who realize the difference between

---

[1] See the author's "War Neurosis," *British Medical Journal*, February 28 and March 7, 1942.

[2] Hill and Watterson, quoted by Sargant and Slater in *Physical Methods of Treatment*.

themselves and normal people and so come to recognize themselves as abnormal. (c) They *may be within the bounds of the normal* as in the optimistic person whose constitutional optimism gives zest to life; or they may be *abnormal* as in the over-optimistic, whose optimism frustrates his aims in life, or the depressed temperament.

In other cases, temperamental characteristics may be *super-normal*, for there are men and women of outstanding personality whose abilities are beyond the average, largely the result of a healthy, strong and balanced physiological make-up. This outstanding general ability persists in some families, generation after generation, producing men and women who would be successful in almost any walk of life, capable in business, skilled in their profession, and in politics, natural born leaders of their fellows. The war has produced such men and women who would make their mark anywhere by the force of their personality. Giotto the painter was chosen an official architect of Florence not because he was a painter, nor an architect (which he was not), but because above all he was a "famous man." And the Medici who appointed him were a family of great eminence.

There are others who are supernormal in *specific qualities* like the genius, whose extraordinary abilities are constitutional and innate. The definition of genius as "an infinite capacity for taking trouble first of all" (Carlyle), or as "one-third inspiration and two-thirds perspiration" (Emerson) is precisely what genius is not! It may produce an outstanding personality, but no man by hard work alone can become a genius. The very point about a genius is that he has the capacity to do these things without correspondingly hard work: indeed, the name implies that these capacities can only be accounted for by his "genius," originally a kind of guardian spirit who is conceived as accompanying him from the cradle to the grave. Genius is something inexplicable and unaccountable, some gift we possess apart from any merit or effort of our own: it is innate and not acquired. Geniuses are often unbalanced because they are of the nature of "sports" and ill-adapted to the environment in which they are called upon to live.

Great artists are always ab-normal, in the strict sense, though not necessarily pathological, because they perceive things in the world around them which "normal" (in the sense of "average") people do not see, as well as having the capacity to give form to that vision which a normal person has not.

Intelligence which is the innate capacity to profit by experience is also an inborn characteristic of a constitutional nature. It varies greatly with individuals, as shown by the intelligence tests, but the capacity remains relatively the same in any individual throughout life, as these tests also show, in spite of his increase in knowledge and experience. This indicates that intelligence, unlike knowledge, is constitutional and not acquired.

The *treatment* of constitutional, temperamental or physiological character traits, which are founded on physiological defects or biochemical disorders, must be along the lines of curing this defect if that is possible, and if not, making the best of the conditions by training as in the case of the dull and backward child.

But it is to be remembered that even when we treat and perhaps cure the physiological disorder, there may still remain the inferiority complex and other psychological disorders that may have resulted from them. The "acidosis" child who is always scolded for laziness develops an inferiority complex which persists even when the acidosis is got rid of. The woman who as an adolescent was very fat continued to be self-conscious even when she became beautiful. Owing to the lack of sympathy to sufferers from allergic conditions like hay fever, or asthma, such disorders may become *perpetuated as hysteric symptoms*, even when the physical condition has been cured. It then becomes a question for the physician to decide whether the patient cannot face life because he has asthma, or whether he has asthma because he cannot face life. In some cases it starts with one and ends with the other.

Mental hygiene in temperamental traits. We must accept our temperaments. For the most part our temperaments are inborn and unchangeable, and whatever they are we must make what use of them we can, finding the right opportunity for the development of whatever qualities and potentialities we are endowed with. It is no use for the gentle feminine type of man to attempt to pose as a Hercules; if he despises his "feminine" temperament and does not use it, he will fail to make the most of himself, and his feminism turns into effeminacy. If, on the other hand, he accepts his temperament, he will use his qualities of intuition and sympathy and develop a strong personality, ruling other men, not by the "iron hand," for that is not his nature, but by understanding them. Again, it is useless for the masculinoid woman to play the fantastic rôle of a sweet little pet to her husband, a rôle she played with her father in childhood. Her marriage can only be made successful by the recognition that she is the stronger partner; she can then appreciate the more sensitive and cultured qualities of her husband, when both are prepared to accept their individual temperaments. The temperamentally aggressive lad, whose high spirits give trouble, may be given outlet and opportunities for the direction of his aggressiveness as in seafaring or farming; whilst the temperamentally timid child may be given confidence, the nervous child given assurance, the sensitive child given encouragement. The sensitive schizothymic child is found a job in a library, the temperamentally gentle individual given work as a gardener, whereas neither of these is likely to make a good foreman in a factory. Vocational guidance and social psychiatry come into their own in the consideration of constitutional and temperamental characteristics, by finding the right job for which the individual is temperamentally fitted: they are of less service in those suffering from the psychoneuroses.

There is no statement more misleading and inaccurate than the slogan that "all men are born equal": politically it may be true, but scientifically it is quite incorrect. Therefore to quote another political slogan, to "give equal opportunity to all" is absurd, for it means failing to give to those most highly endowed, opportunities for the development of their native qualities, and giving to those least endowed what they cannot appreciate and cannot use with advantage. That each should be given the fullest *opportunity* for the expression of his whole personality and whatever latent powers he possesses is not merely political justice, social expediency and economic efficiency, but in accordance with the principles of mental health.

SIMPLE CHARACTER TRAITS

Simple character traits are those which are developed as a result of the direct influences of the environment: they are the ordinary character traits of our daily life, the response of the organism to environmental conditions. It is of course only by virtue of the innate dispositions and potentialities that these environmental conditions can operate, the resulting behaviour being the response of the organism to these external stimuli. But we can distinguish, though we cannot separate, the two factors, for an abnormal character trait like violent rage may be due to an abnormal constitution operating even in a normal environment, or to a normal constitution acted upon by abnormal environmental stimuli. The whole purpose and function of education and training is to determine specific types of response by providing the right environmental influences and training. The naturally sensuous child may be made sensual or he may be made artistic according to the way in which his native tendencies are dealt with, and the temperamentally aggressive boy may be made either strong in will and purpose, or a delinquent, according to his upbringing. Thus acquired character traits are not independent of innate and constitutional factors: nevertheless their specific form and quality may be determined by environmental influences. Depression may be the result of a cyclothymic temperament even under the best of circumstances, or it may be due to adverse circumstances in a person constitutionally optimistic. To say, therefore, that hereditary and environmental factors are all one, or that we cannot distinguish them, is to confuse the issue; we must distinguish them if we are to understand the human personality. They inevitably interact, but one or the other may be responsible for the specific form of a character trait.

The main sources of simple character traits. These are: encouragement, suggestibility, identification and frustration.

(*a*) In their simplest form, simple characteristics are determined by the *encouragement and exaggeration of the innate* dispositions which are present more or less in everyone. A child who is constantly allowed its own way will develop aggressive characteristics; one who is constantly fondled or caressed will develop sensuous characteristics. A child who feels let down by his mother becomes embittered or disillusioned, which may persist as a suspicion and distrust of people in general; constantly scolded he will become over-sensitive; constantly submitted to terrifying conditions in infancy he will develop a timid disposition; given everything he wants he will become intolerant of frustration and will later give up in the face of every difficulty; always praised before others, his self-regard will be over-stimulated and he will become conceited and self-important. Thus simple character traits may be exaggerated by encouragement and become abnormal.

As with tendencies so with the encouragement in *specific interests.* Our interests in engineering, forestry or photography are determined by the encouragement we have been given in these pursuits and the opportunity to satisfy them. Isolated experiences which we have undergone often determine our characteristics and attitude of mind. An artistic temperament may be inherited, but an interest in singing may be derived from "songs my mother taught me." Constant subjection to air raids makes one at first alarmed, then inquisitive; then in some it produces indifference and boredom, in others greater anxiety. Such responses may persist as simple character traits, but as in most conditioned reflexes, simple character traits tend to pass when the stimulus is removed and if the reflex is not reinforced. Being free to express themselves they usually develop into higher and more sublimated forms. Thus an early developed interest in hunting may make a good medical psychologist who ferrets out people's complexes.

(b) The second means whereby simple character traits are acquired is that of *suggestibility*, which consists in the tendency to take over moods, feelings and opinions of others. If the mother is irritable, the child will be irritable; so the child may become affectionate, gay, selfish, mean or sulky, in so far as he spontaneously takes over these characteristics by suggestion from his parents. The mother who is over-anxious to reassure her child that there is nothing to be afraid of when he is ill, will simply make him afraid by suggestibility, in spite of her reassurance, because of her own display of anxiety. Suggestibility is more powerful than teaching.

(c) Still more powerful as a means of developing simple character traits is the process of *identification*, which goes a stage further than suggestibility. The child completely identifies itself with others and absorbs the personality of the father and mother, taking over their characteristics. The process of identification is observable in most normal children about the age of three. "I'm the baker; I'm the engine driver; I am Daddy going to lecture; I am Mummy doing the cooking." This is not mere imitation of action; it is not mere suggestibility to certain moods; it is an identification of the child's *whole personality* with the other person, his actions, moods, ideas, idiosyncrasies, mannerisms, habits and character. The child for the time being *impersonates* the other person. The boy who identifies himself with his pompous father will himself become self-important; the little girl identifying herself with her pretty mother develops vanity, and the girl who though naturally womanly identifies herself with her father, becomes mannish and pursues a man's career. A boy, therefore, may be a "chip of the old block" either because of having the same temperament as his father or because he identifies himself with his father. A child may be shy because she is schizothymic, or because she is snubbed, or because she derives it by suggestion from her mother, or by identification with her. It is on account of these environmental influences that a child's native temperament may be completely swamped by the development of new dispositions. Every individual collects a different set of dispositions and so becomes an entirely different personality.

Such identification is normal and natural: but it may easily take a wrong turn. If the parent with whom the child identifies himself is abnormal, the child's personality will be distorted. This transmission of characteristics from parent to child, from generation to generation, due to identification, is often misrepresented as hereditary. Many conditions like alcoholism, cruelty to wives, linguistic abilities, and a love of travel which may exist in families and are therefore sometimes ascribed to heredity, are found to be due to identification.

The *capacity* for identification, however, itself appears to be a constitutional and inherited tendency (as is imitation in animals), spontaneously appearing in most children about the age of three and onwards. Its biological significance lies in the fact that by identification even the *acquired* characteristics of the parents may be transmitted to the child, which greatly enriches the range and qualities of a child's reaction far beyond those it inherits. We therefore have this curious circumstance: that whereas in the human child there are comparatively few inherited characteristics, *we have in identification an inborn capacity for the transmission of the acquired characteristics of the parent.* So a child's interest in engineering, his prudence, obstinacy, devotion to hard work, or his sociability, as well as his anxiety, depression or dishonesty, may be spontaneously acquired from his parents; they are transmitted from parent to child, not hereditarily, but by the process of identification.

We also identify ourselves with the social life and culture in which we live. This cultural form of identification we call *tradition*, which hands down from one generation to the next the highest standards of honest dealing in business, skilled craftsmanship, devotion to their profession, and hard work in their pursuits; or it may be of military ruthlessness or money making. Thus tradition may be as important a factor in producing culture patterns as hereditary factors, and it is often difficult to say how far racial differences are due to one or to the other.

In the development of the individual, therefore, we have various forces at work, some working towards *uniformity*, the other towards *individuality*. Hereditary and constitutional factors make on the whole for the encouragement of similarities, although even by heredity each individual inherits a different collection of genes from parents and ancestors, so that brothers and sisters may be entirely unlike in appearance and temperament in the same family. Identification and tradition also encourage uniformity by the perpetuation of certain characteristics in a given culture, and indeed largely determine that culture, its habits, tastes and social customs. So by tradition we can profit by the experience of the race, as by identification we profit by the acquired experience of our parents. But curiously enough identification also makes for the development of individuality, for by identifying ourselves with many people, we collect a variety of characteristics from all we meet with whom we identify ourselves. Indeed, the multiplicity of our identifications is one of the richest sources of our individual differences, and largely accounts for the great variation of our character traits. One sociological result of this double motivation, one making for individuality the other for uniformity, is that the younger generation is out for novelty and advance in its early years revolting against the tradition and authority of the old, but as soon as it reaches middle age, it is all for leaving things as they are, and protests in its later years that the younger generation is going to the dogs in straying from the path laid down.

But why does a child identify itself with others? and with whom does it identify itself? *The motives for identification* we shall consider later. But generally speaking we identify ourselves with those we love and with those we admire; and act negatively towards the cruel, unpleasant and undesirable. We may in this fact find a reason why human progress usually takes an upward direction. For those who are lovable and admirable are generally speaking in the higher scale of cultural development; and therefore as long as identification with those prevails, culture pursues an upward course from generation to generation.

But since we may identify ourselves with those we admire, and not necessarily with those we love, identification may be made with those who are ruthless, selfish or dishonest. There are periods in world history, through one of which we have just passed, when a natural admiration for strength and power may lead to an identification with the cruelty and ruthlessness with which that power is associated; in which case there is a regression in the progress of the world and a degradation of its culture. To stray from tradition is not always a mark of progress.

For mental health, therefore, there are certain principles which should regulate a child's identification. First the identification should be with the *right people*; and that is why it is important for the child to choose the right parents. Secondly, the identification should be *multiple*, so that the child can identify itself with many others and take its honey from many flowers. That is why the "only child" who has only the companionship of a governess, however admirable, has an impoverished personality. Thirdly, the identification should be natural and *spontaneous* not forced, so as to give freedom. Fourthly, the identification should not be such as to do violence to the child's native temperament, nor conflict too violently with it; but this is not likely to happen if the identification is allowed to be spontaneous and not under the compulsion of fear: the child will choose or modify its choice according to its temperament.

(*d*) A further type of simple character trait is that due to *exaggeration by thwarting*, the opposite of exaggeration by encouragement. It is a principle of human nature that when a tendency is thwarted it tends to become stronger. What is denied us we want the more. This is no doubt of biological value since it makes for the attainment of the denied object, instead of a too easy abandonment of our desires. Satiation removes desire, deprivation increases it. It is as though the damming up of the energy gives greater force to the impulse and increases its intensity. So the child who is denied mother love develops a mother complex more than the child who is given too much of it, who usually rebels: the child who has a great deal of admiration comes to expect it, but the child who has insufficient attention develops into the "limelight child" who pushes himself forward to get it. Many cases of sexual excess are due to a revolt against a too puritanic upbringing rather than to encouragement in sex. Greed is much more commonly the result of being deprived of food than being indulged with its excess. A patient says, "If I'd had enough love I should not have wanted such a fuss made of me. Now I can't be satisfied with less than that everybody in the world should make a terrific fuss of me. Besides that, I was trying to get out of food what I ought to get out of love: I could never get enough, and became greedy. When I was in love with a master at school, I ate a large suet pudding!"

The principles of exaggeration by thwarting works for good as well as for evil. Strength comes from resistance, a strong character only as we have difficulties to face. Some of the greatest scholars are those who in their early days were deprived of the means of learning. They ultimately overleap the mark of their own ambition and expectation. An inferiority complex may be of great service in achieving success.

So strong is this principle that frustration increases desire, that some people want a thing just because it is forbidden; if it were not forbidden fruit they would not desire it.[1] One of the reasons why people desire to do wrong just because it is wrong, is that the taboo increases the desire, and therefore the satisfaction of the thwarted desire adds a thrill to the wrong doing. But perhaps the

[1] There are those who hold that all pleasure is the release of tension: if so, the greater the inhibition the greater the tension, and therefore the more pleasure at its release.

most potent reason is that the things we have been forbidden are obviously the things we have desired: so we regard all forbidden things as desirable things, and so come to desire them just because they are forbidden, even if we do not really want them, assuming that because they are forbidden they must be desirable! Our only reason for wanting them is that they are forbidden.

The thwarting of a desire may either exaggerate it, pervert it, arrest its development or obliterate it; truly a problem for the parent who sees in the thwarting of a child the only means of bringing it up rightly! Because of this principle of exaggeration by frustration, character traits often go by opposites to what was intended. We were recently consulted by a pious churchworker whose wife had left him to become a prostitute: *he* was the son of a bar tender, and *she* the daughter of a missionary! Identification is obviously not everything. It is the boy who has not had his natural curiosity about sex satisfied who indulges in dirty jokes. So the son of ardent prohibitionist parents became one of the worst alcoholics we have known; and the son of the godly mother became a gunman.[1]

Simple character traits may be normal or abnormal. It is not at all inconsistent with a strong and healthy character that some particular traits should be strongly marked; the development of cheerfulness in one, seriousness in another, love and piety in

[1] This principle raises interesting problems in child psychology. Suppose I wish my boys to like sailing as a manly sport, should I bring them up to it, give them plenty of it and encourage their interest; or should I limit their opportunities so that the desire will be strengthened by denial? The principle which determines which result will ensue is not easy to discover: sometimes a child who is brought up to a great deal of it finds in it his greatest pleasure; whereas too much of it may make him bored. Not having enough may make him long for it the more, but on the other hand frustration may make him lose all interest in it. If a mother is kind and generous to her son he may respond and become generous through identification with her; but it may have the effect of encouraging him in selfishness. If, on the other hand, she deprives him of things, he may become more eager for them by frustration; but he may give up wanting them because it is no use wanting what he cannot get. Being denied affection may make one child sympathetic with others by identification, or it may make him callous and resentful. Who would venture to prophesy in any individual case? But this is the point in which *teaching* the principle of conduct, of consideration for others is of value to the child. One thing at least is obvious; that bad discipline, which constantly tells a child not to and then gives in, is calculated to produce the worst results of both encouragement, thwarting and identification.

The principle also applies to adult behaviour. Is it better for a woman who wants to win the regard of a man to "Keep him waiting" so that he will want her the more (which may only make him annoyed), or to be in time and so indicate her pleasurable anxiety to see him (which in fact may put him off). We can at present only suggest that she proceeds by trial and error, and note the effect!

others, sternness or ambition in others, are all consistent with mental health. A man may be as assertive as he likes as long as this assertiveness does not crush his tenderness, and is directed towards fulfilling the demands and purpose of the personality as a whole: indeed, assertiveness is essential for a strong will and the fulfilment of the personality. Strongly developed tendencies make for a strong character provided they harmonize with the rest of the personality.

Simple character traits tend to develop into higher forms. This is because they are free to develop as we have mentioned. The child whose sensuousness is over-encouraged does not become the pervert, but normally develops into a highly sexed adult type not inconsistent with higher forms of love. The child whose exhibitionist tendencies are encouraged may sublimate these into becoming a public speaker, artist, or actor.

Not only so, but such exaggerated character traits are *modified under the influence of the other dispositions* in the mind, and also by circumstances. The person who is always ingratiating gets himself disliked; the limelight child is boycotted by his playmates; the indolent sensuous person finds it necessary to live; the conceited child is snubbed; the liar discovers that he is never believed. So by painful experience these character traits are transformed or got rid of under the influence of biological and social necessity.

Simple character traits are also *transformed as the result of new identifications*; an early developed cowardice is modified by the desire to be courageous like those he admires, selfishness by admiration of a large-hearted school teacher. Religious identification with Christ is a potent factor in the conversion of many adolescents, transforming the whole character.

We should not, therefore, be too greatly concerned about *simple* character traits in childhood, even abnormal ones, for even exaggerated traits tend to develop both naturally and as a result of environmental conditions into higher forms, *provided they are given freedom to develop*. It is far more dangerous that they should be repressed for in that case they become dissociated, produce complexes and later emerge as neurotic character traits.

Nevertheless the exaggeration and over-development of these natural impulses should not be lightly encouraged, for in the first place their necessary correction under social influences may be a painful process; secondly, they are more likely to come into conflict with the rest of the personality; and thirdly, exaggerated traits are more likely to be repressed, with the production of psychoneurotic disorders. The child who shows off is likely to be snubbed, and so to develop shyness and self-consciousness. Therefore the parents are wise who do not encourage the child to go to extremes.

The characteristics of simple character traits, by which we can recognize them, are therefore:

(a) That they are produced by the *direct influence* of the environment, whether by encouragement, suggestibility, identification, or by thwarting. This we may discover by careful questioning.

(b) They are usually *accepted* by the individual, the bad man accepting his bad ideals and refusing to regard them as abnormal, and the good man his. But they may come to be recognized by the individual as abnormal under the influence of social criticism, and so be changed.

(c) They may be *normal or abnormal*, the criterion of normality being that they are in harmony with the remaining dispositions of the personality as a whole.

(d) Being free, they tend to *develop into higher forms*; but they sometimes persist as abnormalities of character, so that a man may be arrogant and a woman mean all their lives, depending on the way they are brought up.

(e) The most dominant of these simple character traits determine our aims and purposes and therefore form our *character*.

The treatment of abnormal simple character traits follows from the foregoing considerations.

(a) In so far as bad environmental conditions which produce abnormal simple character traits, *a change of environment* may be the most effective treatment. A mere change of attitude in the mother—more affection, less scolding; more firmness, fewer threats—may change the child's whole outlook and behaviour, and in some cases a sense of security will itself cure abnormal symptoms like bed-wetting, arrogance, peevishness and jealousy. We speak of a child's abnormal behaviour; but in most cases the child's behaviour under the circumstances is a normal reaction to abnormal circumstances; change the circumstances and the child will behave normally.

(b) One of the most important functions of parenthood is the providing of *opportunity for the child's development* by providing materials for games, occupations, making things, camping, hiking, boating, and intellectual pursuits. This healthy outlet is itself one of the principle means for the direction of energies, for the development of character and for the correction of abnormalities of character.

(c) *Teaching* right principles and aims in life is valuable, the purpose of such teaching being to direct and so co-ordinate the functions of the personality as a whole towards a common end. Holding up new standards of moral conduct has its place here; and so has religious teaching. But a moral or religious life on the part of the person trying to teach is more eloquent than trying to make the child religious, for teaching is rarely effective unless associated with some degree of identification with the teacher, so that the child wishes to be like the teacher or parent it loves and admires.[1]

(*d*) More effective than teaching, therefore, is the establishment of new ideals by the process of *identification*, and a right personal relationship with parents and teachers based on affection and respect.

(*e*) *Discipline* is necessary, the function of which is to restrain and guide our impulses into right channels, but the only discipline worth while is *self-discipline*; otherwise the child will later rebel against the authority of forced discipline; or if it accepts it, such discipline is apt to be repressive and lead to neuroses. The most obvious treatment recommended for any abnormality of character like bad tempers or sexual habits is *self-control*, and ultimately no form of treatment will succeed without it. For the woman whose marriage is not proving successful, analytic treatment is not necessarily the right treatment; it may be that what she requires is to brace herself up and make it a success; and many have succeeded in such an adventure. Even analytic treatment does not exonerate one from the exercises of self-control and of the will: but what it does is to release the individual from the dominance of his complexes so that his self-control can operate effectively. Therefore for simple character traits in which there is no repression the old injunction to "pull oneself together" may be the best form of treatment, and often the only one to succeed. If it were not successful it would not continue to be so universally advocated. But it applies only to simple character traits, and not to reaction and psychoneurotic, and for the moralist to think that all undesirable impulses can be dealt with by self-control and the exercise of the will is as erroneous as for the psychopathologist to advocate psychoanalysis as a cure-all. We cannot pull ourselves together, as Bernard Hart says, when we do not know what to pull together.

(*f*) Where other methods of treatment have failed, it may be

---

[1] This was recognized by Anytus, an old-fashioned Athenian democrat, who when asked (in the *Meno*) whether a boy should be sent to the Sophists in order to learn virtue, replied that any Athenian gentleman taken at random would do the boy more good.

necessary to resort to *punishment* both for the delinquent's own sake and that of society, and it is only in simple character traits that punishment is called for. But the function of punishment in these cases should be clear; it is to be regarded simply as the *inevitable result* or consequences of the action. Obviously the delinquent regards his delinquency, his stealing, lying or indolence as bringing certain advantages. If these delinquencies are invariably followed by other results, namely punishment, he will come to realize that the disadvantages outweigh the advantages. Thus the punishment is designed to impress upon the culprit that it is not worth while to continue in his anti-social ways, and so induce him to abandon his ways and conform to those of society. Such punishment is neither vindictive nor retributive, but reformatory, and is often most effective. To be prosecuted for a motoring offence will make us more careful on the road and the punishment justifies itself. The ostracism of our friends is often sufficient to make us abandon the undesirable habits of the club bore, the gossiping neighbour, or the aggressive business man. Punishment is the simplest form of correcting undesirable faults, and therefore most commonly used, but it is not always the most effective for it does not necessarily carry a person's will with it. Nor is it any use in neurotic character traits. The simple delinquent may be the unfortunate victim of his social upbringing and to that extent not be responsible for his condition, but he is not the victim of complexes, and is therefore free to change his ideals if he wants to, whereas the psychoneurotic is not: he has freedom of choice and action. By the term "freedom" we mean that *the individual is not prevented by psychological complexes from pursuing right ends* if he wants to, however much he may be by objective circumstances. The trouble is that he may not want to, and the problem is how to make him want to. Punishment may assist us in this where other methods fail. There is a place for punishment even in a psychoanalytic world. The psychoneurotic delinquent, as we shall see, is in different case. He wants to, but cannot.

From all these considerations it will have become obvious that the treatment of simple character traits comes more within the scope of the sociologist, the teacher, and the moralist than the psychopathologist, and it is a course they are all fervently pursuing.

REACTION CHARACTER TRAITS

Reaction character traits are those which are as reactions to an opposite tendency in oneself which they repress. As illustration: the child who has a strong craving for love but feels left out may react by saying "I don't want anybody's love," represses his love and becomes defiant, rebellious and possibly a delinquent. This defiance is a reaction character trait. Adler's stock case of the man who has the feeling of inferiority, represses it and compensates by self-importance is another illustration. It is when he fails to reach this fictitious objective that he resorts to a neurosis to excuse his failure. Other illustrations of reaction traits are those of the ascetic individual who is really repressing a sensuous nature; the coward who hides his cowardice by bullying; the bombastic person who is really timid; the ingratiating person who is latently aggressive, the bright and cheerful person who is compensating for a deep depression.

It should be emphasized again that what we call a reaction character trait is not a mere reaction to the environment, for all simple character traits are that, but a reaction to an opposite tendency in oneself. What is sometimes called "reaction depression" (as distinct from endogenous or constitutional depression) is not a reaction character trait in our use of the term, which conforms more closely to Freud's conception of "reaction formation."

In some cases we may be *conscious* of the tendency we dislike and wish to hide it, like the girl who has been stealing and puts on a face of sweet innocence. Less conscious of what he is doing is the person who, when accused, assumes an attitude of hurt pride or righteous indignation: or the boy who recognizing his temperamental effeminacy puts on a Herculean or tough persona, with deep voice and rough manner, but in a clumsy manner because it is overdone. But what we specifically call reaction traits are those conditions in which *the undesirable qualities are so repressed* that we are quite unaware of them and nevertheless assume an attitude against them. The conceited person, whose conceit is a reaction character trait, may flatly deny that he has any inferiority complex, the defiant rebel that he has any desire for affection, or the jilted girl that she is hurt. They, like some psychotics, have no insight into their conditions.

The reason for such repression is the painfulness of the experience, such as the disappointment of unrequited love, the distress of humiliation, the threat of consequences; and the purpose of the reaction trait is an attempt to obliterate this painful experience, to dissociate ourselves from it, to forget about it, and so to avoid the distress associated with it. We ignore it till we are unaware of its existence, unaware that we are repressing it, and unaware of

F

what we are repressing. All that we are aware of is the necessity
to maintain the compensating attitude. It is such reactions to
repressed tendencies which we specifically call reaction character
traits.[1]

Reaction character traits may be reactions either to temperamental traits (like the temperamentally little man who poses as
self-important) or to simple character traits (like the child who
shows off because of the deprivation of love which he now scorns);
or to other reaction traits (as occurs when such a reaction rebelliousness is snubbed and therefore repressed in favour of
ingratiation).

As in simple character traits we take over by identification other
people's characteristics which we like into ourselves, so in *projection* we ascribe to others characteristics and qualities which we
have repressed in ourselves and take up towards these characteristics in them the attitude we have assumed towards them in
ourselves. We hate people who boast, who are greedy, who are
underhand, because these qualities are in ourselves but repressed.
It is the social climber who accuses others of being snobs. We
identify others with the unpleasant in ourselves and ascribe to
them qualities of which they may be innocent. By such projection
we condemn our own undesirable traits without the pain of
acknowledging them: but in judging others we judge ourselves.
The palmist who said "all men are liars" was writing his own
autobiography. Those nations who constantly accuse others of
war-mongering are often themselves preparing for an aggressive
war.

Reaction character traits are the most misunderstood and
therefore the most wrongly treated of all types of abnormal
behaviour. Therefore it is most necessary that we should clearly
understand their characteristics.

(*a*) They are, as we have seen, the reaction to an opposite
tendency which is repressed.

(*b*) Owing to this repression there is always a *duality in the
personality*, which is divided against itself, since there are two
opposing tendencies, one of which represses the other. There is
a split in the personality, an endopsychic conflict, in which there
is a reaction of the individual against himself. It is no longer a
biological problem concerned with the relation of the individual

[1] This same principle of over-compensation operates in communities and
nations as in individuals, so that, as Jung has pointed out in his B.B.C. talk of
November 1946, it is the revolutionary systems of Socialism and Communism
which when they come to power are the most ardent in bringing about a
planned and rigidly ordered society to which everyone must conform.

to his environment as in simple character traits, but a psycho-pathological problem of a person's abnormal relation to himself. In this respect the reaction traits differ from both temperamental and simple traits in which there is not this conflict or duality. A definite "complex" has now been formed, which thereafter determines our behaviour irrespective of circumstances.

(c) Reaction character traits are therefore *always abnormal* since they involve this duality in the personality. In this also they differ from the temperamental and simple traits, which may either be normal or abnormal. But they are not necessarily recognized as abnormal by the individual himself, and in this respect differ from the psychoneurotic character traits which we shall next study.

(d) This duality in the personality accounts also for many *inconsistencies of character*. Because the daughter is too attached to her mother she has perpetual rows with her. A man is rude to his wife to whom he is otherwise devoted, but charming to everyone else: it is because he has an inferiority complex and dislikes his wife for knowing it; whereas he is charming to everyone else to convince himself that he is not inferior. One patient says, "I go to the dog and pull his hair out which makes him yelp, and then I cry out with pity for him and remorse. I have the thought of committing cruelties to people, combined with the thought of being tender towards them because of these cruelties I have inflicted on them." The sadist is often a masochist, the bully a coward, the god has feet of clay, and the pacifist is often the most bellicose of men in the defence of his pacifism. Such inconsistencies can only be understood when we realize this duality in the personality, in which first one part of the personality is in function, then the other. It is the conceited man who prefaces any remark he makes by apologizing for his ignorance, the object of which is partly to put to shame those who are less learned, but not so humble; but partly to forestall any criticism of himself and avoid humiliation, by verbally admitting his ignorance beforehand. Did not Socrates pride himself on his humility, that whereas nobody knew, he admitted that he did not know, thereby proving his superiority to others. It was hardly surprising that his fellow-countrymen turned against him!

The reaction character is therefore the mask or "persona" we assume which may be quite different and even the opposite of our real self, of which indeed we may now be quite unaware. But other people's intuition is able to "see through us" so that others know us much better than we know ourselves. We complain that we are "misunderstood" when in fact we are understood only too well for our liking.

(e) Reaction character traits are *always exaggerated* because they are under the necessity of living down the opposite tendency which they repress, and must therefore go to the opposite extreme: they not only compensate, but *over*-compensate. The hard-working man who is reacting to a latent indolence will not permit himself one moment of leisure nor let himself relax even in his recreations: the mother who is over-solicitous and over-anxious about the health of the child may be compensating for a repressed wish to be rid of the child. The convert is the greatest bigot because he is still unconsciously attached to the faith against which he is now revolting. On the other hand, Saint Paul breathed out threatenings and slaughter against the Christians because he was already half-way to being a Christian and was fighting against it.

Reaction character traits may be of the same nature as simple traits, though differently motivated, so that kindness, self-centredness, sullenness, revenge, indolence, ingratiation, scorn, jealousy and resentment may be either simple or reaction traits. But the reaction trait may often be recognized by the fact alone that they are overdone, and we become suspicious when a person talks of the social standing of his family, draws attention to his generosity, goes out of his way to tell us what a lot his firm thinks of his work, or tries to impress upon us what a libertine he is when in fact he is probably too afraid to be so. The woman patient who keeps stressing the fact that she is very happily married is proclaiming that she is not. In all these cases the exaggeration is necessary to keep in abeyance the hidden complex.

(f) Reaction traits are also recognized by the fact that they tend to be *fixated and arrested in development*. They remain primitive in character; they fail to develop because they are the products of repression and not free to develop. Simple character traits may also be exaggerated, but being free from repression they usually develop naturally into higher forms. Not so reaction traits which are not free because they are under the necessity of keeping guard over the other tendencies which they hate and repress, like the jailer who is almost as much a prisoner as the man he guards. Reaction traits may therefore be recognized by the fact that not only are they exaggerated, but they are crude and childish, like petulance, obstinacy, boasting and auto-erotism.

(g) Reaction traits are *persistent*. This is partly because they must always be on the watch against the repressed tendencies emerging; for every time even the unconscious tendency say of inferiority or aggressiveness is aroused, it throws into activity the reaction to it. If a child reacts to the need for affection by sullenness, each time the feeling of the need of affection is aroused even latently, he will become more sullen. Thus many children demonstrate their need for affection by being persistently difficult and disobedient and it is not surprising that the nature of their disorder is not always recognized. Reaction character traits are also chronic because they represent an unsolved problem since the repressed tendency is unconscious.

(h) Though reaction character traits are always abnormal they are usually (as we have just implied) *accepted by the individual himself* as justifiable. The child who is difficult for lack of affection, blames others, not himself, and justifies his sullenness and antisocial behaviour: the delinquent is defiant.

(i) Reaction traits may also be recognized by the *occasional emergence of the repressed tendency* (which is in fact a psychoneurotic symptom). The over-compensated gay person will occasionally get moods of depression, the conceited person feels that nobody likes him, the rebellious person reverts to self-pity, the self-righteous person falls into his secret vice, the ingratiating person has sudden outbursts of vindictiveness, the "hard" person becomes sentimental and sheds tears at the theatre, the criminal has moments of tenderness, the man of irreproachable character yields to a sudden temptation, and the Pirates in *Peter Pan* long for a mother! These are all symptoms of which the individual is afterwards heartily ashamed, as they are contrary to his adopted character, but they show up the reaction trait to be abnormal.

It is to be remembered that though we are inclined to condemn these reaction traits as abnormal and vicious, they may be the attempt of the personality to maintain itself against unnatural circumstances, the only means of maintaining one's individuality. A child who is unwanted and feels inferior may have no other option than to be conceited or egoistic if it is to maintain its self-respect and its interest in life at all and not fall into utter despair. Not only so, but these so-called abnormalities of character are a patient's defence against what he fears or dislikes in himself, and lightly to remove them without enabling him to cope with the underlying tendencies may meet with disaster. Merely to abolish his conceit (if we can) without re-establishing his self-confidence, will only throw him back into despair and sense of failure.

Treatment. Of all the types of character traits, these reaction traits are the most difficult to diagnose and the most difficult to treat. The difficulty in diagnosis lies in the fact that they are usually regarded as simple character traits and treated accordingly. Again, on account of their resistive nature reaction character traits are sometimes difficult to diagnose from psychopathic personality, but its causes are psychological not constitutional. It is not that he can't be taught but won't be taught. The difficulty in treatment lies in getting the co-operation of the patient, since as a rule he refuses to admit that his attitude or acts are abnormal. In regarding them as simple traits and failing to recognize them as reactions to other tendencies, we treat them in exactly the opposite way from what is appropriate and effective, and so accentuate the very condition we are trying to cure.

The secret of dealing with reaction character traits and delinquency is obviously to pay regard not to the surface behaviour which is the reaction, but *to the underlying feelings* and emotions to which they are the reaction.

If a man is conceited because of a basic feeling of inferiority, we shall no more cure him by "taking him down a peg" than if he is shy because he has a basic conceit shall we cure his shyness by telling him he is a fine fellow. In each case we must take cognisance of the latent and repressed trait of character which gives rise to the manifest behaviour and treat that: the inferiority in the former case, the conceit in the latter. When a child's lying, truculence, stealing, self-pity or grievance is a reaction to a frustrated need for affection, we do not punish these character traits, or even seek by teaching or identification to change them, but deal with the basic need for affection, and by giving such understanding affection as will give him confidence and the sense of security. But such treatment is not always easy nor immediately successful, because such a child, once possessed by the sense of grievance, will often reject the love it unconsciously craves but has repressed; and the mother, herself rebuffed, is inclined to say "very well then!" But patience and persistence usually win in the end by convincing the child that the love is genuine. Similarly, many a child has been cured of the masturbation which was resorted to as a solace for the lack of love, by being given affection not punishment, for now that the child has found someone who loves and someone beside itself on whom it can bestow its love, it reverts to the natural reaction and abandons the perverted. There are many understanding people who are able to deal with such children *intuitively* without knowing the mechanisms of these conditions: they have a natural understanding of the deeper motives of these rebellious, bumptious, shy, sensuous or difficult children, and know "instinctively" (as people say) the right way to deal with them, and that right way is by recognizing why the child behaves like that.

Such environmental treatment may be permanently successful with small children where the personality is still in a fluid state and the complexes not fixed. In other cases it has a temporary good effect as long as the circumstances last, but as the complex remains the morbid reaction may reappear. That is also why a man will do splendid work in a firm with one kind of chief (who plays the rôle of kindly father) and is hopeless with another; and it accounts for the fact that the children who do excellently with one teacher go all to pieces in their behaviour with another teacher, who may be a better teacher, but "does not understand them."

But the complex may be too deep-rooted to be affected at all by such environmental treatment, and then *analysis* is the treatment of choice, the purpose of the analysis being to discover and *release the repressed emotions* of which the character trait is the reaction, and utilize them for the purposes of the personality. But this, like all analytic treatment, requires the co-operation of the patient, and this is precisely the difficulty in dealing with reaction character traits, since the individual justifies his attitude of mind and admits of nothing wrong; it is society that is wrong not himself. The first essential therefore is to get the patient's confidence, and if this can be won the results of analytic treatment are promising.

The sympathetic understanding of the physician is as important as his skill and patience, and will usually gain his co-operation in the end, for such people in spite of their protestations are not happy. The treatment of delinquents of this type by these means is most gratifying.

In other cases, where the patient will not be treated for his reaction character trait, he is often ready to be treated for the psychoneurotic condition, which, as we have said, often accompanies it, and is the emergence of the repressed tendency. The self-opinionated man has what he regards as irrational moods of feeling inferior, and wants to be treated for that: the individual who is over-compensating for his wounded affection by a contempt for women will not be treated for the latter which he justifies, but will be treated for his psychosomatic indigestion which is the manifestation of his hurt pride. These are psychoneurotic character traits and symptoms due to the emergence of repressed tendencies and are recognized to be abnormal by the patient because they represent in fact what the patient has been trying to repress. The approach to the reaction character traits therefore is often by way of their psychoneurotic counterparts, which we shall now proceed to discuss.

PSYCHONEUROTIC CHARACTER TRAITS

Psychoneurotic character traits are the *emergence into activity of repressed tendencies*. A reaction character trait such as we have discussed is a reaction to an opposite tendency which it represses: the emergence of this repressed function is the psychoneurotic character trait. The man who represses his feeling of failure by a show of over-confidence nevertheless has bouts of despondency. The mechanism of both reaction and psychoneurotic character traits is the same, but in the former it is the repressing, in the latter it is the repressed tendency which provides the symptom. But which of them we regard as *the* symptom is a matter of taste or of emphasis; they are both abnormal. The reaction trait is usually complained of by others, the psychoneurotic trait by the patient himself. Thus if fear is repressed in childhood and an attitude of bravado assumed, the latter is an abnormal reaction trait, though not recognized as abnormal by the patient who adopts the attitude as a defence: but if the repressed fear emerges as anxiety, we have a psychoneurotic character trait of which he complains. If a feeling of inferiority is compensated for by a reaction of self-importance, the latter is the reaction trait, and the former, if it occasionally emerges in spite of the patient's dominant self-importance, is the psychoneurotic trait. Such a patient will come for treatment not for his bravado or self-importance (which others may consider most requiring treatment) but for his feeling of anxiety or inferiority which he regards as his true symptom. That is why it is said that if a patient has an inferiority complex he often has a superiority complex. But it may work either way, for a person with an initial sense of superiority owing to being spoilt, may repress this when snubbed and thereafter suffer from a feeling of shyness and inferiority with occasional outbursts of arrogance. Both are abnormal, but the patient may be treated now for one, now for the other.[1]

Psychoneurotic character traits may be due to the emergence of either repressed temperamental, simple or reaction traits. An instance of the first, to take our previous example, is where a constitutionally effeminate man represses this and reacts in favour

---

[1] Cosmetics, we are told, were first devised by a Spanish Queen who suffered from embarrassing attacks of blushing: this blushing was obviously a psychoneurotic symptom. But it was also associated with the opposite tendency of self-assertive independence in ordinary life; for she was the first Queen who dared to walk or smile in public!

of the Herculean rôle, but the original femininity comes out say as a compulsion to wear women's clothes; a simple hate may be repressed in favour of docility and timidity, but comes out in stealing; in the third case this reaction docility and timidity may be repressed in favour of a show of self-confidence, but emerge as a symptom of hesitancy when it comes to action.

The characteritics of the psychoneurotic character traits, by which they may be clinically distinguished are:

(a) They are the *emergence into conscious activity of repressed tendencies*. It may seem irrational to call these characteristics "repressed" at all, since they are so active and conscious. But the main characteristic of repression is not inactivity, nor even unconsciousness but dissociation, and these symptoms are due to the activity of the dissociated part.

(b) They are, like reaction traits, always *abnormal* because they are the results of repression, and repression implies conflict in the personality. But they are *recognized to be abnormal* by the patient, and in this respect they differ from the temperamental, simple and reaction traits, which are generally speaking accepted by the individual as normal, even though they are psychologically abnormal. No one, least of all the patient, justifies the psychoneurotic traits which appear to him utterly unreasonable, as in the case of compulsive stealing or bad temper.

(c) They are always *exaggerated* because they represent the emergence of tendencies which have been repressed. They were originally exaggerated before repression, and have become further exaggerated by frustration.

(d) They are always crude and primitive because they have been *arrested in development* owing to being repressed, and have therefore been deprived of the opportunity of development. Therefore they emerge as childish irritability, irrational jealousy, crude infantile sexuality, morbid self-pity or clumsy delinquencies. They are even more arrested in development than the reaction traits, because the latter, like the jailer, has a certain amount of freedom to develop, whereas the psychoneurotic tendency being completely repressed and imprisoned, has no opportunity at all for development.

(e) Because they are dissociated, psychoneurotic character traits are *beyond the power of our will* and tend to be compulsive. These people do not want to be like that but cannot help it. The woman who has outbursts of temper against her baby to whom she is devoted has a latent and repressed jealousy of the baby whom her husband loves, but she cannot help herself.

(f) But the most distinctive feature of the psychoneurotic character traits, by which alone it may be diagnosed from the other types of character trait is that they are the *complete opposite of the ordinary character of the individual.* It is the model boy at school who is found to be a thief; the pious, well-behaved girl who is found guilty of writing indecent letters; the quiet, homely girl who gets the illegitimate baby; the apparently indifferent person who flares up. The woman shoplifter is a respectable and well-to-do woman and has no need of the things she takes; the child who is obstinate and defiant during the day is found at night to have moods of weeping, misery and loneliness and despises himself for it; the intellectual feels a fool, the man of steel is moved by a "sob-stuff" story and kicks himself for being so sentimental:[1] the ascetic is often a sex pervert, the devoted wife is unreasonably jealous, the superman suffers from claustrophobia, the frightened man gets the V.C., and the Field-Marshal has a fear of cats. These are not just passing moods, but constantly repeating and compulsive states of mind, completely alien to the individual's dominant character.

It is indeed one of the tragedies of life that so many people find themselves victims of impulses and passions, morbid desires and repugnant thoughts, which are completely alien to their ideals and principles but which they are quite unable to account for or control. They find themselves doing things of which they are ashamed, desiring things they feel to be unworthy of themselves, and which they repudiate. "It is no longer I but sin that dwelleth in me," they cry. It is not surprising that the victims of these morbid impulses often regard them as activated by outside agencies, malign influences and temptations of the devil.

The distinction between the psychoneurotic character traits and the psychoneurosis proper (like hysterical paralysis) simply lies in their complexity. They are both the product of repression, both the emergence of repressed tendencies. But we use the term psychoneurotic character trait when the repressed tendency comes out in a comparatively simple form, as timidity, tempers, self-pity or auto-erotism, the psychoneurotic counterparts of which are hysteria, obsessions and sex perversions. In other cases they emerge in somewhat distorted forms as depression, expressive of a need for love; lying, from a combination of self-will and fear; cynicism, from a combination of superiority and diffidence; ingratiation, from

---

[1] A business man who has served several years imprisonment for embezzling feels quite callous concerning the many families he has ruined, but cannot refuse money to anyone who comes with a sad story.

a desire for love and fear, all of which also may be called psycho-neurotic character traits. The psychoneuroses proper are more complicated, for as we shall see they are a compromise between two conflicting tendencies, *both* of which are repressed and combine to form a symptom. For instance, jealous hatred of a rival may be repressed by fear of consequences, and may emerge as a character trait of irrational jealousy; but it may give rise to an obsessional phobia of hurting people, in which repressed tendencies both of hate and fear find expression. This distinction is arbitrary, like most psychological distinctions, since the personality functions as a whole and even the simplest psychoneurotic character traits often have an element of compromise in them, but the distinction is a clinically useful one, for in the abnormal character traits it is only necessary as a rule to discover and release one trait, whereas in the psychoneuroses it is necessary to release both repressed tendencies of which the symptom is a compromise: failure to do this often results in only a partial cure of the neuroses.

Since psychoneurotic character traits are due to the emergence of repressed tendencies the *mental hygiene* of both reaction and psychoneurotic character traits consists in the avoidance of repression of natural tendencies by a too strict discipline, which results in their being no longer available for the use of the personality, or becoming distorted to become abnormal character traits, and substituting for this the right direction of these impulses. This requires the right use of restraint and discipline by means of which such tendencies are utilized and directed to right ends. This is necessary to mental health, to social adaptation and to personal freedom.

The treatment of psychoneurotic character traits is simply told: analysis such as we shall describe in a later chapter is the only adequate form of cure, the purpose of which is to discover and liberate the repressed tendencies so that they may develop as they would have developed if they had never been repressed; self-pity into sympathy for others, aggressiveness into confidence and will power, auto-erotism into adult love.

Because psychoneurotic character traits are opposite to the ordinary character of the individual, these are the conditions for which the patient most willingly comes for treatment, and gives his full co-operation to get rid of a symptom so revolting and so alien to his normal character. We have then the curious state of affairs that the psychoneurotic character traits which are the most complicated in mechanism are the most straightforward and promising to treat—provided one has the technique.

In the small child, in whom free association is impossible, analysis can be conducted by *play diagnosis*, by means of which the child unconsciously reveals its problems, and *play therapy* by means of which the child automatically works out its individual difficulties in a material medium, for the function of play is not merely to "prepare for life" but a means of working out immediate personal problems. Children who were blitzed in the Bristol raids were first stunned, and then after some days began to play at bombing, obviously not to recapitulate any pleasurable experience, but to attempt to work out a yet unsolved problem of fear, and also to reassure themselves by exercising power over the material situations, and controlling events instead of the events having power over them.

The child who reveals the diagnosis of his problem in play, even his moral problems, may then be left to work them out to a satisfactory solution, also in play; or he may be assisted and encouraged to find a solution in the play; or if he is old enough the play may be interpreted and the problem itself discussed with him. In other cases, having seen from the play the nature of his problems, we may suggest to the parents a change in their attitude which itself would solve the problem, the nature of which they were originally quite unaware. In an older child, of thirteen and upwards, free association may be used as with the adult, provided we can get the co-operation of the patient, which we can usually do in psychoneurotic traits.

It is obvious from our description that in dealing with any abnormal trait of character or a delinquency we are not justified in taking it at its face value and treating it as such: if we are to treat it properly we must distinguish its type. It is obvious that the man who lies because he is a constitutional psychopath and has no sense of right or wrong, requires to be treated differently from the one who lies because he has been taught to lie in childhood, or the pathological liar who finds himself with a compulsion to lie but cannot help it.

This classification of types into temperamental, simple, reaction and psychoneurotic has been found valuable in practice for several reasons. First, the classification is based on a difference in causation and therefore enables us to deal with essential causes, and not simply with their symptoms and manifestations in behaviour.

Secondly, each type may nevertheless be recognized by a study of its manifestations in *behaviour*: for though we are not justified in treating a delinquency or behaviour disorder at its face value, a study of their overt manifestations and characteristics as already described will help to diagnose the type. It is true there are mixed cases where, for instance, part is due to temperamental and part to reaction traits, but it is precisely in these cases that we need to be aware of the distinction in types so as to determine what element and proportion of each is present.

Thirdly, this classification is valuable in distinguishing the form of treatment required, which is different for each type. A smacking will cure one child of bed-wetting but make another worse; belladonna will cure one, whilst telling him not to worry cures another.

Whenever, therefore, we are presented with an abnormal character trait, we find it convenient to ask ourselves in the first place to which of these *types* it belongs, and then what are the *specific* causes in each individual case; and we can usually tell this by the various symptoms presented in accordance with the characteristics we have described. Only so can we treat the condition adequately.

Whatever abnormal characteristics we take therefore, whether laziness, greed, bed-wetting, shyness, cruelty, lying, truancy, arrogance or sexual vice, these may be found to belong to any one of these types, and it might pay the reader to exercise his ingenuity in working out in any particular case how these may be temperamental, simple, reaction, or psychoneurotic, and suggest types of appropriate treatment.[1]

---

[1] By way of illustration:

Indolence. A boy is brought suffering from *laziness and indolence, lethargy and inability to work.* In the first place this may be *temperamental* due to an asthenic constitution, or other physical causes, like anaemia, chronic tuberculosis, or "acidosis," lack of sleep or malnutrition. It may be a *simple* character trait in a child who is accustomed to having everything done for him so that he gets into the habit of leaving everything to others and hopes for the best: he will never do to-day what he can leave till to-morrow. Or he may be normally energetic but so frustrated in spontaneous activity by a possessive mother that he loses heart and does nothing. Such children, however, if temperamentally healthy, will usually rebel against their mothers' coddling and may become delinquent. In another case it is a *reaction* trait in a child who has been pressed to overwork and become over-ambitious, against which he reacts by a refusal to do anything. We have known students of this type deliberately throw up their University careers and refuse to do any study. This is a reaction not against the mother, but against an attitude he had himself previously adapted. He will probably refuse treatment for this. The *psychoneurotic* indolence may be the emergence of an earlier lethargy in a child who was ill and delicate as an infant, but later compensated for this by hard work to overcome the earlier anxiety. But he over-compensates and is over-conscientious, and this proves too much for him, so that he has a breakdown in which try as he will he cannot work at all. He

DELINQUENCY

Delinquency may be defined as *anti-social behaviour*.

It is a condition of the individual's enjoyment of the privileges of society (protection, food, culture, etc.) that he must conform to the demands made upon him by society, to modify and change his conduct in response to its demands. If the individual in spite of his acceptance of the privileges of society refuses to conform, then his conduct is regarded as a delinquency, a vice, or a crime, and meets with punishment, both in order to protect society and to make him think better of it by denying him its privileges. Delinquency is therefore primarily a term of social application; it is a failure in social adaptation.

But it is so often caused by pathological disorders that it requires to be studied also as a problem in mental health. Delinquency may be the manifestation of neurotic complexes.

Some people consider that all delinquents are responsible for their actions, and that they should therefore be punished. The more severely they are punished, the less likely they are to repeat the crime. In point of fact it is found that while this is sometimes successful, many delinquents are made worse by punishment. Others regard all crime as a disease, said to be due to disturbances

sits for hours before a book unable to work or to remember. It is a psycho-neurotic trait for which he is only too glad to have treatment.

The distinction of the character types has social implications, as may be illustrated in those who crave for peace. *The pacifist* may be a man devoid of aggression in his constitutional make-up, the kind who would never kill a fly (temperamental): or he may have plenty of normal assertiveness, but having been brought up a Quaker he is in favour of peace at whatever cost (simple): but he may, and often is, disguising a sense of dispeace in his own soul by a show of contentment (reaction), or failing to solve his own moral problems he projects his need for peace on to the outside world, and tries his hand at the easier task of bringing about universal peace. Finally the psychoneurotic type is the man who, denied the peace he desires, reacts by being the warrior who is all out for conquest, but who has occasions when the longing for peace forces itself upon him, contrary to his settled aims.

Those who have to do with charitable and propaganda societies soon become aware that the members of such societies are divided between those who are genuinely motivated by a love for the cause, and those who are motivated by a hate for their opponents. The women's suffrage societies consisted partly of those who had a genuine regard for women and their place in the world, and those who were activated by a hate of men because they themselves would have liked to have been men: in reality they despise the womanhood they ostensibly defend. They may marry several times with a view to subduing their husbands. Working men's movements consist largely of those who genuinely desire to improve the lot of the working classes, and those who are activated by envy and therefore hate the rich, and have no hesitation in taking their places when they get the chance. They are traitors to their cause, and one finds them in all movements ready to go over to the enemy at a price.

in the physiological make-up of the individual, who can be proved to be a degenerate by the shape of his skull (Lombroso) or his biochemical deficiencies. Others regard most crime as primarily due to psychological complexes, which should be treated by psychoanalysis. Some reformers believe in treating the delinquent humanely in the hope of appealing to his better feelings, so that he may be wooed from his anti-social tendencies back to a more useful life: others say he has no better feelings to appeal to, and the sooner society rids itself of the pest the better.

All these forms of treatment are effective in some cases, but none of them are applicable to all. The answer to the question "Is crime a disease?" is that sometimes it is and sometimes it is not: therefore any form of treatment which is applied to all cases is bound to fail in some. Punishment is remedial in some cases, and does harm in others. Humane treatment which succeeds in winning some back to decent citizenship, is simply wasted on others who take advantage of it. Obviously we must discriminate between the types of delinquency, but especially the types of delinquent, before we can treat them adequately.

Magistrates naturally look to psychologists for some help in this matter, both to discriminate between these types and to help in the appropriate treatment of those who are considered mentally abnormal or psychoneurotic. For they are becoming increasingly convinced that many of the delinquencies which come before them are committed by those who are the victims of diseased states of mind like sexual exhibitionism or psychopathic personality which cannot be regarded as insanity, but require medical treatment. On the other hand, they are naturally suspicious of those psychologists who regard all crime as disease, or all delinquencies as psychoneurotic, since they hold the view, rightly or wrongly, that some of those criminals are responsible for their actions and the duty of the magistrate is in any case to protect the public. They also point to the undoubted fact that punishment often does in fact prove to be a deterrent to crime. But if punishment has the effect of making an individual more anti-social, as it undoubtedly does in certain cases, it obviously fails of its purpose in protecting society. If therefore the legal authorities are to carry out their function of protecting society, it is necessary not only to rid society of the criminal for a period of imprisonment, but to rid the criminal of his morbid propensities for all time if this is possible: and it is possible only in some cases.

Judges and magistrates therefore naturally want to be assured of a rational criterion of judgment by which they may distinguish the ordinary criminal from the pathological criminal, before they are willing to let the psychologist loose upon the prisoner. Much harm has been done in the past by sentimentality.[1]

In investigating the causes of these conditions the physician finds that in many of these cases the delinquent or criminal knows perfectly well what he is doing, knows that it is disapproved by society, and has the power to desist if he wants to; but he does not want to. Whether he *can* not want to, considering the environment in which he was nurtured, is another question, but he can obviously be made not to want to, as proved by the fact that in many cases punishment is enough to prevent him committing the crime again.

But in other cases he has not the power to distinguish between right and wrong, owing to mental deficiency or insanity: in still other cases he may understand well enough the nature of the act, and the distinction between right and wrong, but has not the power to resist certain uncontrollable impulses in himself. Indeed many of the delinquencies are found to be of the same nature as other forms of neurotic compulsion, such as phobias, compulsive thoughts, or actions like the compulsion to put things straight, or to step over cracks on the pavement.

The legal authorities do not worry themselves about people who have to count ten before deciding anything; nor does the policeman haul before the magistrate the man who must *pick up* every bit of orange peel, but looks on with his usual complacency. But suppose he is unfortunate enough to have the obsession to *scatter* orange peel the case is very different. The magistrate is not concerned if you have the compulsion to touch every lamp post, but suppose you knock down the lamp post with your car, he imposes a fine; and it matters little whether it is done from pure devilry or from an obsessional compulsion, as it was in the case

---

[1] Those judges and magistrates who object to the introduction of psychological considerations into legal questions, may be reminded of the fact that psychological factors already appear at every turn; even the act of murder is decided upon psychological issues and not merely on fact, namely the accused's *intention* to kill, and the question whether it is a case of manslaughter or murder is often determined by the jury on what they consider the psychological *motive* for the crime. The question of *provocation*, another psychological concept, is also taken into consideration, that is, whether what the prisoner had to suffer was considered beyond his endurance; or whether he *thought* his life was in danger and so acted in self-defence. The psychological factor is indeed often the deciding factor in legal questions.

Let it be remembered, especially in murder cases, that the fact that the criminal tries to avoid detection does not mean that he necessarily considers it wrong: he may only be aware that others consider it wrong. This sometimes applies to the psychopathic personality who is devoid of moral sense but has considerable common sense.

of the patient who in a borrowed Rolls-Royce car speeded along the highway, suddenly had the compulsion "Now for a bl...dy bump!" deliberately ran into another car, and was then horrified at her compulsive act. This was due to a morbid craving for excitement and we can only hope it succeeded in its aim. The man who was brought to court for cutting off the long hair of girls in street cars (and was defended by a psychiatrist as a moral pervert) was found to sell it for a dollar a tress. He is in a very different case from the University lecturer in Moral Philosophy who did the same under the compulsion of a sex perversion. When therefore we meet with a case of delinquency such as stealing, lying, truancy, violent tempers and destructiveness, the first question that arises in the mind is the diagnosis of the type of case, for it is obvious on the face of it that such conditions may not only be due to a variety of causes, but belong to entirely different categories of behaviour. To the magistrate the protection of the public is the important question: to the psychologist the personality of the delinquent and the nature of his delinquency is all important, irrespective of whether the impulse takes the form of an overt act or not. But a combination of their functions may be of equal benefit to the delinquent and to society.

(a) *Benign delinquencies.* Since delinquency is to be regarded as anti-social behaviour, it is necessary for us first to distinguish a group of delinquencies which may be abnormal from a social or legal point of view, but are not abnormal from the point of view of mental health. Playing truant on a bright spring day to go hiking in the woods is a delinquency; it is against school rules and is punishable. Playing football in the streets is illegal and boys are hailed before the magistrate for it. But no one would regard these acts as necessarily a sign of psychological abnormality: indeed, we have heard even magistrates when giving out the prizes at their old school boast of their early escapades as an indication of what fine fellows they were! The girl who trespasses to get a swim in a private stream, or the boy who climbs over the dock gates on a Sunday to see the ships and even slip off in a sailing dinghy is showing an adventurous and romantic spirit worthy of encouragement and right direction rather than being sent to a reformatory. This does not mean that they should necessarily be allowed to do these things, whether in the interests of their safety or the safety of property, but it is necessary to recognize that in such boys it is neither a crime nor an abnormality and proper outlets for their adventurous spirit should be found. Many mute inglorious Raleighs are to be met with in the dock!

G

These delinquencies, therefore, we call *benign delinquencies*, borrowing the term from "benign" tumours of the body, like warts or fibroids, as distinct from malignant tumours: they ought not to be there, but they do no particular harm. The term "benign" delinquency is also suggestive of the attitude of mind that we should adopt towards them.[1]

But there are many other delinquencies which are obviously abnormal not merely from the social point of view but from the point of view of mental health. These follow the four main groups of character traits which we have already described, which require different types of treatment.

(b) *Temperamental delinquencies* are very common, that is to say, delinquent forms of behaviour based on disordered physiological functioning. Menstrual changes in girls and women are so commonly the prelude to delinquency that Havelock Ellis has said that if a woman is a shoplifter the chances are that she is at the time of her menstrual cycle. This is not universally true even of pathological stealing: but we have recently had a mixed case of a respectable professional woman of ample private means who committed four thefts, three of which were at the time of her period and the fourth within a week of it. But there were also marked psychoneurotic factors present relating to the repressed rebellion against her father. Physiological disturbances of this kind serve to make us less balanced so that psychological complexes come to the surface and make us give way to the uprising impulses to which otherwise we should not have succumbed. Temporary physiological disturbance may be the occasion for the complexes to manifest themselves. Recently a man charged with murder successfully pleaded that his attacks of violence coincided with a low blood sugar.[2]

[1] Stealing is practically normal for the child of eight or nine who is in the "primitive man" stage of development in which he is predatory. It is a benign delinquency—it cannot be allowed, but mothers and teachers should not take too serious a view of it or regard it as moral turpitude. To call such a child a "young thief" may lead him to become one.

[2] Curiously enough, comparatively few delinquencies are found to be due to mental deficiency. Cyril Burt considers that only 10 per cent are so, but 28 per cent of delinquents are definitely dull. Healy considers that there is very little difference between the mental level of delinquents and non-delinquents. Physical defects are more common as a cause of delinquency (170 as against 79 controls) because the physically handicapped have a sense of grievance because they are less able to compete in life; but such delinquencies are not the direct effect of the physiological disorder but the psychological reaction to it. On the other hand, Sessions Hodge (*B.M.J.*, Dec. 21, 1946, p. 966) says, "Of a group of 63 cases referred for examination from Courts of Summary Jurisdiction, 36·5 per cent on complete investigation might properly be considered to suffer from epilepsy or "epileptic equivalents," as judged by the encephalograph.

(c) *Simple delinquencies* are those which are the product of ordinary environmental influences. They do not require detailed description. They relate to the ordinary delinquencies and crimes against which society requires to be protected by the law. They are the product of the conflict between the claims of the individual and the demands of society and probably account for the majority of crimes. They are due to (a) bad circumstances such as poverty, overcrowding, drunkenness and prostitution in the home. But that those are not the only causes of crime is proved by the fact that roughly speaking half the delinquents come from circumstances in which there is *no* poverty and other such extraneous causes (Burt's *Young Delinquent*). (b) Simple delinquencies are more frequently due to bad upbringing, such as spoiling, too strict upbringing, lack of discipline, wrong discipline, too much discipline and frustration: also from identification with bad parents and bad companions. These correspond to the types of simple character trait we have already discussed.

We have just interviewed for military service a "smash-and-grab" expert of the toughest type, who boasted of his exploits. He was the youngest child, doted upon by his parents, and spoilt by his older brothers and sisters; in the eyes of all, so he tells us, he "could do no wrong." His crimes appeared to be partly due to this lack of discipline, but partly a reaction trait to compensate for being a spoilt baby, and playing the gangster to prove that he was not.

A married woman previously honest, stole money from her husband whom she suspected of being unfaithful. There had been aroused in her mind an experience in childhood when her sick mother with a similar grievance against her husband told the girl to take money from a mug on top of the dresser. It was a case of simple identification.

The treatment of these simple delinquents is a sociological and moral one. New environment, new identifications, new purposes in life, new ideals are what is required.

More salutary are those preventive agencies, voluntary or otherwise, which are designed to occupy the leisure time and to direct the energies of youth, such as clubs, social and athletic, playgrounds, not least of all the cinema, which in spite of all that is said, probably prevents far more crime than it ever produces. Creative work, like pulling to pieces and rebuilding engines, making canoes and other activities connected with the world of reality, is best of all. For such conditions encourage the right direction of natural impulses, and at the same time give new identifications.

Punishment is sometimes called for, as we have stated, to convince the delinquent that crime is not worth while: in some cases it is the only form of treatment practicable. But all punishment should be as far as possible a form of "cure" by which we mean "restoration to normality." Punishment is a form of treatment when the conditions we impose are for the definite object of changing the individual himself and curing him of his morbid tendencies of character, and therefore ranks side by side with change of environment, morals, religion, or psychotherapy as a form of treatment. Punishment of the delinquent, therefore, should be remedial. Whether it should ever be retributive is a problem for social psychology, and must depend upon observed results. Punishment is retributive when it is regarded as the penalty that the individual has to pay for his crime, an expression of the vengeance and disapproval of society as well as for the protection of the community. In giving expression to such vengeful feelings retributive punishment may be beneficial to society if not to the individual. This possibility is not to be scouted without further investigation; for if society is not thus satisfied it may be offended by the too great leniency and shocked that a brutal criminal should go unpunished, and thus suffer a rebuff to its sense of justice which may lower the whole morale of the community. Again, if society is not thus relieved by the punishment of the criminal it may release those vengeful feelings on others. The scapegoat is a sinister figure in history and not unknown in our time and generation. Lynching of merely suspected and sometimes quite innocent victims is a case in point, due to the tardiness of justice, and the frustration of a feeling of just revenge. On the other hand, retributive punishment may be merely a means of giving expression to the sense of guilt of the community by projecting the sins of its members upon the criminal who then becomes the scapegoat for the sins of society. Self-righteousness which covers up a sense of guilt may be brutal in its vengeance. This satisfies the self-complacency of the community, but prevents it from rectifying its own sins, since it projects its sins on others and satisfied its sense of guilt by punishing them. This projection of our sins upon others which is a commonly recognized feature of individual psychology may be observed in the behaviour of communities.[1]

Capital punishment is obviously not remedial, though it

[1] Hitler "protected" the countries he ravaged; Russia, with its one party system, claims to be the only true democracy; America's sense of guilt regarding the negro problem projects itself into blaming the British for their ill-treatment of the Indians; and Britain spread her "beneficent rule" throughout the world and made a good thing out of it!—now a thing of the past.

effectively prevents the criminal from committing further crimes and so protects society. Whether it deters others from murder is a question upon which experts differ, and is not easy to determine: but the problem is not made easier by the prejudices, whether sentimental or sadistic, of the contestants. To start a discussion of capital punishment or of corporal punishment is always calculated to produce the maximum of prejudice in which there is so much smoke, not to speak of heat, that the whole problem becomes befogged. Nothing brings out people's complexes in so short a space of time. On the one hand we have those who are great believers in corporal punishment presumably because it has produced such fine result in themselves (or because they are sadists); and on the other hand we have the sentimentalist who assumes that for a child to get a smacking will lead to lifelong complexes and misery. That smacking often produces a sense of injustice, resentment, fear, neurosis and sexual masochism is an undoubted fact, and is therefore undesirable. But to assume that it is always detrimental is to contradict the fact that numerous canings have been and are daily given which are accepted as the just punishment for misconduct and leave no more scar on the mind than they do on the body. Nevertheless we may usually find better ways of dealing with misbehaviour, and the occasions of retributive punishment should continually diminish as the scope of treatment is enlarged.

(d) *Reaction delinquencies* are very common and probably account for large numbers of recidivists owing to wrong treatment. Like the simple delinquencies they have been produced by environmental conditions, usually in childhood, but these conditions have been repressed and developed definite complexes in the mind which thereafter determine the individual's behaviour, whatever the environment. The most common reactions are those due to the feeling of deprivation of love, which is necessary to every child.

A girl at school was very troublesome. She was defiant, rude to her teachers at school and stole things from her schoolfellows. She was born during the war in the absence of her father; and was naturally spoilt and allowed her own way by her mother. When she was three years of age her father returned for good. She resented his intrusion since he now bossed the house which she had previously dominated. Some time after, another baby arrived which she regarded as "another bit of dirty work on father's part," and she was still more furious that the new baby was now getting all the fuss and attention. She reacted to this situation by tossing her head and saying, "be damned to the lot of you!" tore up her parents' photographs (getting rid of them symbolically) and ever after maintained this defiant attitude. She was a rebel, not merely against society, but a rebel against herself, against her craving for love and affection which she unconsciously craved but outwardly scouted. To treat such a child by punishment is precisely the way to perpetuate her resentment and make her more defiant. She was willing to co-operate, being unhappy at school, and was treated by analysis. She came to realize the cause of her defiance, readjusted her attitude towards her teachers who were in fact kind, and was cured not only of her stealing and other "difficulties," but also of this resentful attitude towards life.

That reaction traits and delinquencies are *accepted* by the individual is evident in this case: a youth from public school steals, but is defiant— "I have the impulse to steal money or anything else at the moment; and I don't feel it to be particularly wrong. I know I should be punished, but I don't feel it is wrong and I have no conscience about it afterwards." (A very different attitude from the psychoneurotic delinquent.) This youth's mother died a few months after birth and from infancy he felt himself robbed of the affection he wanted. He reacted by this defiance and rebelliousness. Obviously it was a reaction character trait, a reaction to his own desire for affection. It was difficult to get his co-operation, so we did not treat him for his stealing, in which he felt himself justified and which was not a symptom to him, but for his psychoneurotic depression. In analysis the depression led to the basic need for affection, and this to the explanation and cure of his defiant delinquencies.

A composite case, mostly reaction, was that of a schoolboy, a brilliant classics scholar, who gave great trouble to the masters, broke rules, told lies, and was antagonistic. It originated in (a) *temperamental* instability, for he was fifteen and had the development of a boy of eighteen; (b) a *simple* identification with his father who was domineering and arrogant, so that the boy was arrogant and scornful of other boys, which made him disliked. This was increased by the fact that his father deserted the family and left the boy "head of the home" at the age of five! (c) A *reaction* to a longing for his father's affection, which was denied him, for his father sneered at him and rebuffed him, so that he became resentful, rebellious, anti-social and ultimately delinquent. This situation was perpetuated at school, for owing to his arrogance he was unpopular, and failed to get the friendship of the other boys for which he longed, so that he turned against those whose friendships he wanted, masters and boys alike. Such a psychological tangle was beyond the environmental treatment that his house-master could provide, and obviously punishment would only make him worse in giving him a greater sense of grievance. His condition required expert analytic treatment and by this he was cured.

Sexual reaction delinquencies are very commonly due to the feeling of deprivation of affection. Protective love and sensuous pleasure are so intimately associated in infancy that it is not surprising that one is easily substituted for the other; so there are those who are deprived of affection who turn to find in sexuality a solace, and like all reaction traits this is obstinate, crude and exaggerated. Many of those who take to prostitution are of this type; deprived of affection they become completely disillusioned and cynical about love, and then find a temporary though not permanent satisfaction in sex. Many "mistresses" are of this type; the real need was for affection, not for sex, in which in some cases they took no particular pleasure, but being friendless they accepted the situation in return for what love and companionship they could get.

Treatment of reaction delinquencies. It is a matter of common observation that there are some delinquents and even ordinary "naughty" children who are made worse by punishment. A boy who is delinquent and steals because he feels the sense of injustice through the favouritism of his young brother, is not likely to have his resentment removed by what he considers to be a further injustice. The first effect that punishment has upon such a boy who steals is to make him steal the more, and this we have often found to be the case. That is why they become recidivists. It is not by any means only the mental deficients "upon whom punishment has little or no deterrent effect," but also those suffering from reaction character traits. They are made chronic criminals by treatment which increases their sense of grievance and impels them to resort to further crime to express their increased resentment. They are the most difficult to treat of all forms of delinquency.

A boy of fourteen, a weedy bespectacled youth, constantly stole, and as constantly was beaten by his father, a Sergeant-Major in the regulars. The more he was beaten the more he stole. It transpired that his buccaneer spirit which made him steal was a compensation for his feeling of physical inferiority. The more he was beaten, the more the spirit was crushed, the more he had to assert himself by stealing. Without treatment he might have become a chronic criminal.

The case of "simple" delinquency is so different; the act is deliberate and due to bad training or low standards of social conduct. The forms of treatment, therefore, suitable for a child with a simple delinquency is often exactly the reverse of what is suitable for a reaction delinquency. Punishment as we have seen is sometimes useful in a simple delinquency; it is worse than useless in a reaction trait because it only makes the child more resentful. *Kindly treatment* has been tried in some prisons, but without distinguishing the types for whom such treatment is appropriate, it would often lead to failure. It is useful where the delinquency is based on a need for affection, and is also of the greatest value if it succeeds in effecting an identification with those in authority: but kindly treatment, as we have said, is only regarded as "weakness" by others, and advantage is taken of it. In psychoneurotic cases it is appreciated by the delinquent, but it requires more drastic treatment than that to cure him. Failure to distinguish the types has meant that this method has had less encouraging results than its advocates hoped, though better than its opponents expected. Indeed, a uniform method of treatment of any kind is bound to fail in some cases, whilst succeeding in others, and only a study of the individual as well as his type of disorder can provide the right type of treatment, and make it more universally successful.

Analytic treatment, as we have stated, which discovers the latent cause of the reaction and releases the repressed feelings is the most adequate form of cure.

Psychoneurotic delinquencies are those most frequently met with by the psychopathologist, to whom they are constantly referred by the social worker, schoolmaster or magistrate. For they are the ones most easily detected as abnormal, since they are so inconsistent with the youth's normal character. But for one that is so sent by an understanding teacher or magistrate, there are numbers which are undetected and become victims of punishment for conditions for which they are not responsible. Psychoneurotic delinquencies are *the emergence of repressed impulses in the form of anti-social behaviour.* They are mostly due to latent resentment.

Delinquencies are often put down to "adolescent instability." Such instability may be constitutional, for we often find that endocrine disorders of development producing overgrowth, undergrowth, over-development and under-development are common causes of delinquency. Indeed, it appears that any incompatibility between mental and physical development makes for lack of balance, or is an indication of it.

But "adolescent instability" may also be due to complexes already present, which are particularly liable to surge up in the changing scene of adolescence. Unsatisfied sexual cravings may take the form of taking things of sexual significance. But stealing in adolescence is often due to the need for love and security, especially in girls at puberty, which is different from sex craving. Money is the symbol of security, and stealing is often of things belonging to the person most loved. Truancy is often a primal tropistic urge to wander, to migrate, to get free and independent which matures at adolescence: in most cases, however, it represents rebellion against authority. Fire raising is often symbolic of this release of suppressed sexual passion; in other cases it is the morbid craving for repressed excitement, as well as of pure devilment.

The following is a case presenting all the characteristics of a psychoneurotic delinquency, the latent causes of which were revealed in analysis.

A sweet charming girl, a probationer nurse, was to everyone's surprise found to be taking stockings which she did not in any sense need (this was pre-war!) from another nurse. It was obviously due to repressed resentment. This led us back to the age of three when she, a temperamentally assertive child, was made to stop playing to go out to tea. She rebelled and when dressed was put in the hall whilst her mother dressed; she got her revenge by pulling up all the tulips in the garden. These tulips lying on the grass looked "so darned complacent" that she did the same with the next garden and was well on to the third when a hue and cry was raised, she was caught, shut up in her room, and beaten by her father when he returned home. This broke her defiance and she became the sweet girl, a Sunday school teacher, beloved of all. When she left home her independence again began to assert itself, and when another nurse tried to set the others against her, her repressed resentment again emerged, and she had this compulsion to steal. When she was charged with this and with many other crimes she had not committed, she admitted them all, to show her defiant attitude. Her repressed aggressiveness being released in analysis developed into self-confidence. She became a person of stronger character, though perhaps less sweet, and her stealing propensities, derived from her previously repressed resentment, disappeared.

Another patient, this time an adult married woman, was a notorious shoplifter who reckoned that she had stolen over £4,000, was diagnosed as a simple thief by the magistrates who in previous convictions had sent her to prison, and diagnosed as an epileptic by a doctor on the grounds that she had an "aura," becoming flushed and hot in the head before precipitately, and with little precaution, going forth to steal things for which she had no use. In fact the case was neither, but a true case of psychoneurotic or pathological stealing, the "aura" being a reproduction of an experience in childhood. As a small child she was terribly spoilt by her father, which developed her self-will, but was disliked by her jealous mother, who in revenge made her dress in ugly clothes. This filled her with such resentment that she became defiant till her father thrashed her and she became terrified of him and of God. (So far a reaction character trait.) But still defiant she had to lie even about the most trivial things. Sometimes she would get away with it, and then felt that God wasn't so all-powerful and all-seeing as she was given to understand, "and it gave me the idea that God was something dopey and didn't know what was going on." This encouraged her to take further risks. Her rebelliousness was finally crushed when her mother, to punish her (unjustly as it happened) for breaking a vase, put her head under the bath tap and nearly suffocated her: and said, "Now will you admit that you did it on purpose, or do you want more punishment?" This effectively "cured" her of her naughtiness. "I was such a coward that I had to say I had done it on purpose, though I hadn't. Then I felt I'd jolly well wait and would do something on purpose. But I felt utterly beaten—by people, by circumstances, by everything. I always felt in the way; I was not wanted. I longed to change with other people's mothers who were nice." So she repressed all her rage. Her shopliftings in later life were always found to coincide with contact with her mother, whom she hated but of whom she was afraid. They were partly motivated by the unconscious desire to disgrace her mother who was a Society woman and her father who was a magistrate, and who would be affected by his daughter being sent to prison, as she had previously been for six months. That explains why she stole things she did not want, and also why she did not take particular precautions against detection—both signs of "pathological stealing." The flushing before she stole was a reproduction of the intense feeling in her head when it was put under the cold tap, which brought her to heel. It is obviously a psychoneurotic symptom, being quite alien to the woman's moral character, as she was a charming wife and devoted mother. In this case the magistrate put her under probation for treatment: she was cured and no further incidents have occurred for the last twelve years.

In other cases where the sex cravings are repressed, they emerge as "substitute delinquencies," taking a symbolic form because of their repression. Fire raising is a case in point, symbolic of the sexual passion; stealing without any specific desire for the object itself is frequently an expression of repressed sex, and the object is often though not always a sex symbol. It signifies taking the forbidden thing.

A girl was taught by an unscrupulous gardener to handle him sexually. When she went indoors she tried to do the same thing with her father, a clergyman, who was naturally shocked: so she had to repress such desires. But she went on: "If I can't handle my father sexually I'll get my gratification by handling his papers and things in his study: so I went and messed my fingers about in his papers and then went into his drawers and took out some money. (Symbolic of her sexual desire.) And then I thought how nice it would be to run away and spend it— so I rushed out of the house and down the street and spent the money."

It will be obvious that the study of the *type* of delinquency as well as the individual case is necessary in the diagnosis and treatment of delinquency, as of all other types of character traits.

CHAPTER IV

THE PSYCHONEUROSES BIOLOGICALLY CONSIDERED

THE PSYCHONEUROSES AS BIOLOGICAL RESPONSES

THE psychoneuroses may be regarded as a failure in biological adaptation. Whenever an organism is faced with any critical situation, say that of danger, it responds by producing an amount of energy to cope with the situation and releases this energy in the form of an impulse.

These reactions are specific to the particular situations which call them forth: fear reactions, if the situation is one of danger; pugnacity, if the individual is thwarted or attacked; sex, if aroused by the appropriate stimulus; tenderness in the presence of a helpless offspring. The whole activity then ends with the achievement of the goal, the satisfaction of the impulse aroused, the release of tension and the restoration of the whole organism, body and mind, to a state of equilibrium.

Associated with these activities are certain changes in the organism itself to enable it to carry out the necessary action.

There are, in the first place, changes in the *autonomic nervous system*, and the viscera: the heart beats more rapidly to give a greater supply of blood to the muscles; the breathing is deeper to refresh the blood with oxygen; the digestion ceases and thus allows a greater supply of blood to the tissues; sugar is released into the blood stream which makes more energy available; the adrenal glands pour their secretions into the blood to aid these visceral processes and the whole body is thrown into a condition we call excitement.[1]

All these movements, as Cannon has shown, represent *preparedness for action*.

These activities are further associated with *mental changes*; we become more alert, the senses are more acute, eyes, hearing and touch are accentuated, perception is keyed up to appreciate the danger, to distinguish prey from foe, and to be mentally prepared for appropriate action.

---

[1] It is found, however, by experiment (*Journal of the Royal Society of Medicine*, October 1945, p. 675) that some people instead of having excess of sugar in the blood when in a state of anxiety, have a deficiency of sugar owing to the secretion of insulin, which utilizes the sugar to produce energy.

Finally, the energy thus accumulated normally discharges itself in *voluntary motility*, such as running away, crying out, attacking the enemy, seizing the prey or pursuing the object of love; all of which are functions of the *central nervous system*.

These are all normal processes, the function of the central nervous system being to enable the organism to adapt itself to the outside world; the functions of the autonomic nervous system being to adapt the organism to itself and its functions; and the mental functions being directed to appreciate the situation and devise appropriate means to cope with it.

But any of these functions may be disordered, usually as the result of frustration, and these disorders constitute the psychoneuroses, which are therefore disorders of biological function.

If the functions of the *central nervous system* become disordered we have disorders of voluntary motility such as paralysis of arms or legs, or disorders of sensations like blindness or pain. These correspond to *Conversion hysteria*.

If, on the other hand, the functions of the *autonomic nervous system* are frustrated, we have disorders of the viscera, such as nervous indigestion, violent palpitations, disorders of breathing, sweating and trembling, fatigue from the exhaustion of sugar, sexual impotence, the cessation of menstruation, headache from the congestion of blood in the cranium and more subtle disorders of the liver or the functions of the thyroid gland. These are the *Psychosomatic disorders*.

Further, if there are disorders of *mental function*, such as when escape is impossible, we are thrown into a state of apprehension, dread, and anxiety. Such are the *Anxiety states*. Or it may be that the hopelessness of the situation makes us give up hope of escape, and we suffer from *depression* and other affective disorders of mental functioning.

But man lives in a *social* as well as a material environment, and needs to conform to the demands and *mores* of society, not only for his comfort, but because his safety and security depend on others. Morality is the penalty which society demands of its individuals in return for the security it affords. The conflict between the individual's desires and the demands of society give rise to serious individual as well as social problems. Failure to accommodate himself to the demands of society may lead to anti-social behaviour and *Delinquency* on one hand, where the individual demands are predominant; and to *Obsessions* where the demands of society are uppermost and being accepted by the individual leads to the repression of his natural impulses. The guilt arising from the rebellion against society makes it imperative that the individual should propitiate for his forbidden desires and impulses in order to avert the consequences of his wrongdoing; hence the handwashings, ceremonials, over-conscientiousness and other propitiatory acts. Delinquency and obsessions may therefore be regarded as a failure in adaptation to the social environment, and failure to solve the moral problem in oneself, respectively.

Finally, the physiological functions already referred to are usually associated with *sensuous pleasure* in their successful fulfilment; it is a pleasure to eat as it is to escape from danger. The function of this pleasure is to encourage the biological processes, and pleasure is therefore a means of adaptation to life. This particularly applies to the reproductive functions, which because they do not subserve any individual advantage require to be encouraged by the heightened pleasure associated with them. But these sensuous pleasures may be divorced from the biological functions of reproduction they naturally serve and give rise to *sex aberrations*. Moreover they are liable to come into conflict with the biological demands of reality as they are to come into conflict with social demands; and as a result they are frustrated. Sex perversions are always the result of the repression of early sensuous activities. The result of such frustrations can be observed even in animals, such as rams which can be made permanently homosexual if kept too long segregated from female society of the ewes.

Certain characteristics of these abnormal reactions have already become apparent. (*a*) It is of interest to note that these abnormal reactions are most commonly due to the *thwarting* or frustration of the natural impulses. It is not the natural expression of anger, fear or sex which produces pathological effects like palpitation, headache or hysterical paralysis, but it is when rage is thwarted that it gives rise to indigestion; when fear is frustrated that it gives rise to anxiety. This gives a biological setting for the psychological theory of repression. Bacon says: "We know that diseases of stoppings and suffocations are the most dangerous in the body; and it is not otherwise with the minde"[1]. (*b*) In the second place it is important to note that these psychoneurotic disorders are not disease entities in themselves, but *reactions*, responses of the individual to certain abnormal conditions.

The psychoneuroses may therefore be regarded as a failure in biological adaptation, and it is not surprising that some people have regarded psychoneurotic symptoms as nothing else than

[1] Quoted, E. Jones, *Papers*, p. 490.

abnormal biological reactions to objective situations in life. Is this then a sufficient explanation of psychoneurotic disorders as we find them in human beings?

The first fact that strikes us is that these objective situations of crisis and danger such as give rise to these abnormal reactions are rarely met with in civilized life except in war, in accidents, or in illness; and therefore cannot account for the vast majority of the psychoneuroses met with in ordinary life, most of which occur without any marked precipitating cause of this kind. In hysterias and obsessions of ordinary life there is as a rule no objective danger, no external crisis, and no external inhibition to the expression of the emotion.

Most of the problems of life are not concerned with objective dangers, but with dangers and doubts arising from our own complexes and impulses. Our fear is not so much of bombs and illnesses, but a fear that we shall prove cowards. The stimulus of danger comes from within.

Not only so, but the frustration and inhibition come from within. The man with the hysteric paralysis is not the one who is paralysed with fear because there is no escape; he is one who will not allow himself to escape. The obsessional is not merely one who has to perform propitiations because of the demands of society, but because he accepts them and places these demands on himself. It is a child's own guilt which makes him repress his sex desires and so later produces a sex perversion. In brief the crisis may be a purely subjective problem.

But curiously enough, although the dangers are from impulses within, and although the inhibitions to these impulses are also from within, the patient reacts in precisely the same way as if they were external dangers. The very thought of making a fool of himself will make him sweat as if he is afraid of an objective danger. In such cases there is no biological stimulus, but there is nevertheless the same bioligical response of paralysis, sweating or indigestion. The individual is not in any actual danger but his body behaves as though he were. Or if he is in danger it is from impulses from within himself threatening the integrity of his personality: but what is the use of sweating in such a situation? He gets blind because he cannot bear to look at himself, sick because he is disgusted with himself, develops aphonia because he dare not speak, and pains to call for sympathy and attention. Such physical responses to mental and moral situations are obviously inadequate.

Nevertheless the hysteric symptom which was originally purely a biological response, comes to serve very much the same purpose as the biological response, namely to get him out of the distressing situation, even if it is a moral situation, and to excuse him from facing his responsibilities, even though these are responsibilities and tasks he has imposed on himself. His symptom has now become purposive.

So we pass from a biological to a psychological consideration of the psychoneuroses, using the term "biological" in a somewhat arbitrary fashion to express the individual's response to the environment. The former explains abnormal behaviour in terms of an individual's adaptation to objective life, whereas the latter finds that whilst some of the psychoneuroses, like the traumatic neuroses, are so conditioned, most of them are determined by an individual's failure to adapt himself to himself, to his own impulses, and to the demands he makes on himself.

An appreciation of this fact is of the great importance in treatment; for if we explain abnormal behaviour in terms of an individual's adaptation to his environment, we shall treat his condition by changing his environment, a method which is found to have very limited success. But if we regard the essential feature of the psychoneuroses to be man's maladaptation to himself, we shall seek to discover the basic subjective conflict and eradicate the complexes which are at once the source of danger and the cause of the abnormal responses.

THE PSYCHONEUROSES AS ALLERGY

The neuroses may further be considered in terms of *hypersensitivity or allergy*.[1] As we may be hypersensitive to nicotine or quinine, so we may because of earlier experience become hypersensitive or allergic to fear, to criticism or to frustration, and react in an exaggerated or an abnormal manner to these stimuli. Moreover such mental hypersensitivity follows very much the same principles as a physical hypersensitivity.

For when we are subjected to an unusual or noxious stimulus like nicotine, our first reaction is to reject the stimulus, so that the boy's first smoke makes him sick. If the stimulus persists, the organism gradually becomes acclimatized to it, until it can tolerate doses so large that they would originally have harmed or even

[1] The difference between the two terms, which we may ignore for the time being, is that "hypersensitivity" means an exaggeration of a normal response, whereas an allergy means a response "other" than the normal one. Both of these types may appear in the neurosis: one man may be exaggeratedly terrified of bombs, while another may under the same circumstances develop homosexual episodes.

killed us. So we get immune to large doses of arsenic, high alti-
tudes, or to morphia: and the savage can drink water from the
village pond, which would kill those of us not accustomed to it.
But ultimately there comes the time when we go a step too far, and
a violent reaction sets in: after which we react so violently to these
objects that even the most minute doses will produce a reaction
far beyond its normal effect. The smoker who becomes acclimatized
to smoking a large number of cigars a day may suddenly get
"smoker's heart" with palpitations after smoking even one.

The biological value of this series of responses is obvious. The
organism is so devised as first to reject, and then to accustom
itself to unusual experiences; but if the noxious stimuli continue
and are likely to become a real menace, the physiological organism
turns against it and avoids it altogether by the violence and
exaggeration of the response.

Hypersensitivity and allergy may thus be regarded as a defence
against the dangers of an overdose of any noxious stimulus.

Psychological allergy follows the same principle. In the London
blitz, most of us were afraid of the first air raid: then we acclimatized ourselves to them and went out of doors to watch them with
interest or slept through them. Then one "near miss" or the
shattering of our home, although we were unharmed, might
thereafter make us panic-stricken, after which even the back-fire
of a car sets us in a state of dread. We have become hypersensitive
to noise. The neurotic is one who because of childhood experiences
has become hypersensitive or allergic to certain situations; over-
sensitive to criticism, to humiliation, to hate, to lack of affection,
to frustration, so that he reacts exaggeratedly or abnormally in
such situations. To the neurotic, every pin-prick is a dagger
thrust, every molehill a mountain, every sound the threat of
doom: he cannot bear to face strangers, he "goes off the deep
end" if thwarted, he becomes depressed if the slightest thing goes
wrong, he "loses his nerve" when there is nothing to fear. In both
the physical allergies and the neuroses the predisposition to the
exaggerated response is usually more important than the precipitating situation. This conception of the neuroses in terms of
allergy is illuminating, but it is incomplete as an explanation, for
we have still to ask, what produces this hypersensitivity? What
determines this mental allergy? what are the conditions which
originate "the neurotic constitution" which predisposes the individual to act in this exaggerated fashion? The answer can only
come from a study of the deep-seated causes of the neuroses, which
it is now our purpose to discuss.

CHAPTER V

GENERAL AETIOLOGY OF THE PSYCHONEUROSES

BEFORE proceeding to study the particular types of psychoneurosis it would be as well to discuss the causation of psychoneurotic conditions in general.

The psychoneuroses are psychogenetic, that is to say disorders due to mental and emotional causes. They are of various types:

Conversion hysteria are psychogenetic disorders, manifesting themselves in physical symptoms, mainly of the *central* nervous system, like functional paralysis and blindness.

Psychosomatic disorders are psychogenetic disorders, mainly of the visceral and *autonomic* nervous system, like nervous indigestion, palpitation of the heart, and sweating, many of which are of neurotic origin.

Anxiety states are a motley group related to hysteria on the one hand, and to obsessions on the other, which are characterized by morbid anxiety.

Sex perversions are those conditions in which the sexual functions, instead of being directed to the normal sexual *object*, are directed to an abnormal object like a fetishistic shoe, or someone of the same sex; and those in which there is an abnormal sexual *activity*, such as exhibitionism or sadism, which takes the place of normal sex desires.

Obsessions are morbid mental compulsions, such as compulsive tics, compulsive propitiatory acts like hand-washing, or compulsive character traits like over-scrupulousness, religiosity, and moral punctiliousness.

Finally, there are what for the sake of distinguishing them we may call *Personality disorders*, such as dual personality and fugue states which are due to a mass dissociation of the personality, in which one well-organized part of the personality acts automatically and independently of the other.

Apart from these there are the *Behaviour disorders*, already discussed, some of which are psychoneurotic.

All these psychoneuroses are to be regarded not as entities, but as *reactions of the personality*; they are morbid responses of the organism to life and to its own problems: they are not diseases but

H

disorders. Under certain circumstances the personality reacts hysterically, at other times by obsessional reactions; sometimes by anxiety, and at other times it resorts to aberrations and perversions to satisfy its desires. Sometimes it reacts in several of these ways at once, so there is no absolute dividing line between the various types of psychoneurosis; it is only for clearness of diagnosis and treatment that we so distinguish them.

The problems confronting us are, first, to discover in what way these psychoneuroses differ from organic diseases; secondly, what it is that determines that the personality reacts in a specific type of neurosis, now in a hysterical way, now in an obsessional way: and finally what is the cause of the specific symptom, that is to say, why one hysteric person develops a paralysis, and another blindness; why one's anxiety neuroses takes on the form of an agoraphobia and another a claustrophobia; why one obsessional says prayers and another washes his hands. There must be a specific explanation for all these facts.

Psychogenetic nature of the psychoneuroses. The main feature of the psychoneuroses distinguishing them from organic illness, is that they are psychogenetic, that is to say, originate in mental and emotional disturbances. Man adapts himself to the environment in two ways, by physical adaptation and mental adaptation. In organic illness it is the physical adaptation which fails so that he falls victim to bacterial infection or heart disease: in the psychoneuroses it is the mental adaptation which is at fault, so that although he may be physically fit, he is incapable of responding adequately to his responsibilities.

Proof of the psychogenetic nature of the psychoneuroses, say of a paralysis of the legs, is to be drawn from the following facts: (1) In many cases of these disorders *no physical cause can be found.* It is possible that an examination of the body may reveal some toxic or other physical condition, but not enough to account for the disorder: in many cases the examination is quite negative. As an illustration: an athlete who was a fine specimen of a man, captain of his county cricket, and of his town in football, suffered from claustrophobia which produced in him a dread of travelling by train. In the absence of any discoverable organic cause for his condition, the assumption that it "must be" organic is pure conjecture and the evidence that it is psychogenetic highly probable.[1]

---

[1] This argument, it is true, is not conclusive, for the fact that we cannot find an organic cause does not prove that it is not there: and there are many cases referred to the psychophysician as functional, which prove to be organic on

(2) In the second place, these psychoneuroses are commonly *precipitated by purely psychological experiences*, like bad news, mental strain or emotional shock. A cabin boy goes blind on seeing a huge oncoming wave in a storm; a man develops labour pains when his wife is in labour; a man has his first attack of claustrophobia on entering an underground tube station after an argument with his directors; another suffers nervous dyspepsia from the moment he heard of his appointment to a responsible post. The determining factor in each case was undoubtedly the psychic shock. We should, however, keep in mind that, as in many cases of asthma, the psychic shock may merely be the precipitating factor in an underlying constitutional disorder.

(3) A further proof of their psychogenetic nature is the fact that these conditions can be *cured by psychical means alone*; a patient paralysed for two years is cured in a few minutes by the recovery under hypnosis of the experience of being blown up and the release of emotion occasioned by it, and walks out past the four men who are waiting to carry him back. A patient suffering from headache, depression, anxiety, indigestion or claustrophobia, relives in analysis the infantile experience which originally distorted his reactions, whereupon the symptoms immediately disappear. Indeed, there are cases in which the therapeutic result is the best and sometimes the only means of diagnosis between organic and psychogenetic disorders.

The cure of these conditions by mental means alone puts in a dilemma those materialistically minded physicians who insist that all mental diseases are of organic origin: for either they are compelled to admit their psychological origin, since they are cured by psychic means, or if they insist that these conditions are organic they are driven to the conclusion that an organic condition can be cured by psychological means. The immediacy of the result following the treatment rules out chance and coincidence.

(4) There are other characteristics of the disability pointing to a diagnosis of a psychoneurosis as psychogenetic. One woman gets

deeper investigation. Indeed, cases are sometimes diagnosed as neurotic on no other grounds than the failure to discover an organic cause. This is not justified since the psychoneuroses should be diagnosed on a positive basis not merely on a negative inference. In many of these cases the medical psychologist of wide experience can often say that from his observations this case does not conform to the picture of a true psychoneurosis as he knows it, although he may not be able to say what is the specific organic cause. For instance, the very manner of speech an approach of a patient to his complaint is often the indication of this: the patient with the organic complaint describes it as something he *has*, the neurotic as something he *is*. Nevertheless, the absence of any organic cause, so far as it goes, is a presumption in favour of the condition being psychogenetic.

sickness and fatigue whenever she has to look after her children, and on no other occasion. She could play golf, move furniture, preside at meetings, and take long walks without effort, but if the walks were with her children the tiredness and sickness resulted. Some patients get their symptoms at definite times; one patient gets a headache at 11 o'clock every morning, irrespective of where he is, what he is doing, or what he has eaten; because, as it was discovered in analysis, this was the hour when his regiment was ordered over-seas. Another develops a morbid sense of guilt and suspicion whenever he goes to Northampton for no known reason, but in analysis it was discovered that it was because he felt he had disgraced himself when serving with the Northampton regiment in the war.

(5) Finally, all these psychoneurotic conditions can be *produced artificially* by suggestion, with or without hypnosis; and the paralysis, pain or indigestion thus produced can in no way be distinguished from the corresponding hysterical symptom. We have produced by suggestion, paralysis, blindness, positive and negative hallucination, a bilious attack with severe sick headache, and compulsive acts; and all of these in waking suggestion apart from hypnosis, in suggestible subjects. The only difference between these experimentally produced disorders and the psychoneurosis proper is that the symptoms are produced by the suggestions of the physician, whereas in hysteria they are usually the result of the patient's own auto-suggestions. It was the great neurologist Charcot who originally demonstrated the psychogenetic nature of hysterical disorders by reproducing them experimentally. "We have here," he concluded, "a psychical affection; it is, therefore, by a mental treatment that we must hope to modify it."

These then are the facts which lead us to accept the psychogenetic nature of neurotic disorder, and justify us in regarding them as a separate entity from ordinary organic disorders. They also justify us in regarding them in a different category from psychotic disorders which are mainly the result of physical and constitutional causes. (See note at end of this chapter.)

From the point of view of diagnosis, therefore, we may distinguish four types of disorder. (i) *Physical causes* may give rise to *physical disease*, like pneumonia or tuberculosis. These are the ordinary organic ailments. (ii) *Physical* causes may give rise to *mental* disorder, such as the grandiose ideas of general paralysis due to syphilis, the reserve of the schizothymic, the hallucinations from physical exhaustion, or the "brain fever" of the novelists. These are psychoses. (iii) *Mental causes* on the other hand may produce *mental illness* like morbid anxiety, obsessions, and sex perversions. (iv) But *mental* causes may produce *physical* disorders like conversion hysteria or psychosomatic disorders. So that whenever the medical man is presented with any symptom, whether mental or physical, such as a headache, indigestion, depression or anxiety, he has to answer the question (*a*) whether it is primarily due to physical causes, or (*b*) whether it is due to psychological causes, or (*c*) how far both factors play a part.

Methods of treatment must obviously be based, not on the manifest symptom, but on the nature of the cause whether mental or physical. The problem confronting the general practitioner whose task is far more difficult than the consultant who sees only advanced cases, is that the earliest symptoms of many *physical* diseases manifest themselves in mental and emotional disturbances, like lack of interest, irritability and depression, and the only symptoms in many *psychogenic* disorders are physical conditions like indigestion, headaches from worry and other psychosomatic disorders.

Precipitating and predisposing causes. We have already indicated that the psychoneuroses are found to have both precipitating and predisposing causes. The precipitating causes may sometimes be of the greatest importance, as in *traumatic cases* of car accidents, shell explosion, death of a fiancé, failure in business, sexual assault, or, as in one case, the sudden death of a father during a heated argument. In such cases the precipitating cause may for practical purposes be regarded as the essential cause of the breakdown. In these cases it may have been that these patients would never have broken down had it not been for these traumatic experiences, and when these precipitating causes alone are dealt with, the patient may be cured of his symptom, as happened in so many cases of "war shock" which recovered sufficiently fit for civilian duties, after a few treatments by the abreaction method. Nevertheless, as we shall see, there is good evidence to show that there are predisposing causes even in these cases, however severe the shock, and it is these factors which determine that one man breaks down, whilst another blown up by the same shell recovers after the initial shock.

In most civilian cases the precipitating causes are of a trifling kind, quite incapable in themselves of producing a breakdown. A girl breaks down because of disappointment in love, but whereas the healthy-minded girl would accept the fact and look for someone else, this girl feels that life is not worth living, and tries to commit suicide, which points to the existence of predisposing causes. A woman developed a bad anxiety state which persisted for years because her husband went away for the week-end on business, the first time they had been separated since marriage; another developed a chronic anxiety state when the car in which she travelled swerved to avoid another. A man is carrying on with his ordinary occupation and not conscious of any particular worry, but suddenly goes off into a fugue state and is found with loss of memory in Edinburgh, where he had never been; another is looking at a stained-glass window of the Virgin and Child in a cathedral and finds himself going blind. It is evident that these circumstances are not sufficient in themselves to produce a breakdown; they happen to everybody. It must be that these patients are already predisposed for so slight an experience to produce so permanent a disorder.

Since the precipitating causes are insufficient to account for the disorder, we must obviously ask, *what are the predisposing factors* which make one person break down under certain circumstances, whereas another does not? Why, when two brothers are involved in a business crash one starts afresh, whereas the other develops an anxiety state? Why does one girl in a factory with a rough foreman break down with depression and weeping, and another says "Who cares?"

The most common answer to the question is that it is because of a *neurotic constitution*. True! but what do we mean by a "neurotic constitution"? This popular term usually covers two quite different conditions, the neurotic temperament and the neurotic disposition.

A *neurotic temperament* depends on the physiological and constitutional make-up of the individual: a *neurotic disposition* is determined by earlier experiences affecting his attitude towards life. One man is a weakling and cannot face life because he is asthenic and weedy, the other because he has never been taught to accept responsibility. These types must be clearly distinguished.

The neurotic temperament. It is obvious that the individual who is constitutionally sensitive and highly strung will be less capable of standing up to adverse conditions, and will be more predisposed to break down because of his instability, than the robust or the phlegmatic. Instability makes of one man a genius, of another man a neurotic. A mild psychosis may be a predisposing factor in a neurotic breakdown.

Therefore, we often find that those who have nervous breakdowns are the highly strung and sensitive: indeed, it is usually the interesting people who get the neuroses. But it is not necessary for sensitive people to break down: to be highly strung it is not necessary to be abnormal; to be nervous is not to be neurotic: one may be sensitive without ceasing to be sensible. Temperamental sensitivity may even be an asset enabling us to appreciate the subtleties of science, the beauties in art and the goodness of common life. But the temperamentally nervous and sensitive person is predisposed to breakdown and is less capable of adapting himself to the rebuffs of life, and when he cannot do so his breakdown is the more catastrophic.

Thomas Huxley writing of genius says, "On the general ground that a strong and therefore distinct abnormal variety is, *ipso facto*, not likely to be so well in harmony with existing conditions as the normal standard, which has been brought to be what it is largely by the operation of these conditions, I should think it probable that a large proportion of 'genius sports' are likely to come to grief, physically and socially."[1] This general principle applies to the psychoneuroses to which many people's sensitive temperament predisposes them.

A child of nervous temperament, therefore, though more liable to be neurotic, is also capable of achieving greatness provided he is given a stable background. The trouble is that so often the unstable child has the constitutionally unstable mother or father, so that the child not only inherits an unstable temperament, but is subjected to a disturbed atmosphere least calculated to give him the stability he needs. But the child who inherits its highly strung temperament from his father, and is cared for by a serene, affectionate and common-sense mother, may develop into a capable and healthy individual.

But there are men and women of robust constitution, athletes and climbers, who suffer from all kinds of neurotic symptoms and silly phobias which suggest that temperament is not the sole factor in the psychoneuroses. In these people, it is not a neurotic temperament which predisposes them to break down, but a neurotic disposition.

The neurotic disposition differs from the neurotic temperament in that it depends not on physiological but on psychological factors; it is due to untoward experiences in childhood, especially of insecurity and fear, which form themselves into morbid dispositions or complexes and predispose the child to react abnormally to life. These experiences quite apart from constitutional factors produce in the child a nervous disposition, and make him hypersensitive to the rebuffs and difficulties of life, so that a relatively mild disturbance later will precipitate a nervous breakdown.

[1] Quoted by Nisbet, *The Insanity of Genius.*

Most psychopathologists are agreed that what makes a person hypersensitive to these rebuffs are predisposing conditions in the early formative years of childhood. These may require untoward conditions in later life to precipitate them into a breakdown, but they are as a rule the essential causes of the psychoneuroses. What then are these early experiences?

Freud, as we all know, derived the psychoneuroses from infantile sexual wishes, especially of an incestuous kind. These infantile sexual wishes are repressed by a fear of castration, and the psychoneurosis represents the emergence into activity of the repressed sexual wish in symbolic form. "Neurotic symptoms are substituted for sexual satisfactions."[1] The specific form of psychoneurosis depends on the type of sexual fixation, such as the oral or anal-sadistic. In his later years, he recognized a primary aggressive factor as well as the sexual.

Jung has emphasized the fact of the present-day moral problem as determining the psychoneurosis, but even so he recognizes a predisposition to this, owing to the arrest of development by infantile fixations. "The neurosis," he says, "is the result of the characteristic influences of the parents upon the children," such as the over-fondling of parents, or disagreement between parent and child. This results in fixation of the libido, which makes the neurotic regress and seek refuge in the past when faced with the difficulties of life: the neurosis is an escape from an intolerable moral situation.

Adler also finds, or originally found, the root of the trouble in childhood, in the inferiority complex which he derived from the sense of physical or "organ" inferiority. This leads the patient to over-compensate by the development of fictitious goals, and compels him to pursue exaggerated ideals, which he naturally finds beyond his strength. Failing to achieve them he is precipitated into a neurosis, which excuses him from having failed to achieve his fictitious goal. Latterly Adler emphasized the lack of co-operation as the essence of neurosis, and regards the pampered child with his "desire to be first" as the typical example of the child who breaks down because he expects too much. Adler's is the "psychology without tears."

Using Freud's method of free association, but pursuing an independent investigation, we have come to a different conclusion.

In our experience *the basic cause of the psychoneuroses is the feeling of deprivation of love, the repressed craving for love.* This is

[1] *Introd. Lectures*, p. 259.

reminiscent of the Freudian formula that the psychoneuroses are due to repressed sexuality. But love is not merely sexual; love is protective as well as sexual, and *the need for protective love and security is of far greater importance in the development of the psychoneuroses* than the sexual.[1]

The most fundamental need of every child is for protection and security: this is involved in the very nature of childhood itself, for during infancy the child is helpless to care for itself and must have the protective love of others. This need is *biological*, for the child is in fact dependent upon others for its very life, for its food, its warmth, its safety from danger. But this need is also *psychological*; for the child not only needs protection but *feels* the need of it.

This need for protection and security is normally provided for in the care and tenderness of the mother, who responds to the child's helplessness and dependence by surrounding it with the atmosphere of love. The child therefore experiences the need for security as a craving for love. So the mother's love becomes the central fact of the child's life, providing him with the satisfaction of his bodily needs. But because this protective love is first experienced in close contact with the mother, it is also associated with sensuous pleasure, so that the mother becomes the main object of pleasurable desire. The main function of maternal love is to satisfy the child's need for protection and security: the sensuous pleasure accompanying it both in mother and child encourages the mother to give such love and the child to seek it.

It is a strange thing that the higher in evolution we go the more helpless is the offspring. We should have expected it to be the other way; that the higher the stage of evolution, the more capable the child would be to protect and defend itself. But in fact the human child is far more helpless than the newborn lizard or fly. But there is a biological reason for this. Insects and reptiles have no childhood; they are born with a ready-made mechanism for meeting the ordinary contingencies of life, fixed reflexes in full working order. But because of this, there is no elasticity in their nature and little variability in their actions, so that if any

---

[1] Freud identified sex and love, for he states that by sex he means all that we can include under the word love, making both terms synonymous. It is true that he recognizes other love tendencies besides the strictly sexual, such as respect and admiration, but even these he regards as "aim restricted," that is, sexual tendencies which have been bereft of their aim. Later, however, he contrasts the need of "love" in the girl with the "sexual" wish in the boy, and so begins vaguely to distinguish them.

change in circumstances occurs, they cannot cope with it, and die, as we say, like flies.

The human infant with his helpless childhood is far less capable of fending for itself than the insect; he is born with fewer fixed responses, and is therefore not immediately capable of coping with the difficulties of life. Not only so, but he has a much longer childhood. He therefore requires to be protected, or else in his helplessness he becomes a prey to untold enemies and is in danger of immediate extinction. Briffault speaking as an anthropologist says "The attachment of the young to the mother consists in a sense of dependence which gives rise to panic and fear when that protection is withdrawn, and to a dread of solitude."

There are, however, distinct advantages in a childhood with fewer fixed reflexes, provided it is given the atmosphere of protection. This lack of fixity in its responses means that the child is capable of developing a far greater *variability of response*; and is far more capable of profiting by experience than the insect. The child is therefore not limited to one form of reaction in any particular situation, but can learn by experience and profit from the experiences of others, by imitation and suggestibility, and so can build up innumerable dispositions or *potentialities of response* which ultimately enables it to cope far better than the insect with all kinds of new experiences in life. Such elasticity and variability of response makes for the survival of the individual. It means also that ultimately the child is able to respond adequately to a much larger number of situations, varying its responses to each as circumstances demand. The moth with its fixed reflexes flies time after time into the candle until it is burnt to death, urged by its fatal reflexes: the human child whose reflexes are not so fixed, touches the light once and never again. The insect with its fixed reflex is well provided for all the ordinary circumstances of life; but if anything unusual happens it cannot deal with it, and dies off: the human child with its variability of response and its capacity to profit by experience is more helpless in the beginning, because it has fewer fixed reflexes, but in the end is far better able to cope with new experiences. Further, the longer childhood gives *opportunity for experimentation* in an atmosphere of security, so that the child develops new adaptations to life. Thus the species with the longest childhood has the greatest chance of survival, and has risen to greater heights in evolution and in the development of personality.

But for this, as we have indicated, an atmosphere of protection and security is demanded, which is provided for in the protecting love of the mother. So that whilst the higher in evolution we go the less capable is the offspring of looking after itself, the higher we go the more necessary is maternal love and care. The very helplessness of the child means that if that atmosphere of protective love is not forthcoming, *the human infant is far worse off than the insect*, more incapable of meeting the dangers of life, and more liable to develop abnormal responses. That is why the human being is so much more prone to nervous breakdown than the lower animals, and why neurotic disorders are so much more prevalent in the human species, as compared with the animal. Neuroses are found amongst mammals like rats and dogs and sheep, all of whom depend on their mothers for security, but to nothing like the same extent as is found in human beings, few of whom have altogether escaped from some form or other of neurotic reaction or morbid fear. Childhood is therefore at once the greatest achievement and the greatest risk of evolution: it carries with it the greatest potentialities of development, but also the greatest possibility of disaster.

Protective love is therefore the greatest need of the child, both biologically and psychologically, and the deprivation of love the main cause of disaster. Consider the child's reactions.

Given love, the child has the sense of security and develops self-confidence: so that he can go out to face life with confidence. *Given love* and an atmosphere of protection and security, the child can experiment and so learn to adapt himself to life. The normal and healthy child naturally loves the thrill of adventure, the taking of risks, which he does with confidence when assured of protection and security from others. Later when he has developed his self-confidence, he will throw off this protective cloak of his mother and achieve his own freedom and independence. Indeed, the healthy youth, especially in adolescence, likes to impose hardships and disciplines on himself, working, training, riding, sailing, hiking, overcoming difficulties, enduring hardships, seeking adventures, exercising courage in the doing of them, and finding confidence in his own achievement. But he cannot do so unless he first has the sense of confidence in himself. Such confidence can only be established in the first place by the sense of security which in early childhood comes from the assurance of personal love. To impose independence on a child before he is prepared to face life and to deprive him of the sense of security before he has established his self-confidence, is to throw him into a state of anxiety, and to make of him a coward. *Given love*, a child learns to love; for the characteristic of a child is to be loved, that of an adult to love.

The child who is given love can afford to love, to give of what he has received, so that he grows up to be sociable, affectionate and a good companion in marriage. *Given love,* the child identifies himself with those he loves, and so gets from them a stable ideal by which he can co-ordinate, direct and harmonize his energies for the purposes of life. So he becomes healthy-minded, strong in will and determined in character.

If however the child is *deprived of love,* or, what is the same thing from the child's point of view, *feels* himself deprived of love, he reacts abnormally to life.

Deprived of love the child falls into a state of anxiety; he lacks confidence to face life; he is filled with a sense of apprehension and insecurity, which makes him incapable of facing his difficulties, unable to accept his responsibilities, and a promising candidate for neurosis.

Deprived of love the child is *arrested in development.* Living in an atmosphere of insecurity he cannot experiment, nor express himself spontaneously; filled with apprehension he has no freedom nor exercise for the development of his natural tendencies; he remains a child. Neurosis itself is a childish reaction to life.

Deprived of love the child falls into *self-love*; failing to receive love he cannot afford to give love and so becomes selfish, self-centred, narcissistic, and auto-erotic.

Deprived of love and the means of identification the child has *no stable aim or purpose in life,* except that of his own self-preservation, no guiding principle to co-ordinate and direct his native tendencies: or if he has they are motivated by fear which tends to repress his native tendencies, such as the sexual and aggressive, and so threaten him with further disaster from within.

It may however be objected that many children become neurotic not because they have too little love, but *because they are given too much love.* This is true and we often find, as Adler says, that it is the pampered child who becomes neurotic. But it is precisely such a child who feels most the deprivation of love. Nevertheless, it is not the pampering which produces the neurotic reaction; it is the subsequent feeling of deprivation which makes the child depressed, auto-erotic, full of self-pity or afraid. Not all pampered children become neurotic. Pampering alone produces abnormal character traits like conceit, selfishness, self-centredness and self-willedness: it does not of itself produce a psychoneurosis. The temperamentally healthy child becomes tired of the pampering and breaks away from his too possessive mother; or later conditions such as meeting with other children compels him painfully to correct his idiosyncrasies. But if there have been earlier fears, and the child after pampering is then deprived of love, he clings overmuch and becomes neurotic. Spoiling and petting alone will never give a child a hysterical pain, but the petted child will be the first to develop a hysteric pain when it feels neglected or left out. It is the withdrawal of affection, not its surfeit, which makes the child react neurotically, just as it is the withdrawal of light not its absence which makes us experience blackness. Whether or not the child was justified in feeling itself deprived of affection is another matter· but it was the deprivation not the love which makes him react neurotically.

It is therefore important to realize that it is not necessarily a real deprivation but a felt deprivation which makes the child react abnormally. That is why in our original statement we emphasized that it is the *feeling* of deprivation of love which produces neurotic reactions. Sometimes it is an *actual* deprivation, sometimes an imagined or *relative* deprivation which produces the psychoneuroses, for if a child feels deprived it will react as though the deprivation were real, although in fact it is only relative, or even not at all.

Common instances of *actual deprivation* which have been found to originate psychoneuroses, are when the mother is harassed with too many children, worried financially, or is herself neurotic, depressed or ill. Or it may come from the child being unwanted, or from the neglect of nurse or mother, or the indifference of a mother who wanted a boy and a girl arrived, the jealousy of the parents or other children, the concentration of the mother on a favoured child or new baby, or the necessary absorption with a sick child. The child who is in robust health is often psychologically neglected—"there is never anything wrong with *him*," and so is left to himself in favour of the delicate child and feels left out. The healthy child may have all he needs but not all he wants. These and many other circumstances may cause the child to feel neglected, because in fact it is neglected, and so reacts abnormally.

In other cases there is not a real but only a *relative deprivation*, the most common instance of which is jealousy of a younger child. When a child has been accustomed to a great deal of love it expects too much and is proportionally rebuffed at failing to get all it wants. If he is the only child for three years and accustomed to 100 per cent of the parent's affection, he *feels* ignored and left out at the coming of the new baby, even if he still has 75 per cent of their love, and still more if, as is so often the case, most of the attention is turned towards the baby. Sometimes it comes from an *imagined lack of affection*, as when the child is ill, and even the most devoted mother can do nothing: where the mother is over-anxious about the child's illness, and transfers her anxiety to her child; where the mother herself is absent through illness; where the mother, however affectionate, lacks understanding of her child's wants; or where the mother is naturally undemonstrative, and the child feels the need of mothering. These situations are sometimes unavoidable, as in the case of the child periodically terrified at the heart attacks of his mother, which made her faint as though dead. In many other cases it is due to a *misinterpretation of the situation*, as in the case of a child who thought that the mother had deserted him for a new baby, when in fact the mother had died in the childbirth, and he was not told for some years. In these cases there is no actual lack of affection, but the child has felt the sense of deprivation, which produces the same reaction.

The feeling of deprivation of love is most accentuated when the child is subjected to both experiences at the same time or alternately; when for instance the child is unwanted by the mother, but for that very reason pampered by a nurse: or when the petting by the father calls forth the jealousy of the mother and *vice versa*, a common situation not always appreciated by the jealous partner who usually objects that it is "bad for the child." Frequently the child is pampered by the mother, and therefore like Joseph ill-treated by his brothers or sisters. Delinquency is often found to result from a combination of spoiling on the one hand and harsh treatment on the other: when one parent is strict and the other lenient; the one lets him feel he can have what he wants; the other threatens him and makes him rebellious.[1]

Real love. But when we speak of protective love as the fundamental need of the child we mean real love, an essential element of which is concern for the well-being of the person loved.

What passes for love is often not real love at all, but merely

---

[1] Foundlings and children brought up in Institutions may get very little personal affection, yet because they expect very little have less feeling of deprivation. Such children are often somewhat joyless in their attitude to life, but if they have the necessary sense of security even without much personal affection they find they can cope with life. They have sufficient for the needs though not for the enjoyment of life. On the other hand there is no reason why children in Institutions may not receive love, although it has to be shared by so many, and may come off better than a wealthy and pampered child entrusted to the care of a loveless nurse by parents who are too busy to devote themselves to him. It is surprising how many children of such homes of luxury have everything they want, but feel the sense of deprivation of love.

vanity, or sensuousness, or possessiveness, or anxiety on the part of the mother.

Some mothers pamper their children, show them off, give them nice dresses, the most expensive toys, without any true regard to their child's real happiness and future welfare but merely to gratify their own *vanity*, to enjoy the reflected glory. The child himself is not deceived, as his mother is, into thinking that this is love. A pretty boy with a mass of curls, shown off by his mother on the sea-front every morning for the gratification of her vanity, remarked: "I am bored to death of my beautiful curls; I wish that my mother would love *me*." Indeed, the preoccupation of so many parents and others with the looks of children, whether pretty or plain, gives a child entirely false values, and is fraught with as much danger to the pretty child who relies upon this and therefore has no need to make any effort, as to the plain child who is given an unjustifiable feeling of inferiority, a lack of confidence and a feeling of being unloved for something for which she is in no way responsible. A child wants to be loved *for itself*. An instance of mismanagement due to vanity is that of a stepmother who was very anxious to do her best by her foster-children to show people how well she could bring them up, and avoid the reputations of bad stepmothers. But her "corrections" of them in company, to prove how efficient a mother she was, simply filled them with humiliation and anger, and they became delinquent.

Again, what passes for love may be mere *sensuous gratification*. This happens particularly in widows, in mothers who do not get sexual satisfaction from their husbands, and those who are not in love with their husbands: also in mothers who are sexually frigid, but are nevertheless sensual, and satisfy their sensual feelings in pampering and fondling their children, without realizing what they are doing, attach the child sensually to themselves, and so arrest the development of adult love. This may appear to be "love," but it is only sensual love and does not seek the welfare of the person loved so much as its own self-gratification. Such mothers often fall in love with their sons, consciously or unconsciously, and produce in them an Oedipus complex. This indeed in our experience is the most common origin of the Oedipus complex, the initiative coming from the mother's (or father's) devotion to the child, not primarily from the child's sexual wishes towards the opposite parent. Most children break loose of this sexual attachment, though often with bitterness and hate against the parent; but this attachment is particularly accentuated if it is combined with an earlier fear perhaps from illness, which makes the child then cling to the parent both for sensuous and protective reasons. On the other hand, such precocious stimulation of the child's sexual feelings may itself arouse fear, so that we have an attachment which is both binding and terrifying, the mother protecting the child from the terror she has herself produced.

Further, what often passes for love is often merely *anxiety* on the part of the mother, who worries over her child, is over-careful of his health, anxiously picks up every bit of child psychology that she can lay hands on, and applies it however inconsistently. She thereby produces an anxiety state in him. A child is extraordinarily suggestible and absorbs the anxiety of the mother even in the first year of life. Having herself a morbid fear of thunder she rushes to the child to ask him if he is afraid, and immediately fills him with apprehension. Many a child feels no alarm until the mother says, "Don't be afraid." Many a child who is ill or in an air raid is not anxious until he sees the mother anxious. In other cases, however, the anxiety of the mother is an over-compensation for an *unconscious* dislike of the child who was not wanted, and a desire to be rid of him, so that her guilt makes her over-anxious about his health. Far from being a sign of love, it is a manifestation of unconscious hate; and the child senses this.

Again, what passes for love may be *possessiveness*. The so-called "maternal instinct" is a sentiment, a group of tendencies surrounding the object of maternal care, the main feeling of which is tenderness, but which may include the feeling of self-importance. The possessive mother has a morbid craving to mould the lives of her children, to do everything for them, to be essential to them, to hold them so that they cannot do without her, are rendered unfit to face life and become hopeless husbands and wives. A classic instance is the mother of Mary Rose in Barrie's play. Such a mother does everything for her children to make herself indispensable instead of allowing them the joy of spontaneous development; she cannot leave them alone even when they marry, becomes the terrible mother-in-law, and ends her days grumbling at the ingratitude of her children, whose lives she has done her best to ruin. That is not love, though it may pass for devotion. The more fortunate of such children rebel; others like Mary Rose become hopeless neurotics, incapable of facing life, afraid to grow up, afraid of marriage, and escape into a world of ghost-like unreality, because they cannot face reality. Even small girls can be seen exercising their sense of power by such "meddlesome motherhood" over their younger brothers or sisters, and their dolls. Let the mother watch her small girl playing with her dolls if she wants to see a reflection of herself.

Further, when we speak of the need of a mother's protective love as being the first essential for the child, we do not mean *over-protectiveness*. We may best protect a growing child by letting it learn to look after itself. There are many mothers and nurses who "protect" a child when it has no need of protection. The healthy child loves to experiment, to fall, to take risks, and hates to have the mother or nurse surrounding it with a "loving care" that it neither wants nor needs, protecting it from "dangers" which are not in fact real, and which in fact the child does not fear. On the other hand, one of the surest ways of making a child over-reckless is by warning him of dangers which when he experiments he finds to be untrue. Once again the situation is gravely accentuated if there has been an earlier invalidism or anxiety, say from illness, for then such a mother makes the most of her opportunities to gratify her protectiveness, by keeping her child a baby.

It is necessary to mention these bogus forms of love; for whilst true love is necessary to the healthy development of the child, these spurious forms of perverted "love" are often the cause of the neuroses, in that they deprive the child of the real love it needs. The function of love from the biological point of view is to provide an atmosphere of protection and security in which the child may gain confidence and normally develop. Yet merely giving the child security is not enough for what the child looks for is the *personal* devotion of the mother, which not only provides it with present needs of food, warmth and clothing, but gives assurance of continued care and protection. A patient said, "I wanted my mother to feed me; but it was not so much that I wanted her to feed me but that she should *want* to feed me." Not only protection but protective love is required for healthy development. If there had not been some reason in biology for love as distinct from mere protection, it would not have arisen nor have been perpetuated in human evolution: it is love that provides the security and gives it permanence.

Specific reactions to the deprivation of love. Let us then consider some of the more specific reactions to the deprivation of love. Suppose a child feels left out and unloved, how will it react? One child reacts by *depression*, another by being *anxious*, another by resorting to *sensuous gratification* as a solace, like thumb-sucking. These are typical reactions in the first year of life. Another finding the world of reality unpleasant, escapes into a world of *phantasy*, and it depends on later circumstances whether he becomes an imaginative artist, a writer, a neurotic, or a pathological liar who, like the mediaeval lady, spins coarse yarns. Another child feeling unloved develops a feeling of *inferiority*; indeed, the feeling of being unloved is, in our experience, the most common cause of the inferiority complex. A child a little older will react to the withdrawal of love by *showing off* or calling attention to himself and becomes the "limelight child"; another, feeling deprived of affection, will be angry and jealous, spiteful and *aggressive*, which is at the root of obsessional phobias like the fear of poisoning. Another, still older, will react by *self-pity*, and say "I have a pain in the back," or "I feel tired," to get sympathy; this is a typically hysteric reaction. Another child, perhaps at the age of four or five, feeling deprived of his rights of love becomes anti-social, independent and defiant, says "I don't care for anybody, I'm going to to be bad," and ultimately may become a *delinquent*. Yet another becomes *very good* and ingratiating, in order to win back the lost love.

The following observations may be made on such reactions:—

(*a*) All these reactions correspond to the psychoneuroses; and given certain later conditions may actually develop into neurotic depression, anxiety, sex perversions, inferiority, hysteria, the obsesssions and delinquency.

(*b*) They are all reactions to the feeling of deprivation of love.

(*c*) These psychoneuroses are not disease entities but *reactions of the personality* to certain situations.

(*d*) Since they are reactions of the personality, we may have a number of these disorders in the same person, or at one time, as we shall see. The psychoneuroses are therefore not mutually exclusive, nor can they be based wholly on innate temperamental differences between individuals.

(*e*) This conception of the origin of the psychoneuroses as due to the feeling of deprivation of love was derived in the first place *from the analysis of neurotic patients*, in whom we invariably discovered the need of protective love as the basic cause of their neurotic reactions.

(*f*) But all these reactions to the deprivation of love may also be *directly observed* in any nursery, with the minimum of interpretation, which confirms the findings of analysis. We may actually see the child who is bereft of love and feeling left out, behaving in these ways, now by anxiety, now by depression, now by anger, now by showing off or ingratiation.

(*g*) These psychological reactions are also in line with biological considerations, for they are all based on the organism's fundamental need for safety and security. They are the natural responses to untoward conditions.

Commonly a child reacts in one way or another of these ways according to the circumstances, but in other cases the child responds by a number of them at once. The following case illustrates the various reactions to the deprivation of love (the reactions are in italics):—

It is that of a school-teacher suffering primarily from depression, hysterical symptoms, a fear of hurting the school-children and failure to discipline them. She had been the only child and being spoilt felt antagonistic to her mother when a new baby arrived: so she tranferred her affection to her father. "I was sitting on father's knee: he was putting on my socks, making a fuss of me. Mother comes in and wants her dress buttoned: father puts me down. I am *angry* at this and said I wanted my socks on—*my feet were cold*. No notice—then I get angry and say, 'Nasty Mummy! go away. I hate you. Nasty Daddy,' and hit him. He takes hold of me and puts me out. *I feel sorry for myself* (self-pity) and think they don't mind whether I have cold feet or not. Then feelings of *resentment* and I say I don't care for them. I would not sit on my father's knee even if he wanted me to (repression of love). I hated them all, and have done with them. I have feelings of independence, of ambition (over-compensation), and when I had achieved, then they would be sorry that they had been unkind to me: I would be *very clever* (limelight) and could do anything I wanted to do: I now wanted their *admiration*, to win that, not their affection, I didn't want that. I'd be more like a grown-up than a child: they would be sorry for what they had done and I'd forgive them: they had not recognized my merits. I'm frightfully *jealous* of my mother: who was she that she was preferred to me? Myself and my father are the only important people. Then my father comes and talks to me—I mustn't be a selfish little girl: he will be very angry when I lose my temper and asks if I am sorry. I say nothing, I feel *defiant*, I'm not sorry and I don't care, and I'm not going to care what he thinks any longer. Then I think it *is silly of me* (super-ego and guilt) to have made such a fuss about such a thing and shall not do it again because it is so humiliating, rather babyish, and would not do it again from that point of view. He tells me to ask God to make me a good girl. I don't see what God has to do with it. God is a person who backs up my father and mother, and nothing to do with me; he is on the other side. I've got all my battle to fight myself and nobody on my side at all. That was the end, but I maintain my point and *go off on my own* to play (independence): don't want to play with him or mother. I'm sitting on the floor playing bricks, feeling *miserable and depressed*—I've got what I wanted and did not like it, I did not like being alone; wished I could get back where I started from: but it is irrevocable. *I would like to say I was sorry*, but I wouldn't and couldn't. Then I say *I've got a headache and I'm put to bed* (a hysterical reaction). If I had a headache nobody would think anything of it—quite in keeping with my pride. I think of a headache, and wish it, and then I have one (hysteria). It is not humiliating to have a physical pain, but I *get attention*. So I begin to cry and say I've got a pain in my head: they say I can't be well, and that is why I am naughty, and put me to bed. I feel at first they were wrong and then I feel they were right because I liked the explanation, because I feel the getting in a rage was childish, so if it was not my fault so much the better."

In such an instance we have a series of neurotic reactions as a result of the feeling of deprivation of love: anger, self-pity, hate, independence, power fantasy, humiliation, depression, loneliness, pride, fantasy of goodness (I'd forgive them), guilt (it is silly of me), hysteria (cold feet and headache), and finally rationalization. By repression the hate later turned into a fear of hurting; and her failure in discipline was due to the repression of her aggressiveness.

It may be objected that all these reactions may occur not only as reactions to the deprivation of love but to the frustration of other tendencies. Frustration of our assertiveness may give rise to depression, anxiety, or even sex. Frustration in sex may give rise to anger or to depression. We frequently found in the last war that many men broke down especially with depression, not because they had too much responsibility, or felt helpless, but because they had not enough to engage their powers and abilities.

That is true, but although the morbid reactions in these cases may not be due to the deprivation of love, it is very commonly *because of the need of love that they are repressed*, which is the second stage in the development of a neurosis. The arrogant child is ostracized and feels lonely, the sensuous child is threatened. Fear, which is the most common expression of a need of security, is the most common cause of repression; indeed, the usual method of forcing a child to be obedient is by threatening him with terrifying consequences, the disapproval of the mother, and the loss of her protecting love. This threat may force a child to repress even natural and normal tendencies, which are not in conformity with the demands of the parent upon whom depend his safety and security; how much more abnormal reactions.

The deprivation of love, therefore, acts in two ways: (*a*) It gives rise to abnormal reactions such as we have described. (*b*) It is on account of the fear of such deprivation that the child is compelled to repress these abnormal reactions. There are very few neurotic cases therefore in which we do not find this fundamental need for love as an essential feature, whether in the production of abnormal reactions, or in their repression.

Mechanism. These reactions to the deprivation of love do not of themselves constitute the psychoneuroses, but are reaction character traits which may persist; so that the patient may continue all his life to suffer from self-pity, resentment of a sense of grievance, which he feels to be justified, but the causes of which may be unknown to him, as they lie in those early experiences. They are definitely abnormal but not neurotic, if we take this to mean the emergence of dissociated tendencies. To constitute a true psychoneurosis *these reactions must themselves be repressed,* so that when they later emerge as symptoms they appear to be irrational and abnormal to the patient who comes to be treated for them.

We therefore have a twofold repression in the psychoneuroses. The situation is as follows: there is the natural craving for affection, which is repressed in favour of an abnormal reaction of self-pity, resentment, sensuousness and the rest. But these reactions being threatened or being found disappointing are in turn repressed in favour of a moral super-ego to conform with the demands of others. This means that in the psychoneuroses there is a conflict between two forces, *both* of which are repressed and unconscious, and the super-ego which keeps them repressed.

The repression, therefore, results in a *duality or split in the personality,* in which one part of the personality is dissociated from the rest, the natural self and its impulses being repressed by the demands of the moral self or super-ego. Thus repression is a source of great weakness in the personality, for not only is the personality robbed of those forces by means of which it can face life, but these forces, denied expression, revolt and cause disturbance in the personality. Not only so, but the moral self, being falsely motivated, is inadequate when called upon to undertake the responsibilities of life. The symptom, as we shall see, is a compromise between all these forces; and the specific nature of the disorder depends on the nature of this compromise.

It is important therefore to understand the meaning of repression.

The essential characteristics of repression in the technical sense and as used by psychopathologists are: (1) that it is *always by oneself.* Therefore the mere restraint by a parent is not "repression" in the technical sense: the child must accept it and himself repress the undesirable qualities; (2) that is is an *unconscious process*; we do not know why we are repressing; we do not know what we are repressing or that we are repressing it; (3) that it leads to *dissociation,* which in our opinion is a more important feature of repression than unconsciousness.

When a mother forbids a child to do something, that is not repression in the technical sense. The child who says "I cannot have the love, so I must do without it, but will get it when I can," is not repressing its craving for love in the technical sense of the word. Repression takes place when the child, being deprived of love, represses the desire, and says "I don't want anyone's love, I can fend for myself." It is then that a duality is formed in the mind between the repressed desires and the attitude assumed, and the conditions of a true neurosis are developed. It is true the child who represses his love still strongly craves for it, but denies that he does: but that is why the need for love has to emerge in some substitute form such as a hysterical pain.

We see this process of repression even in a simple form of hysteria in the child. When the child, feeling left out, comes saying "I've got a pain in my foot," why does he not openly ask for sympathy, instead of using this indirect method of getting sympathy? It is because he is too proud to ask and refuses to admit that he wants it.

Transition from a biological objective to a psychological subjective problem. The result of this repression and the establishment of the super-ego is that the problem is no longer the conflict between man and his environment, but between conflicting forces in his own personality, between the man and himself. From being a biological problem it becomes a psychological problem; from being objective it becomes subjective. One of Freud's most important discoveries was that in the neuroses the conflict is always "endopsychic." To this we have already referred.

Man lives in a society and the price he has to pay for the protection and security afforded by society is that he must concede to its demands. Some people frankly refuse to be bound by them; they are the delinquent and criminal. Others realize that it is for their ultimate good and happiness that they should conform to the society in which they live and on which they depend not only for their protection but for their happiness: they are the social and the truly moral. Others are *forced* to be moral from fear, and they often become the neurotics.

This conflict between the desires of the individual and the demands of society is at the root of most social and moral problems, which neither sociology, religion or politics has yet been able to solve: it is the basic problem of civilization. Such moral conflicts are inevitable and indeed necessary to human progress and where the elements of the conflict are conscious, the problem can only be solved by the moral self directing the impulses of the natural self to its will and purpose, or if this is too severe a demand, by a modification of the moral self to meet the demands of the natural self.

But when, because of biological necessity, the individual is forced to accept the demands against his own judgment, these demands become incorporated within him as the super-ego, and there is set up the duality in his personality between the ego or natural self, and the super-ego.

This conflict between the ego or natural self, and the super-ego or moral self, is the basic conflict in all the psychoneuroses, and the nervous breakdown is the refusal of the natural self to conform any longer to the too rigid demands of the super-ego.

This conflict between the natural desires and the demands of society takes place very early in life, when the child is being trained to be obedient, to be sociable, to behave itself and be good. That is why we have to look to the first three or four years of life for the origin of the conflicts which later produce the psychoneuroses. These result from the failure of the personality to organize itself aright, and to bring about that co-ordination of the dynamic function of the personality which is the essence of mental health and happiness.

The super-ego. Since the conflict between the ego and the super-ego is the basic conflict in all psychoneuroses, it is essential to consider the nature and sources of the super-ego as we see them.

It is convenient to divide, as Freud has done, the functions of the personality into the Id, the Ego and the Super-ego, as long as we regard them as ways in which the personality functions and not as entities in themselves. (*a*) *The Id* may be regarded as those functions of the personality which are *potentially active at birth*, whether we regard these as primitive impulses, as the effects of the genes, or as reflexes of the organism. But the Id is in fact a pure abstraction, for as soon as the innate tendencies have once been activated and come in contact with the environment which calls them forth, they immediately become modified as experiences to become part of the ego. (*b*) The term *Ego* may be used of the native potentialities in so far as they are modified by environmental conditions. It includes the "conditioned reflexes" of Pavlov, the "sentiments" of Shand, the "complexes" of Jung, and the dispositions as we have defined them.[1] (*c*) *The Super-ego* is a convenient term to describe those reactions of the personality which are developed in response to the social environment: it is

[1] P. 39.

the incorporation into the individual of the demands of society; it is the representation of society in the personality of the individual. It derives much of its strength from the impulses of the Id, and its nature from the experiences of the ego. But it is more than the mere response of the individual to the environment and the dispositions resulting therefrom, for once adopted, these demands of society become the standards upon which we base our modes of behaviour, and towards which we direct our action. It therefore deserves special consideration as a specific function of the personality. Whilst the ego deals with the objective world of experience, the super-ego is concerned with social and moral values.[1]

The sources of the super-ego. (i) First of all our standards of life are derived to some extent as the *result of experiences.* If impulses like venturesomeness lead the child into danger it develops an attitude of caution: if sex stimulation leads to sickness, sex is inhibited and regarded as "wrong." (ii) Secondly, standards are adopted because of positive *threats*: If a child is disobedient it is slapped; if it makes a noise it is shut up and made lonely. So the child becomes obedient and learns to behave as it is supposed to behave. That indeed is the object of punishment. (iii) Many of these standards are due to *teaching*; we are taught that it is right to be unselfish and kind, wrong to be greedy and cruel; or we may be taught that we have to think of ourselves first or no one else will. But teaching has little effect unless the child loves or respects the teacher. (iv) But of all the sources of the super-ego, *identification* is the most important. Freud[2] says, "The ego ideal or super-ego (it is to be observed that Freud uses these terms interchangeably) is the representative of our relations to our parents." By identification the child not only imitates others, and takes over the moods and feelings of those around, but by *intro-*

---

[1] *Sociologically*, and politically, the basic problem is how to accommodate the individual to the demands of society without doing violence to his individuality. It involves the problem of the freedom of the individual in an ordered state. It is obvious that everything will depend on the nature of these standards, whether they are such as can be willingly adopted so that there is no clash between the individual and social demands. The function of those in authority is to provide incentives capable of inspiring the individual to act for the common good. For if these demands are forced on the unwilling individual he rebels against them and becomes a delinquent. It is of the greatest importance therefore that those who make the laws should carry the public with them; otherwise, if the laws go beyond the consensus of opinion, it results in general slackening of morals, black-marketing and the rise of an army of spivs. Similarly it is of the greatest importance that the super-ego, which is the incorporation of the will of society in the individual, should not go beyond the capabilities or else it results in psychoneurosis or revolt depending on the strength and severity of the super-ego. [2] *Group Psychology*, p. 45.

jection of the personality of others into himself, takes over his whole
personality so that the child *is* for the time being that person.
When the boy says "I am Daddy going to lecture," or the girl "I
am Mummy doing the cooking," they are not only imitating, but
for the time being *are* the persons of their parents. In this way
the child takes over not only the actions, but the attitudes of mind
and moral standards, whether kindness or cruelty, bad temper or
calmness, cheerfulness or depression, greed or generosity, vanity
or modesty, from their parents. This capacity for identification
appears to be in all normal children, so that by identification we
have an *innate capacity for the transmission of acquired characteristics*, as we have previously observed.

What then are the motives which lead a child to identify itself
with parents and incorporate their personalities into its own?
(*a*) In the first place the child tends to identify itself with those *on
whom it depends* for safety and security. He must keep close to
them, imitate them, take his cue from them, and thereby adopt
their personalities. (*b*) The second motive appears to be the
opposite; the child naturally wants to be grown-up, and is filled
with admiration for those who are big, and wants to be like them.
The function of identification is therefore fundamentally a biological one, satisfying in the first place the need for safety and
security, and at the same time preparing the child to be grown-up
and independent. These two are normal motives of identification
which the child willingly and naturally adopts, and are in conformity with mental health. (*c*) *Fear* is a false motive of identification when the need for safety and security compels a child,
under threats, to adopt the parents' standards against his true
nature, and therefore causes him to repress his natural self in
favour of a false super-ego. (*d*) The *sexual motive*, namely the
child's desire sexually to possess the opposite parent and therefore
identify himself with the parent of the same sex, is in our experience an artifract and abnormal (see p. 385). It is not surprising
that it gives rise to abnormal modes of behaviour and to the psychoneuroses, as Freud has maintained.

The results of the incorporation of the personalities of others into
the individual as the super-ego produces far-reaching changes in
the personality. Indeed, this is perhaps the most important
moment of life in the development of the child from the point of
view of mental health, since it is at this time that the personality
is organized for good or evil.

In the first place, there is formed a *duality in the personality*
between the natural self as organized from native tendencies on

the one hand, and the super-ego or impersonation of the personalities of others on the other. The child's whole future, happiness and mental health will depend upon how far the super-ego is able to co-ordinate these two aspects of the personality. In the second place, this duality gives rise to *self-consciousness*, which is the consciousness by one part of the personality of the other part of his personality. Thirdly, it provides the means of *self-control*, because the super-ego can now control the impulses of the ego. Because we are brave we must control our fear, because we are unselfish we must control our greed. Finally it produces *self-criticism*, for the super-ego criticizes the desires and impulses of the ego, and in extreme cases produces a sense of shame and guilt.

Conscience, psychologically speaking, is the judgment which the super-ego or moral self passes on the ego or natural self. When this is adverse we experienced a sense of guilt. Self-criticism and conscience are of the greatest social value in that they encourage man to change his conduct in conformity with social demands and towards a better life. But conscience may be morbid. When it is due to identification with a severe and threatening parent, conscience may be so tyrannical a master that it may completely incapacitate an individual, compelling him to do things he does not wish to do and preventing him from exercising his will. He becomes so completely hag-ridden by his morbid conscience that it renders his whole life a misery: instead of leading to right action it may stifle all action since it is better to do nothing than to risk doing wrong. Conscience is by no means an infallible guide, since it may be morbidly motivated, and a morbid conscience may be the cause of many disorders of character like self-righteousness and bigoted condemnation of others, on the one hand, and psychoneurotic disorders, particularly the obsessions, on the other.

The conditions of a healthy super-ego. The natural function of the super-ego, or its more conscious counterpart, the ego ideal, is the co-ordination and direction of the native and acquired potentialities to a common end and so bring about the mental health of the individual. But this can happen only when the parents with whom the child identifies itself are themselves tolerably mentally healthy with *sane standards*: when they allow *spontaneity* in the child, so that he can develop his own personality; when the standards are *voluntarily adopted*, and not forced upon the child; and when they are *healthily motivated* in the child, that is to say from natural love and admiration of the parents and not from fear nor from prematurely aroused sex attachments.

Abnormality occurs when the parents set wrong standards and

ideals, incapable of harmonizing the personality, in which case the child is *lacking* in stable standards so that it becomes the victim of its own impulses; or on the other hand, when the standards are *too rigid* so that they repress the native impulses of the ego, which leads to psychoneurosis.

The morbid effects of the super-ego may be observed in the case of the three brothers, which illustrates the relative influences of the ego and super-ego: the oldest completely adopted the rigid and narrow religious super-ego of his parents, became excessively severe with himself even to the extent of marrying a very unattractive woman so that he should not be guilty of having any sexual feelings towards her; the second became a bad obsessional, resulting from the conflict between the ego and the super-ego; the third brother elected on the side of the ego, left home, became somewhat of a rake, and distinguished himself in the war! But we shall deal with the pathological aspects of the super-ego in later chapters.

The breakdown is precipitated when the moral problem is reactivated. That is why it is that a man may get a nervous breakdown from apparently trifling causes.

The illustrations given (p. 118) will make this clear. The woman who developed a persisting anxiety state when her husband went away for the week-end, discovered in analysis that the real cause of her breakdown was that she was secretly in love with another man, and the thought that the absence of her husband would give her the chance to meet him clandestinely filled her with guilt, horror and anxiety. But as the moral problem remained, so did the anxiety persist, and became a chronic symptom. The man with the fugue state loathed and detested his life at the desk, though he refused to admit it to himself, as he had to support a family: the repressed natural self took the matter into its own hands and decamped to Edinburgh. The man who went blind looking at the stained glass window at the Madonna and Child had aroused within him buried sexual attachment towards his mother. He desired still to gaze but his sense of guilt obliterated this forbidden desire to gaze by making him blind.

In all these instances there are unresolved moral problems, and the precipitation of the breakdown is when the crisis is brought to a head. We must recognize, therefore, in the production of a psychoneurosis two separate factors: the early *objective* experiences which produced the abnormal reactions, and the *subjective moral conflict* in the personality arising from these conditions, the precipitation of which produced the actual breakdown.

Jung in particular has stressed the importance of present-day moral problems in the production of the neuroses. He says: "The pathogenic conflict exists only in the present moment; only in the actual present are the effective causes, and only here the possibilities of removing them."[1]

We agree there is always a present-day moral conflict, but we maintain that *there would not have been this present-day moral conflict were it not for the experiences of the past.* Indeed the moral conflict itself originates in the past. The man who went blind looking at the Madonna was obviously suffering from a present-day sexual attachment to his mother, of which he was unconscious, but of which he felt guilty. But there would not have been that problem were it not for the development of the abnormal sexual attachment towards her in childhood; nor indeed was the sense of guilt a modern development but was formed in childhood. The more effective treatment would be to discover the original reasons for this, which turned out to be his widowed mother's sexual attachment to him which produced in him both fear and devotion. Even if we regard the essential conflict as that between his infantile fixation and his development into adulthood, it is still these early experiences which prevent him growing up.

The woman who developed the phobia for travelling in buses was actually on her way to an important interview, and at the moment had omnipotent phantasies as to how this new job would give her power to revenge herself on her family for not appreciating her importance. Her reverie was suddenly cut short by the swerve of the car, which put a sudden end to the phantasies and aroused her sense of guilt. But the fear was the reproduction of an objective fear and rage in infancy when her mother, whilst feeding her, was suddenly alarmed by the entry of a drunken father, and "swerved" the child into the cot. The fear automatically repressed the aggressiveness, so that whenever her assertiveness was aroused as on this later occasion the fear of consequences was aroused. There was a present-day moral problem, concerning her assertiveness, a basic fear of her aggressive phantasies of omnipotence, but she would not have developed the problem had it not been for the experiences of childhood which were repressed by fear of consequences.

These past experiences, therefore, are not merely incidents from which (as Jung says) the patient borrows his symptoms: they are *causal factors in the production of the psychoneuroses*, which must be taken into consideration if we are to cure the patient radically.

[1] *Analytical Psychology*, p. 271.

The recognition of these two basic factors has led to two approaches in analytic treatment. There are those psychotherapists who deal primarily with this moral problem in its present-day presentation, interpreting to the patient the unconscious motives of his actions and feelings, especially as revealed in dreams. There are others, like the writer, who consider that the most effective means of dealing even with the present-day moral problem, is to discover its deep-seated causes in childhood, and so to eradicate the complexes from which the present problems spring. For whilst the analysis of the precipitating causes may reveal the problem, the discovery of these early experiences reveals the origins of the problem, and the causes of the moral conflict, the precipitation of which produces the breakdown. An understanding of these predisposing causes in childhood is also, of course, of the greater importance for the *prevention* of the psychoneuroses which is our main concern. That is why it is with the predisposing causes of these disorders in early childhood that we shall most particularly deal in the following pages.

The precipitating causes of a neurosis are innumerable, some of which will be mentioned as occasion arises, but there are some which are consequent upon certain biological phases of life, such as adolescence and the menopause. In adolescence not only the sex impulses but love impulses, especially in the girl, and aggressive impulses, especially in the boy, are strongly aroused and precipitate a conflict previously latent. If the main repression has been of sex impulses, these may precipitate a sex perversion; if the repressed impulses was the need for sympathy and affection, the resultant symptom is more likely to be a hysteria; if a sense of guilt has been repressed it may produce an obsession. A specific hysteric symptom characteristic of girls at this age is pain at time of menstruation, which gynaecologists now recognize to be frequently of hysterical as well as of endocrine origin, the causes of which must be discovered to be eradicated. They are frequently combined so that an endocrine pain may be used as a means of getting love and sympathy at an age when the love craving is particularly active. So the depression of a girl at the menstrual periods may be due to the thwarting of love or to pituitary gland deficiency, or a combination of both.

The thwarted love craving also happens in women about the age of 28–30 whose natural desire to be married seems less likely to be fulfilled and who are getting bored with a "career" which is losing its attraction. The healthy-minded woman frankly accepts the thwarting of that desire, adapts herself to life, and finds other though perhaps less perfect forms of interest. But if she has not learnt to tolerate frustration, or if she has an old repressed yearning for affection, the resultant conflict may produce either unsatisfactory illicit affairs, restless depression, or hysterical symptoms.

The woman at the menopause is also liable to hysteria because she feels her attraction going and her love functions both as wife and mother passing. The age of 55–60 is a common time for breakdown in men, especially the successful man, for he finds his power waning and is confronted with having to yield to younger and more energetic men. It is the too great urge to power and achievement that produces both his success and his breakdown; but that urge, as we shall see, is often based on a more deep-rooted anxiety. So this loss of power most commonly takes the form of anxiety hysteria whereas in the woman in the menopause the disorder more commonly takes the form of conversion hysteria owing to the loss of affection.

There are *three main types of psychoneuroses*: Hysteria, Obsessions and Sex perversions corresponding to the reactions of the personality to the deprivation of love. The hysteric responds to life by *dependence*; he desires to escape from life, he shrinks from life. The obsessional responds to life by *aggressiveness* and self-will, and it is these forbidden impulses, the consequences of which he dreads, which compel him to propitiate. The sex pervert is characterized by *sensuousness* and the resort to sexual pleasure apart from its biological functions. In each case these modes of response have first been highly developed, and then repressed, and finally emerge in their specific forms of neurosis.

We may regard the three main forms of neurosis as the three primary colours of the spectrum which may appear in pure form but which more often appear as mixtures: or again, as a wave of sound which varies not only in volume, but the *shape* and overtones of which determine the timbre by which we can distinguish the violin from the flute. So the timbre of an obsessional, both in character and symptom, is quite different from that of the hysteric, and the hysteric from the sex pervert.

NOTE ON PSYCHOSES AND PSYCHONEUROSES

The distinction between the psychoses and psychoneuroses is not yet clearly defined. There are some who regard the psychoneuroses simply as mild forms of psychoses. But there are many severe psychoneurotics whose state is much worse than, say, a mild schizophrenic; and most people regard these two conditions as different in kind as well as in degree.

Many other criteria of the psychoses have been suggested, none of which are satisfactory. The most common one is that of "insight"—that the insane patient has no insight into his condition, whereas the psychoneurotic has. It is an important distinction from the point of view of treatment since where there is insight we can get the co-operation of the patient, whereas where the patient denies that there is anything wrong with him we cannot do so. But it is not a true distinction for some psychotics (e.g. G.P.I.) have insight and know they are going insane; whereas there are a number of people like the conceited man who is obviously not psychotic, but has no insight into his condition and even regards himself as modest.

Another criterion of the psychotic is that of a person who is *completely dominated by his morbid state*, whether depression, rage or delusional ideas. This is true of the advanced psychotic, but there are psychotic people who have delusions but are very skilful in keeping a check on them during an interview with a doctor looking for evidence to certify them. On the other hand, even psychoneurotics often "go off the deep end," fall into deep depression, become hysterical, and the obsessional is often completely dominated by his compulsion or contamination complex, for the time being. It is this criterion which leads some psychopathologists to say that "all children are psychotic." But this is also a misrepresentation, for every being must be judged by its own standard of normality, and uncontrolled behaviour is normal to a child at the age of two, who has not yet co-ordinated his personality under the control of the will. The psychotic, like many others, suffers from lack of control; but his lack of control is due to constitutional weakness; he suffers not only from loss of control but from the *capacity* of control; whereas in the psychoneurotic, the disorder is due to too great repression of natural impulses, which therefore surge up as neurotic symptoms. The treatment is therefore different: generally speaking, the psychotic needs to be given more power of control; the psychoneurotic needs to relax the control of his morbid super-ego so that these repressed impulses may be released and be utilized for better purposes.

Another criterion suggested is the *sense of reality*; the diagnosis depending on whether the patient is in touch with objective reality or whether his mental condition alienates him from his surroundings. But this again is only a matter of degree, for many psychoneurotics because of partial dissociation have "the feeling of unreality" and detachment from objective reality; and if this were taken as an absolute criterion, the sleep-walker and the man in a fugue would be psychotic.

These distinctions have their value for clinical purposes but none is adequate as a distinguishing mark of the psychoses.

Since there are, in the main, two main sources of mental disorder, *it is better*, as we have said, quite frankly *to regard as psychotic those mental disorders which are the result of organic and mainly constitutional causes; and the psychoneuroses those which are determined by abnormal psychological experiences*. The psychoses are fundamentally *somato-*

genetic, arising from bodily conditions; the psychoneuroses are predominantly *psychogenetic*, arising from mental disorders. One man is depressed because he is cyclothymic, the other is depressed because circumstances are against him, and a third, the psychoneurotic, because his inner inhibitions frustrate the expression of his personality. One man has a fugue state because he is epileptic, another because of an unconscious escape from intolerable circumstances.

In actual fact this distinction corresponds fairly well with the criteria of the psychoses already referred to, because it is the person who has a weak constitution or is in a toxic state who is *overwhelmed* by morbid thoughts and feelings; who is so confused that he has *no insight* into his mental condition; and who is so absorbed with these emotions as to be *out of touch with reality*. The basic factor in all these cases is the physiological instability.

On this criterion we include as psychotic not only *constitutional* and often hereditary disorders like cyclothymia, and acquired conditions like general paralysis of the insane, exhaustion psychoses, and toxic psychoses like delirium tremens, but we shall also include as *temporary psychosis* the hallucinations and delirium of the patient with fever, and as *mild psychosis* such conditions as irascibility from toxic states or acidosis, elation from alcohol or cocaine, and depression from jaundice. These are all mild disturbances arising from somatic causes which in more exaggerated forms may become certifiable psychoses, and there is no reason why we should not classify them as such, however mild. The moroseness due to limited amounts of alcohol are only different in degree from the delirium tremens which comes from taking more doses of alcohol. The one is a mild the other an advanced psychosis. The term "insanity," however, does concern itself with the severity of the condition, and not merely with its nature. It is a legal term referring only to the more advanced cases of psychosis who are a danger to themselves and others and who can therefore by certification have their personal and civic liberties legally taken from them.

Because of mixed aetiology an apparent psychoneurotic may turn into a psychotic, not because these are different degrees of the same disorder, but because, although the psychogenetic factor may have been the first to appear, the constitutional factor is the predominant one. Indeed the psychogenetic symptoms may be the earliest manifestation of a constitutional breakdown, and determine the form which the psychosis takes. Religious mania is a case in point: there are commonly religious problems such as a sense of guilt, but these are not the true cause of the breakdown; no one gets religious mania unless he is constitutionally unstable. On the other hand, bad psychological experiences such as shocking news may precipitate a constitutional condition otherwise latent and produce a psychosis, as in many war cases who were constitutionally predisposed but broke down only under the stress of war.

In such cases of mixed aetiology the patient may sometimes be saved from complete breakdown into insanity by dealing with the psychological factors and straightening those out, even when nothing can be done to change the constitutional factor. This of course can be done only when the patient is well enought to co-operate. Thus in favourable cases psychological treatment is effective even in psychotic cases, for when we have removed the psychological or moral problems, the patient is then capable of coping with the constitutional part of his disorder, and a permanent recovery, though not a complete cure, is effected. Great care, however, is required in analysing the mild psychotic, lest by arousing repressed emotions in a patient constitutionally lacking in control, we unbalance him still further, and precipitate in him a deeper psychosis. In other cases, even in mild psychoses the patient who feels he is losing control may be given suggestion treatment to quieten his mind, and to give him confidence and stability, whilst an attempt is made by analysis to unravel his difficulties. The psychological treatment of such cases requires much care and patience, and is not to be lightly undertaken: it is also very time-consuming and for the present must be regarded in the nature of research rather than a matter of clinical expediency.

PART II
CLINICAL

CHAPTER VI

PSYCHOSOMATIC DISORDERS

VISCERAL NEUROSES

Psychosomatic medicine is concerned with the body-mind relationship in the production of disease. It represents the interaction of body and mind, as against the too-exclusive dualism which regards disease as being either organic or psychogenetic in origin. Our personality reacts to a situation as a whole, and this reaction involves both mental and physiological changes. Psychosomatic medicine regards the personality as a functioning unit.

The term *psychosomatic disorders* is therefore sometimes used of all those disorders of the personality in which the body-mind relationship is the dominant feature. But so used it covers the most of medicine; for there are few physical diseases which have not their mental effects and few mental disorders but have some, though not necessarily a corresponding effect on the physiological organism. It means that we should have to classify tuberculosis or beri-beri as psychosomatic disorders since they give rise to mental and emotional disturbances, as well as conversion hysteria since the physical symptom of paralysis results from an emotional cause. This is to render the term useless since it is made to explain too much, for according to this definition almost all medicine is "psychosomatic medicine."

By others the term "psychosomatic disorders" is restricted to these disorders in which both mental and physical factors *combine in the production of the disorder*, a typical case being that of asthma, in which there is frequently a constitutional predisposition, but the attacks of which are often precipitated by emotional disturbances. In such cases the cure of either one or the other factor may be sufficient to "cure" the whole, by removing one of the essential causes. On this criterion such conditions as duodenal ulcer may be called psychosomatic in so far as both mental and physical factors contribute to the production of the disorder. But to limit the term psychosomatic disorders to those conditions in which there is a combination of physical and psychological causes, excludes conditions such as a simple nervous indigestion or headache due to worry, in which the causal factors are entirely psychological.

Whilst, therefore, we shall use the term psychosomatic medicine to express the broad relationship of body and mind in the production of disease, we shall use the term *psychosomatic disorders* in a more restricted sense of those physical disorders like nervous dyspepsia, nervous headache or palpitation, which are the immediate effects of emotional disturbances and manifest themselves especially in *disorders of the automatic nervous system.* Since the effects of emotion are to be found mainly in visceral changes, the term psychosomatic disorders corresponds most generally to the so-called "visceral neuroses."[1]

We have seen that when the organism is faced with a critical situation such as that of danger, changes take place first of all in the autonomic nervous system and visceral organs to prepare the organism for action, after which the energy liberated is normally discharged in voluntary action, as running away or fighting.

But if the energy thus released cannot be discharged in voluntary action, as when escape is impossible, it is dammed back into the organism so that these visceral activities are greatly exaggerated and we have violent palpitation of the heart, pressure in the head, breathlessness, faintness, sickness, trembling and perspiration. These are typical psychosomatic or visceral disorders, which are as varied and as numerous as the functions of the autonomic nervous system itself; other instances of which are nervous indigestion, nervous headache, constipation, diarrhoea, vomiting, blushing, angio-neurotic oedema, some cases of asthma, incon-

[1] The theory of body and mind which seems best to fit the psychosomatic disorders is that of *psychophysical interaction*, namely that bodily functions and mental functions may each act upon the other, and yet may function independently, that is to say without any *corresponding* effect on the other. The body, for instance, may function without any effect on the mind, as when we are deeply under chloroform. On the other hand, conscious states like the appreciation of music or religious faith may affect us physically but there are, so far as we know, no physical states corresponding to their "meaning" or "significance." From the practical point of view the theory of psychophysical interaction, therefore, seems to have advantages over that of *epiphenomenalism*, which regards mental processes as being merely the product of physical changes, the foam of the wave, the smell from the flower. This theory, which denies that mental process can have any influence upon physical processes and therefore that all mental as well as physical disorders must have a physical basis, is no longer tenable if we accept the fact of "psychosomatic disorders." Psychophysical interaction also has advantages over the theory of *psychophysical parallelism*, in which body and mind are conceived as running parallel to one another but without any causal relation. The psychosomatic disorders suggest that, the personality being a unity, there is a two-way system of causal relationship, the possibility of which we have discussed in dealing with consciousness (p. 49), in which mental states and processes can affect physical, and physical can affect mental processes. The conception of psychophysical interaction gives independent functioning to mental and physical processes and yet relates them so that they can work together in the production of a common disorder. That indeed is what is commonly meant by a psychosomatic disorder.

tinence of urine, sexual impotence, ovarian and uterine pain and disorders of function in the liver and other organs whose functions are affected by the autonomic nervous system. These changes in turn affect metabolism of the whole body and give rise to general ill-health; thus many a man gets "run down," and literally loses weight from worry and anxiety.

The *mechanism* of these simple psychosomatic disorders is not difficult to undersand if we take a particular instance, say that of nervous indigestion. It has been proved (Cannon, Pavlov and others) that when we are in an emotional state, say of fear or rage, the flow of gastric juices is disordered, and the function of digestion almost ceases. This inhibition is brought about through the medium of the adrenals and the sympathetic nervous system.

Biogolically, this arrest of digestion is valuable in that it conserves our energies and utilizes them to meet the immediate situation in question for which all available energy is required. If, therefore, a man is in a state of worry, anxiety, irritability, or is frustrated in love, the flow of gastric juices is disturbed, the food in the stomach remains undigested and the individual suffers from "nervous indigestion." This, be it noted, is a real indigestion due to deficiency of the gastric secretions, and not an hysteric indigestion developed in order to get sympathy or to escape responsibility: nevertheless it is caused by mental worry or anger.

Now it is obvious that such a condition of nervous indigestion, originating in an emotional state and ending with a somatic disorder, is the "no man's land," or every man's land, between the organic physician and the medical psychologist. The former treats the end result by giving the patient digestives and may cure the indigestion, and therefore naturally claims that the condition is obviously physical. The medical psychologist goes further back and cures the emotional worry which started it, so that the indigestion disappears, and he therefore claims that the condition is psychogenetic. So the unnecessary quarrel goes on. But there is no doubt which treatment is the more radical and scientific; for the somatic approach cures the end result but not the worry which causes it, so that the symptoms may return, and the patient becomes a chronic medicine-taker, the curse of the general practitioner: whereas the psychological approach, by dealing with the worry which originated the disturbance, and giving the patient confidence, releases the energy in purposive action and cures both the indigestion and the worry of which the indigestion was the direct result.

CLINICAL TYPES OF PSYCHOSOMATIC DISORDERS

Psychosomatic disorders may be of a simple, symbolic, or psychoneurotic type. A case will illustrate all three. A man suffers from pressure in the head especially round the temples, and he cannot see clearly. He had a nagging wife who would keep him awake till two or three in the morning and sleeps it off while he has to work. This he bore like a Christian martyr and mentioned it to no one out of loyalty. When he was encouraged to let out in analysis all his feelings of rage and resentment against his wife, his symptoms completely disappeared. The pressure in the head due to suppressed rage was a simple psychosomatic disorder: the difficulty in seeing was symbolic of the fact that he was refusing to "look facts in the face": it was not a simple but a symbolic psychosomatic disorder. But there was a neurotic element in that he unconsciously used his symptoms to escape from these responsibilities, and to indulge in self-pity.

A. Simple psychosomatic disorders

Simple psychosomatic disorders are those which are the *direct somatic results of thwarted emotion*, whether of fear, sex or anger, the causes of which are *conscious* and usually of an *objective nature*. Headache due to worry, and loss of appetite due to anxiety, are cases in point. So a business man can suffer indigestion from having a row with a partner: a workman in an uncongenial job in which he feels his personality stifled may suffer from asthma; brooding resentment may cause pseudo-angina, with pain at the heart; and a girl, unwillingly kept at home, suffers from nervous headaches due to frustration, whilst her sister whose sexual cravings are aroused and not satisfied suffers from pain in the back from uterine congestion. Many girls in adolescence go "off their food" because of physiologically aroused but frustrated love.

These effects of emotion are not only observed clinically but they can be experimentally established; for under hypnosis we may produce artificially induced emotional states like fear and anger, and under these "laboratory conditions" can observe and test the bodily effects (Wittkower). The heart rate is affected and the blood pressure raised even under an imaginary fear. A condition of annoyance produced under hypnosis checks the flow of bile, with all the physical consequences of this. Constipation can be induced and is often cured by hypnotic suggestion; menstruation can be checked or postponed by suggestion (it used to be done before Balls); and amenorrhoea can be produced. Everyone knows that the fear of getting a baby in an unmarried girl may itself be enough to stop her periods.

The characteristics of simple psychosomatic disorders are as follows:

(1) They originate in *mental and emotional causes*: they are therefore psychogenetic. In this respect they resemble the psychoneuroses, but differ from disorders of organic origin.

(2) The causes of the emotion may be quite *conscious*. We are quite aware of the emotions of fear or rage producing them; and in this respect they differ from the psychoneuroses which always have an unconscious motivation. A timid person may be sick with fear, develop palpitation or sweating in a bombing attack or at receiving bad news, the causes of which have no relation to any unconscious conflict. The unmarried girl who is worried about the possibility of a pregnancy may get a cessation of her menses, not from the pregnancy but from the worry, and the cessation further adds to her worry, thus creating a vicious circle and perpetuating the amenorrhoea, although she is quite aware of the cause of her worry. A man who receives news that his wife has left him develops a severe headache and knows why; the swain who has been rejected in love may lose weight; and the torpedoed petty officer, worried at the possibility of going back to sea, develops a chronic sweating which immediately subsides when he is told he will not be sent to sea. These are the cases of simple psychosomatic disorders, but not true psychoneuroses: for in all these cases there is consciousness of the emotional cause. They are neurotic only if we are to use the term in the popular sense of all abnormal emotional conditions, but not if we reserve this term for those more complicated conditions in which there is repression, dissociation and unconscious motivation.

(3) In all these cases it is the *frustration* which causes the headache or indigestion. It is when we cannot adequately express our fear that we get indigestion, when our anger is checked that we get a headache, when we worry about a problem we cannot solve that we get constipated, and when we are hopelessly in love that we lose our appetite. This approximates to Freud's theory of repression, but in these cases there is only frustration and not repression which is an unconscious process.

(4) They are the *direct physiological effects* of these emotions. In this respect they differ from ordinary hysteria which is indirect and purposive. The psychosomatic vomiting is the simple result of emotional disturbances and has no "purpose" except the purely biological one of emptying the stomach in preparation for

action. The psychosomatic headache is due to pressure from a congested circulation; the hysteric headache is devised as a means of escaping responsibility, and is the result of an unconscious wish, not of pressure.

(5) Moreover they are *real somatic* disturbances. The psychosomatic indigestion though caused by worry is a "real" one due to deficiency in gastric secretions. The headache is probably due to actual pressure in the head, perhaps from the congestion of blood. The constipation may be due to actual atony of the bowel or the lack of bile; in psychosomatic amenorrhoea there is actual, not an imaginary, cessation of menstrual flow. They are in the true sense of the term "functional nervous disorders," in that there is primarily a change of function in the nervous system, but not a change in organic structure. Nevertheless there is evidence to show that if these functional psychosomatic disorders continue long enough *they may culminate in real organic and structural changes*, as in some cases of duodenal ulcer, or whitening of the hair from mental strain, commonly seen in young women in London during the war.

(6) Psychosomatic disorders may arise from *any emotion*: so we may get nervous indigestion from thwarted anger, sex or fear; both the angry person and the person in love loses his appetite. Nervous headaches are as often due to the arousal and frustration of resentment as of worry. Breathlessness can come from anger as well as from fear. Disorders of blushing, sweating, palpitation, liver or ovarian function may likewise result from the frustration of any emotion, since any emotion can set going the adrenals and autonomic nervous system which in turn affect the heart, breathing, capillary circulation and other visceral functions. These *autonomic* functions are "preparatory to action," but to no specific action: it is the function of the central nervous system to direct the energies in a specific direction.[1]

Differential diagnosis. Simple psychosomatic disorders are often confused with *conversion hysteria* like hysterical paralysis in that the symptoms in both cases are physical. But the psychosomatic disorders may be due to conscious worries whereas conversion

[1] Psychosomatic disorders used to be called "Anxiety Equivalents" (Freud, *Introd. Lectures*, p. 334), a term used to cover shuddering, faintness, palpitation of the heart, and inability to breathe, which are the results of anxiety, but in which no conscious anxiety is recognized. "They have," he writes, "the same clinical and aetiological validity as anxiety itself." It is true that these psychosomatic disorders are frequently associated with anxiety, but this is an unfortunate limitation of their scope, for they can be and often are produced by other emotions. Moreover we can get these somatic equivalents from anxiety consciously induced.

hysteria is due to unconscious conflicts: and psychosomatic disorders are mainly visceral and autonomic, whereas conversion hysteria is mainly of the voluntary nervous system. This differential diagnosis, however, depends somewhat on our classification: for if we take as our criterion the *anatomical distinction*, we regard conversion hysteria as a disorder of the central nervous system, and the psychosomatic as a disorder of the autonomic. But if we accept the *criterion of purposiveness*, we regard hysteric symptoms as representing an unconscious wish and devised for a purpose, such as escaping responsibility, whereas the psychosomatic disorders are simply the physiological results or effects of emotional disturbances. But in either case there is some overlapping: for a visceral neurosis, though the immediate and direct result of the emotional state, may, as we shall see, come to be used purposively as a hysterical symptom to get attention and sympathy. On the other hand, a disorder of the central nervous system may be the direct result of the emotional state, and not have any element of such intent or purpose, such as trembling, stiffening of the neck and immobility. There are patients who suffer from torticollis (wry-neck), expressive of "turning away" from an unpleasant thought or an experience which they are unwilling to face. This involves the central nervous system but is nevertheless the physical expression of an emotional state. There are, we believe, paralyses of this simple type, especially in traumatic neuroses, which are purely biological reactions, and have no element of the "wish to be ill." As a rule, they soon pass away and constitute some of the "rapid cures" claimed by doctors who work near the front line in war. But if too much fuss is made of them, they may come to be used by the patient, and be transformed into a true hysteria. That is why it is advisable to treat them early.

Many psychosomatic disorders are temporary because the situation which caused the emotional upset, whether domestic worry, failure, disappointment in love, business anxiety or air raids, is temporary. All of us have gone through these experiences. Most of us know what it means to be sick with disappointment, to have a sinking feeling in the pit of the stomach with fear, to feel hot about the neck with anger or to feel the heart jump into the throat. In these cases the symptoms usually pass off themselves when the crisis is over and the objective stimulus passes: the stomach quietens down, we cease to perspire, appetite returns and the heart returns to its normal position!

Chronic psychosomatic disorders. But there are circumstances which tend to make these conditions chronic. (*a*) In the first place, psychosomatic disorders may persist because the *cause of the emotional state* persists. It stands to reason that if the business man's worry continues it will cause him chronic indigestion: the wife who is dissatisfied in her marriage suffers from a chronic headache: and the professional man who is constantly trying to attain what is beyond his capacity will suffer from chronic palpitation. But there are reasons of a more specific nature.

(*b*) One is the *persistence of physiological excitation*. When, on account of the emotion, physiological changes have taken place it takes time for the products of these changes to be thrown off and for the organism to settle down into a state of equilibrium. Therefore for a time after the shell has burst and the danger is over we continue in a state of trembling anxiety. These conditions are analogous to the "after images" of sight which are caused by the continued chemical action in the retina for some time after the light itself has been removed. Thus the thyroid gland may continue in a state of activity for long periods after the shock, and its continued secretion may perpetuate the excitement even when its objective stimulus is past. This is liable to create a vicious circle between the mental and the physical, for the mental excitement stimulates the thyroid and the thyroid perpetuates the excitement, so that the condition may apparently last for years. An illustration in point is that of a girl undressing in a bedroom, who looked up to see a man looking in at the window. She dare not scream: but rapidly developed a hyperthyroidism which persisted. Airmen who have crashed often suffer from this combination of anxiety and hyperthyroidism which is much more difficult to cure than a simple anxiety neurosis because of the physio-psychological vicious circle produced. We have found these conditions resistive to psychotherapy alone.

(*c*) In other cases it is the after-thought of a distressing experience, the *memory of what has happened*, which causes the palpitation or other psychosomatic disorder to persist. Indeed, such anxiety tends to become worse in retrospect, because we imagine what "might have been," which is much worse than what was. These experiences may become still more terrifying by being reproduced with even greater terror in dreams and nightmares, the function of which is to stand in the place of experience and warn us of possible coming dangers. This apprehension, together with the physiological accompaniments already mentioned, serves a useful biological purpose, for if once a specific danger has threatened, it may come again and the organism therefore continues in a state of preparedness of body and apprehension of mind to meet the return of the danger. But what is biologically useful may be psychologically very distressing.

(d) Very commonly another type of vicious circle is formed, a psychological, not a psychophysical one as previously described. A woman in the bombing naturally developed palpitation. Thereafter the more the heart palpitated the more she feared: and the more she feared the more the heart palpitated. Her condition was not improved by being told by her doctor, ignorant of the psychological factor in these disorders, that she had heart disease and would have to be careful all her life, adding yet another anxiety and more palpitation which seemed to confirm his false diagnosis.

(e) The most persistent of the psychosomatic disorders are those in which *an old repressed complex is reactivated.* This was the case in the man who suffered from suffocation after being buried in debris in a railway smash, and whose experience revived a suffocation in infancy. These emotions once aroused cannot be so easily allayed. In those conditions a temporary psychosomatic disorder is transformed into a psychoneurotic disorder, by the arousal of an old complex, to which we refer later.

Simple subjective psychosomatic disorders. We have so far discussed those psychosomatic disorders in which an emotional state has been aroused by an objective and conscious situation, and being thwarted produces visceral disturbances, which persist as long as the stimulating cause persists.

But emotions may be aroused from subjective causes within ourselves, fear of our impulses, fear of our fear, feelings of guilt or shame, sex feelings from imagination, resentment arising from some memory of the past, annoyance with ourselves for making fools of ourselves. Curiously enough, as we have already mentioned, *these subjectively-produced emotions may give rise to precisely the same physiological effects as though the situation were objective,* and call forth all those autonomic responses which we call "preparedness for action," although in fact there is no objective situation to meet, no occasion for their use. When we feel the sense of guilt or shame at some remembered sin of the past, we perspire and the heart palpitates, just as much as when we are faced with an objective danger. An emotion has been aroused, and it does not seem to matter whether it is subjective or objective, it automatically produces the physiological effects. Even with subjective danger the body stupidly prepares itself for action which cannot be carried out, and for an objective emergency which does not exist. The bodily reactions are quite inappropriate, and we are left with a lot of useless physiological responses on our hands which, having no adequate outlet, are readily transformed into psychosomatic disorders.

Subjective situations, therefore, are more likely to give rise to chronic psychosomatic disorders than objective ones for various reasons. First, the cause is *within us*; we carry our fever about with us; we cannot escape from it by flight or change of circumstances, as we may from objective danger. Secondly, the physiological reaction is *inappropriate to the situation* because it was designed for an objective situation; so the girl who has a sense of shame about sex desires blushes when she meets people, although the blushing serves no other purpose than to call attention to what she wants to hide: far from preparing her for defensive action, it puts her at a disadvantage and perpetuates the trouble. Finally, subjective problems are more likely to *remain unsolved*, and as long as the cause remains the psychosomatic result will remain, as in the case of the man who is perpetually harassed by shame or anger against himself for some past folly.

We still regard such psychosomatic disorders as "simple," though subjective, for the causes of the emotion may be quite conscious; and although there may be emotional conflict, there is no repression or dissociation.

The treatment of simple psychosomatic disorders follows upon their nature. They are always due to frustration, with the result that there is an *excess of production* of emotion and *inadequacy of discharge*. The condition may therefore be cured either (i) by *checking the production* of the emotion or (ii) by *finding outlet* and discharge for the emotion in voluntary action.

(i) The simplest way of bringing about the first is by the removal of the cause if it persists or by *changing of circumstances*. Removing a man from a tyrannical boss, taking temporary charge of the children of a harassed mother, solving the marriage problem, relieving a business man's strain by temporary financial help, removing causes of irritation in work; these by removing the stimulus will get rid of the emotional worry and so of the psychosomatic disorder. One of the functions of "social psychiatry" is to cure such disorders by changing the relationship with the environment. But all psychosomatic disorders cannot be cured in this way, for sometimes we cannot change our circumstances, and at other times the cause of the trouble is subjective, from which we cannot escape: we merely carry our fear with us.

In other cases, we may check the emotion by getting the individual to react differently to the situation: when we cannot change the circumstances we may be able to *change our attitude* towards them. This is brought about by persuading the individual to abandon his resentment, his pride, his anxiety: the business man is encouraged to "cut his losses"; and the woman unhappily married to put up with what she cannot avoid, and make the best of other things. Or we may bring about the same result of checking the emotion by giving *suggestion treatment* of quietness and calmness, so that the anger and fear being allayed, there is no more congestion in the head to produce the headache, or disturbance of gastric secretion to produce the indigestion. Suggestion is often immediately effective and many a worry headache can be cured by such soothing and quietening treatment, the object of which is not to repress the emotion, but to allay its production. Such first-aid treatment of these simple psychosomatic disorders provides a tempting field for the physician in his first essays in psychological medicine, who claims to cure without resort to deep analysis, and then may regard analysis unnecessary for the cure of the deeper psychoneuroses. But what is effective in simple psychosomatic disorders is of no effect in the more complicated psychoneuroses. We should not cure an acute appendicitis by a fomentation; operation is the only procedure.

(ii) The second general method is by finding a *discharge for the emotion*. After all, emotions are aroused for some purpose and that purpose is action: it is their frustration which has caused the disorder. It may not be right that the patient should cease to strive, or that his fears should be allayed. The right treatment may be to encourage the patient to do something about it and not to take things lying down; to tackle the problem, not to evade it; and it may be our function to help him to do it. The emotion discharged in voluntary action is no longer frustrated, so that the tension ceases, and the symptom disappears.

But short of complete and purposive action, even giving expression to the grievance or other emotions *in words* is often sufficient to provide the necessary outlet, as we find in analytic treatment. In one case, for instance, a lady who had a "pseudo-angina pectoris" was cured when she acknowledged the fact that she was jealous of her husband's attention to her sister, and gave verbal expression to her resentment instead of keeping it bottled up. We saw how the man with the nagging wife got rid of his headaches when he gave expression to his bottled-up rage and hate. It is a common experience that people feel much better when they have "talked things over" or got some resentment "off their chest." The tendency of people to talk over their fears or to air their grievances is a natural and, from the therapeutic point of view of their mental health, a healthy reaction, however annoying to others. The authorities in London invited psychosomatic disorders when they discouraged people in air-raid shelters from talking of their experiences. Fortunately people ignored their advice!

In other cases, *making a decision* will be a sufficiently active method of facing the situation and is enough to resolve the symptom, even though immediate action is impossible, for decision is a form of mental action. The human mind can stand anything but doubt. Those who are ill and are anxious about death are those who are in doubt about it; most people who know they are to die are calm. So with the problems of life; to decide things one way or another, even if our decisions are not the right ones, allays the immediate anxiety.

Physical treatment. Since the emotion works through the medium of the autonomic nervous system, to produce indigestion by inhibiting the gastric juice, headache by producing pressure in the cranium, constipation by relaxing the bowel, these physiological effects can obviously be counteracted by the *use of drugs* which will produce contrary effects—stimulate the gastric juice and so cure the indigestion; stimulate the circulation and so cure the headache; tone the muscles of the bowel and so correct the constipation. By such means we allay the symptom, but do not cure the dsorder; we get rid of the end results, not the cause. The danger of these methods of treatment is that they give the patient the impression that these are organic conditions correctly treated by physical methods, and many a hypochondriac has been produced this way. Nevertheless a drug like belladonna which will abolish sweating and thus remove the *immediate cause* of the anxiety may break the vicious circle. Permanent results are therefore sometimes obtained by such means.

As regards treatment, the same principles apply to the moral problems as to the objective difficulties: we can either *check the production* of emotion by removing the stimulus or *give outlet* for the emotion. If the patient can be brought to face up to the problem and *decide the moral issue* one way or another the situation is relieved and the psychosomatic symptom disappears. If he can be persuaded to do something about it he may not only get better of his symptoms, but become better adapted to life in general. This indeed is the proper treatment of such disorders. There are numerous people who take aspirins for their headache when they should be facing up to their responsibilities: others take soda mint for their indigestion when they should be examining their consciences.

The youth, therefore, whose idealism will not permit him to have extra-marital sex relations, but who constantly subjects himself to sex stimulation in phantasy is looking for trouble, and should not be surprised if he suffers from psychosomatic discomfort such as restlessness, palpitation, sleeplessness, headache, indigestion and other visceral disturbances. This may account for the common but erroneous idea that sexual continence as such is physically harmful, for erotic emotion like any emotion without outlet often produces such disorders. But even a superficial glance at the cause of such a situation makes it clear that he can solve the problem not only by giving outlet to his sex (which he is often advised to do, but which may arouse deeper moral conflicts and guilt, and which Freud has specifically stated is bad psychotherapy), but by removing the constant stimulation. The youth who has many interests in work, hobbies, sports and friendships has little to worry about with regard to sex. But even here early training is an important factor: for numerous people are sexually continent without suffering from either psychosomatic disorders or anxiety, since in their earlier years *they have learnt how to tolerate frustration.*

Mental hygiene in simple psychosomatic disorders. All parents should be made familiar with the fact that children may suffer these psychosomatic disorders as a result of emotional "upsets," especially nausea and sickness, headache, loss of weight from worry, tiredness from frustration and boredom, eneuresis from anxiety and constipation from stubbornness. A child is not always shamming, nor trying to get sympathy when it says it has a headache after a scolding: it may in fact have one. Any condition of emotion, anger, irritability, resentment, as well as worry and fear, may make the child feel sick. The mother excuses the father's temper to the children on the ground that he suffers from indigestion, when it would be truer to say that he suffers from indigestion because he is bad tempered! The mother who scolds the child and makes him sick, may herself then suffer from headache because of her frustrated annoyance; but she can retire with her headache and be sorry for herself that she has such a trying child.

B. Neurotic psychosomatic disorders

These are characterized by three things. (a) They are *subjective*, the cause of the emotion being within ourselves, whether shame at what we have done, fear of our impulses, rage at having made fools of ourselves, or depression at our failure. (*b*) These emotions are not only thwarted and frustrated but *repressed*. (*c*) Unlike the simple subjective disorders their *causes are unconscious*. For all these reasons the disorders they produce are persistent. Nor can they be treated by the first-aid methods already described, but like all psychoneuroses, require specific analytic treatment first to make the problems conscious, to find outlet and expression for the repressed emotions, and to readjust ourselves to the situation.

The following is a case of neurotic psychosomatic disorder.

A children's nurse has such severe indigestion with swelling of the stomach after meals that she cannot wear ordinary clothes, and cannot sleep if she has a meal after mid-day. It originated at the age of thirteen when, left with a helpless widowed mother, she rushed home from school at mid-day, got the meal, ate it, washed up, and rushed back to school. The rush and excitement no doubt caused a simple psychosomatic indigestion. But she was beginning to resent this life and being a slave when all her schoolfellows were enjoying themselves. Yet she could not give it up for she had voluntarily taken up the job of looking after her mother at the age of eight, when her father died a drunkard, not because she loved her mother, but because it gratified her self-importance. Her history as revealed in analysis was that she had in fact been jealous of her baby brother and had attacked him; for which she was shut up in a room, and decided thereafter to be the "good girl." Hence her taking over responsibility for her mother when her father died. But a still earlier memory appeared: in infancy, whilst her mother was feeding her, her mother suddenly put her down, and the baby was furious. The result was she developed a violent indigestion and flatulence which the patient recognized as precisely the same as the present attacks. The realization that her mother's action was not due to unkindness but to her alarm at her father's drunkenness, gave the patient an entirely different reaction, made her sympathize instead of resenting her mother and abolished the hate. The repressed hate and anxiety had been revived at the age of thirteen, and precipitated the symptom; but now that they were entirely released and abolished, her attacks ceased, nor have they returned in 20 years.

In such a case the causes were entirely unconscious. There are, however, varying degrees of unconsciousness of the causes. In the mildest cases the patient is conscious of the worry, say a disappointment in love, and of the dermatitis which results from it, but is unconscious of the connection between the two. Or he may be aware of the situation, but denies that he is worried; he scoffs at the idea that he minds being jilted in love, pretends not to care that he has lost his job: nevertheless the repressed anger produces a headache, the frustration an asthma, the humiliation a blushing, the worry a constipation, the fear a trembling of the limbs which he tries in vain to control. In other cases the patient is altogether unaware of the cause of the worry and will stoutly deny it, in which case the unconscious worry manifests itself only as the psychosomatic disorder. So the patient may honestly believe that he has nothing to worry about, and the physician's question "Are you worrying about anything?" will elicit no satisfactory reply because the patient is unaware of it. The fact that the patient denies having anything on his mind, must not therefore lead the physician to assume that the physical symptom is not a psychosomatic disorder, as the mental conflict may be repressed and unconscious.

Because in these cases the cause of the anxiety which produces the psychosomatic condition is unknown, *the anxiety may then become transferred to the symptom itself*, and the patient will say that all he is worrying about is his palpitation, that all he is depressed about is his digestion, and he feels ashamed because he blushes whereas in fact it is the repressed shame which produces the blushes, not the blushes the shame. The effect of the emotional state is thus taken to be its cause.

By this time we have transferred the whole of the repressed emotion to the symptom. We have now got into a vicious circle, in which the palpitation makes us anxious, and our anxiety makes our heart palpitate; we are ashamed because we blush and we then blush because we are ashamed of blushing.

This transfer of the emotion to the symptom it causes means that the symptom is greatly exaggerated since all the emotion which is aroused by the mental problem becomes discharged in the visceral symptom which is now dissociated from the original cause. Thus people's worry about blushing is out of all proportion to the fact.

Hysteric and obsessional psychosomatic disorders. The transition to a neurosis becomes complete when, once formed, the psychosomatic disorder is *utilized for the purpose of an hysteria*, in which case we have not a simple but an *hysteric psychosomatic disorder*. So the love-sick swain who goes off his food, the direct result of his being thwarted in love, may proceed to make use of his sickness to appeal to the pity of his lady love in his sad state. Indeed this is very liable to happen, for a person who is in the state of emotional distress is precisely the one who will readily use his symptoms as a means of getting sympathy and help. This may of course be quite purposefully and consciously done; but in our case he may be quite unaware of the motives for the perpetuation of his symptoms, which are therefore as unconscious as any other form of hysteria. We then have the complication of a psychosomatic disorder utilized for neurotic gains; for there is nothing to prevent a person of hysteric disposition unconsciously utilizing his psychosomatic blushing which arose from a feeling of inferiority, as a means of avoiding the company which makes him feel inferior, or using his psychosomatic headache as a means of escaping responsibility, in precisely the same way as he uses any other illness in conversion hysteria; but the psychosomatic indigestion is one thing, and hysteric utilization of it another. A tyrannical and jealous mother developed a psychosomatic headache as a result of suppressed anger because of her husband's attachment to the daughter and then used it as a means of paying the family out by making them attend to her. The man who because of worry in his job got nervous indigestion, then used his indigestion as the hysteric uses any other physical symptom as a means of getting out of his job. That is probably one reason why these psychosomatic disorders are so often called hysteric; and the fact that they are both physical gives encouragement to this idea: but in their simple form they are merely the results of the emotional state and may only later be used for hysteric purposes. We are therefore not justified in calling a simple psychosomatic disorder by the name of hysteria, even though they are both somatic in nature and of psychogenetic origin.

A case of hysteric asthma. This was the case of a boy of sixteen who had suffered from asthmatic attacks since an early age—about four or five. He was found to be allergic to dust, etc. His father was also a life-long asthmatic pointing to an hereditary predisposition. It was said that he was spoilt and used his symptom to get his own way and to avoid unpleasant duties, which he stoutly denied, saying, "Do you imagine I would have asthma if I could help it?" In the early analysis the following facts were revealed by the patient. He had one older sister, and the pet of his mother, and felt left out. At Christmas everyone watched his sister open her toys, no one watched him: he cried, only to be asked, "Whatever did he cry for with all these presents? So ungrateful!" He noticed, however, that when his father had asthmatic attacks it called forth the sympathy of the mother: so the boy tried gasping. It was immediately successful, "Poor boy; he is developing his father's asthma." On his birthday he had another attack. Why was this, we asked, when he was getting all the attention? "Because," he replied, "I thought I would get all the sympathy I could while the going was good!" Then he had a cold and some bronchitis and got his mother's attention; but when his mother left him he got an asthmatic attack again to get her back. The doctor was sent for who duly diagnosed "bronchial asthma" —another victory, for now it had a proper name. The asthma was then used not only to get sympathy and attention but *to get his own way*. If he was out and did not want to return home he would get an attack. If the pony had got loose and had to be caught he developed an attack to get him out of it. But after a time the asthma got little attention since he always recovered from the attacks; it no longer served its purpose.

But by this time he had become the victim of his asthma, the unconscious motives of which were now forgotten. So that now even when he *willed* to do something, like studying for matriculation, a latent resentment against it would precipitate an attack of asthma, which now thwarted him in many things he wished to do in life. It is not surprising that he denied all wish to have asthma: but now the asthma had become fatally associated with any occasion when he wanted his own way or wanted more attention—an almost chronic state producing a chronic symptom. There was probably a physiological predisposition to asthma, but the asthmatic attacks which were at first conscious and purposive were now unconscious but still purposive. They were, in fact, hysterical. Such psychogenetic disorders represent the most typical illustration of a body-mind relationship.[1]

[1] Allergic conditions are closely related to psychosomatic disorders. Both physical and psychological factors are found to be operative in many cases. (a) The allergies, though (as we believe) constitutional, may be *precipitated* by emotional disturbances, frustration producing an attack of asthma (symbolically representing the feeling that one's personality is being stifled) or sexual stress producing migraine. (b) Emotional disturbances make an individual already prone to allergy more sensitive, lowering the threshold of resistance and therefore subject to attacks. This is proved under hypnosis, when a hypnotically induced state of emotion is found to predispose the individual to more frequent attacks. (c) One can get asthma, hay fever or migraine of an entirely hysteric type exactly simulating a true attack, since a hysteric may use any symptom allergic or otherwise to stage his need for attention. (d) The allergic patient who is hypersensitive to certain physical stimuli is usually also mentally hypersensitive, and therefore more liable to neurosis, but there need be no connection between the allergic attacks and the neurosis except the hypersensitivity upon which they are both based. It is, however, natural that a neurotic person who has a ready-made allergy will seize upon this to serve as his symptom. (e) But there are many mixed cases in people who are constitutionally allergic to asthma, but whose attacks are brought on by emotional disturbances, frustration of anger, repression of fear. In such a case psychological treatment for the removal of the frustration may cure the attacks leaving only the constitutional predisposition behind. This gives rise to the commonly held opinion that asthma is psychogenetic.

Psychosomatic attacks are often *precipitated* by emotional causes, but that is not to say that the causes are basically psychological; and in our opinion the psychological aspect of many of these psychosomatic disorders is often overstated. Because a man has five attacks of peptic ulcer, each associated with some marked emotional worry, that does not prove that his peptic ulcer is purely psychogenetic. It merely indicates that the psychological factor is an important one in its production, but it may be only the precipitating factor of a condition basically organic. Nevertheless the removal of the psychological irritant may prevent the recurrence of the attacks, or reduce them to a

Psychosomatic anxiety hysteria may arise in the same way. A man gets a psychosomatic indigestion with "heart burn." He then gets the fear that he has heart disease. The condition may stop there, and reassurance may cure the fear. But in this case it linked up with a latent fear of illness developed in childhood (when he was often terrified by his mother's heart attacks) in which case the fear is not dispersed by reassurance, and becomes a typical case of anxiety hysteria with accompanying psychosomatic symptoms.

In other cases the psychosomatic disorders may link up with *Obsessional* conditions.

A schoolboy, who had carried all before him in work as in athletics, was waiting to read the lessons in Chapel, and being nervous began to sweat. This was natural, but in his case it touched on an old complex of masturbation guilt which he feels to be thereby exposed to the whole congregation by his blushing: therefore sweating continues as a psychosomatic sign of his unconscious guilt. He continues with his masturbation because of an unconscious refusal to give it up. Therefore the sense of guilt and the sweating becomes not only chronic but obsessional. He then develops the idea that his sweating makes him smell, and unpleasant to others, a further relic of his earlier guilt; and the idea that he smells then becomes an obsession. Indeed, it has now become symbolic, the idea that he smells symbolizing his moral repugnance at his sex guilt. Such a psychosomatic symptom may go a step further and be utilized as an expression of self-punishment for the guilt.

What then determines the *choice of symptoms?* Why does one person suffer from a nervous headache, another from vomiting?

Some physiological changes are more expressive of certain emotions than others. Worry and anxiety, which put a strain upon the mental functions of the brain, are more liable to produce a headache: fear affects the solar plexus and has an immediate effect on digestion, and so with anger. Blushing is naturally associated with sex feelings (as with girls in adolescence in which blushing biologically reveals rather than hides sex feelings). But when sex is regarded as shameful the response of blushing becomes exaggerated and morbid.

But more commonly the emotional disturbance fixes itself upon the physiologically "weakest spot"; for after all, the physiological effects of emotion are more likely to affect most the part of the autonomic nervous system which is most sensitive and unstable. That is why allergic conditions like asthma so often become the

minimum. In one case of idiopathic epilepsy the attacks were reduced to one out of nine by the removal of an emotional irritant. The one was true idiopathic, the rest hysteric epilepsy.

focus of a psychosomatic disorder, but the constitutional allergy must be distinguished from the psychosomatic utilization of it, and it is in our opinion false to say that allergies as such are psychogenetic. If a patient has a subacute condition of his maxillary sinuses, it stands to reason that when his head is congested with rage, this will produce pain in his sinuses. If a person has a poorly functioning liver it is natural that when he is subjected to emotional strain the liver function will be more affected than the heart which is healthy. It is natural to assume that if a patient has a tendency to gastritis, the irritable stomach will be more affected to produce peptic ulcer. This fact alone often leads to a diagnosis of organic illness, whereas the organic cause may only be a minor factor contributing to the psychosomatic disorder.

C. Symbolic psychosomatic disorders

In symbolic psychosomatic disorders there may be all degrees of suppression or repression. A case in point was that of a soldier who was so sick that he could take no food. In battle he had acted in a way he felt to be cowardly: he was disgusted with himself but was unwilling to accept the fact of his moral disgust with himself so this disgust found expression in vomiting from which he nearly died. He was "sick with himself" morally, but refusing to admit it, he became physically sick. The discovery of the cause and adjustment of the moral problem cured him of his sickness. The patient with the nagging wife could not see properly; when he was led to "look things in the face" he recovered his sight. Another patient could not bear to look at the idea that he was going insane, and partially lost his sight. The choice of symptom in such cases is determined by a symbolic representation which utilizes the so-called "organ language," that is to say, expressing in physical symptoms what the mind wants to say, but does not want to acknowledge. This opens out a wide field of speculation of which some psychopathologists, e.g. Weiss and English, have taken full advantage. There is symbolism in all types of psychoneurosis, but in psychosomatic disorders the symbol becomes a reality in the form of a physical symptom.

The various processes involved in such symbolism are interesting. In the first place physiological functions like sickness are closely associated with mental experiences just as blushing is associated with shame. Thereafter the mental and emotional states may be called by the name of the physiological changes with which they are associated: so we say, "you make me blush" instead of "you make me ashamed." Instead of "you surprise me" we say "you took my breath away!" Instead of "I dislike it," we say "I cannot stomach it." This is "organ language" and is commonly based on a physiological correspondence. We say "he has got cold feet" to express cowardice, because when we are anxious blood leaves the extremities and the feet get cold. So we say "he made me feel hot about the neck!" because the circulation is congested in the neck in states of frustrated anger. We say "my heart stood still" because the heart does so in states of alarm: and "you could have knocked me down with a feather" because this represents the helplessness of surprise. But in using such phrases these mental states are not necessarily accompanied by the corresponding physiological manifestation. The phrases are now used only symbolically. My breath is not actually taken away, nor are my feet in fact cold.

Thus the mental state is expressed in physical terms but is detached from the physiological condition from which it took its name. But if for any reason the mental component is repressed the process goes into reverse and the physiological state which was originally the expression of the emotion is then *substituted for it*. This was so in the case of the soldier who refused to admit he was sick with himself, and instead became physically sick, and in the case of the man who could not see clearly because he refused to look facts in the face. When we refuse to admit that we cannot stand up to things we may get paralysed. The organ language, therefore, occurs especially when for any reason the mental state is repressed; we are then not aware that we are afraid or angry but merely suffer from sickness or pressure in the head; we deny that we are fussed about anything, but suffer from palpitation; we suffer from blushing but are unaware of anything of which we are ashamed.

At this stage we have dropped the consciousness of the mental state and are conscious only of the physical symptom which is now its only expression. We will not admit to ourselves that a task is too great, so we suffer from an inability to swallow instead. This, let it be observed, is not simply an analogy, it is not a "mere symbol" or figure of speech, but a reversal to the actual original physiological expression of the selfsame emotion, from which the emotion took its name and which has now become substituted for it.

As an illustration we may take the case of a man with a "pain in the neck." There must be some reason why people use such a phrase, and the reason is that when they experience a feeling of bored annoyance they sometimes actually do get a pain in the neck. Why pain in the neck? Because when an animal is faced with its foe, it not only bristles, but stiffens its neck in preparation for the attack. So when we resent something we automatically go on the defensive and stiffen the neck, and the muscles, kept in a state of constant tension, begin to ache. This ache may then be used figuratively of a state of stubbornness or chronic resentment. This man in question had an obstinate partner, and he might have said, "You give me a pain in the neck." But he had to continue to work with him, so his feeling had to be repressed, with the result that the suppressed resentment found expression in a subconscious stiffening of his neck and he suffered from actual pain in the neck. Just as a hysteric expresses his repressed craving for sympathy by getting a pain, so this man expresses his resentment by a physical symptom which was originally the natural effect or result of that emotion. Massage may relax and smooth out his neck muscles and give him temporary relief, but it will not smooth out his feelings. We observe then that this "organ language" can find expression in the voluntary as well as the autonomic functions of the body and is often confused with a conversion hysteria, which in fact it may become.

But other forms of psychosomatic symbolism are purely representational, mere figures of speech. Pride has nothing directly to do with swallowing as such, the refusal to swallow merely symbolizing rejection. But when we cannot bear to swallow our pride it may give rise to an inability to swallow food.

The question as to why a symbol is resorted to at all is answered by a consideration of the meaning of symbols in general. The functions of a symbol are:

(1) To encourage or *arouse the feeling* it represents: so kneeling helps us to be reverent, a flag arouses our patriotism; and many symbols are specifically used for this purpose.

(2) Symbols are also used to give *more forcible expression* to an idea or feeling by an appeal to the more primitive expression of the emotion. To say "You make me sick" is more forceful than to say "You displease me." To say "He spat on me" is a more expressive way of expressing a humiliation. To say "You can't make me swallow that" is more forceful than to say "make me accept that." That is obviously because the visceral functions have so much more feeling tone (see p. 235) than the cognitive functions and can arouse stronger emotions. To say "You give me a headache" is more forceful than saying "you bore me!" but to *have* a headache when someone worries you is still more effective. So psychosomatic disorders are a forcible way of expressing feelings which have been frustrated.

(3) The third use of a symbol is as a *substitute for the feeling*. So we kneel to give the appearance of reverence to save us the trouble of being reverent: we give money to excuse us from being charitable. The danger of religious ceremonial and ritual is that instead of encouraging and eliciting the feeling it represents, it is the outward and visible sign of a *lack* of inner grace. So symbols are often intended not to express but to disguise our meaning, in these cases our irreverence or want of charity. This is in line with psychosomatic symbolism, for the physical vomiting of the soldier had the advantage that it enabled him to avoid the more unpleasant experience of thinking himself a coward; but the moral problem persists nevertheless and insists on pressing its claims for expression.

CLINICAL NOTES

We may now refer to some common clinical examples of psychosomatic disorders.

Chronic sweating may be the result of chronic anxiety, which in turn may be due to causes of which we are quite unaware. There may already be a constitutional predisposition due to autonomic imbalance, which, however, only manifests itself under the stress of emotion. A vicious circle is produced in which the anxiety produces sweating and the sweating produces further anxiety and sense of inferiority. We may give first-aid and effective treatment by giving atropine to paralyse the vagus and so check the sweating, and this may produce permanent results by breaking the vicious circle: but in most cases the patient is left with his tense emotional state, and requires more radical treatment of causes.

Blushing is an allied psychosomatic disorder usually representing a sense of inferiority, the cause of which, however, is often repressed and so transferred to the blushing itself, so that the patient usually declares that his feeling of inferiority is only because he blushes. But in all the cases we have analysed, a curious circumstance has revealed itself, namely that the blushing represented not merely the blush of shame but the flush of anger. This is not surprising for the symptom usually originates in some humiliation, when the patient would have a feeling of rage as well as shame at being made to feel inferior, so that both motives are operative in the symptom.

Difficulty in swallowing is a not uncommon psychosomatic symptom. "Yesterday," a lady has just remarked, "I found that I could not swallow my food for the first time." She discovered it was because her husband was trying to make her do something repugnant to her pride, but she had to yield because of her need of his protection. But she would not admit that she had to "swallow her pride," so it expressed itself in physical inability to swallow. A similar case was that of a man who was offered promotion and a job for which he felt he was not fitted. He did not wish to admit that the responsibility was too great, and his ambition compelled him to take the job, but this strong feeling denied conscious expression came out in his symptom. He "couldn't swallow it," so his symptom took the form of taking his food in little pellets, i.e. taking the job a bit at a time. Secondarily the symptom also served as an excuse to escape from the responsibility, as an hysteric symptom. He could be cured either by getting him to abandon the job voluntarily or by removing the causes of his lack of confidence, which is better.

Palpitation. The effect of emotion on the heart is everyone's experience; it makes the heart beat faster to prepare for the emergency: and if voluntary action is checked, but the stimulus continues, the heart's action becomes irregular, and the patient suffers from "disordered action of the heart." There are numerous people going about fearing they have heart disease and taking precautions when there is nothing wrong with the heart; it is only functioning wrongly. The cause of the disturbances may be so repressed that the patient is completely unaware of anxiety but suffers only from palpitation and irregular throbbings.

Disorders of breathing. Some people suffer from breathlessness, from air hunger and from the feeling of suffocation, which are again the direct results of sympathetic stimulation from emotion and anxiety. It is probable that the condition of "globus hystericus" is due to the actual pressure upon the windpipe, but it is nevertheless psychogenetic. We speak of being "choked with emotion."

Headache. A very common accompaniment of frustrated emotional states, especially worry and anger, is that of a headache. Whenever we are emotionally aroused blood surges to the head, as to other parts of the body, to prepare us for action. When action takes places, circulation is restored and the cranial tension ceases. But if the emotion cannot get an outlet the head is congested with blood (we become "purple with rage"), we feel a throbbing in our heads, and we get a headache from the pressure. The patient feels that his "head is going to burst," which he describes as an ache or feeling of pressure, not as a pain. It is significant that the typical headaches from this cause are at the occiput (or nape of the neck), on the top of the head, a band round the head (the *casque* or helmet type), positions which roughly correspond with the blood sinuses in the skull, which if congested would naturally produce pressure. It seems most likely, therefore, that these headaches are due to the actual pressure of blood in the cranium but that this pressure is produced by the arousal and subsequent thwarting of emotion. Experiments have proved that both increased and decreased cranial pressure may produce headaches.

Indigestion. In states of emotion the digestion ceases, because some of the gastric juices stop flowing owing to the action of the autonomic nervous system, which also gives the patient a "sinking feeling in the stomach." The result is that food is not digested. Cannon says, "the conditions favourable to people's digestion are wholly abolished when unpleasant feelings, such as vexation, worry, anxiety, and great emotion, such as anger and fear, are allowed to prevail."

Sickness and vomiting may come under the same category. These may be physiological conditions of biological significance in that they empty the stomach in preparation for action. They may be symbolic, as we have already illustrated. But frequently they are merely the physiological manifestations of an anxiety state. A person, as we all know, may be "sick with horror" and actually vomit at the sight of an accident. Frequently it is an hysteric condition to escape from responsibility: or it may be due to the sense of guilt say for repressed sexual desires, getting rid of them. Indeed almost any emotion may produce it.

Constipation is another condition that is caused by worry, as is well known. Worry relaxes the bowels and stops peristalsis: it also checks the flow of bile. The result is stasis, and this stasis may give rise to toxic absorption with the result that the patient becomes physically ill. Constipation often symbolically represents *stagnation of the personality* due to frustration. It used frequently to be cured by suggestion, by removing anxiety and producing confidence of mind, so that with the restoration of the functions of the personality the bowel resumed its normal activity.

Fatigue. A sense of disappointment often causes physical fatigue. Where there is no incentive there is no release of energy, so we get tired. One person instead of saying "your conversation does not interest me," says more effectively "you make me tired," but another who does not want to be so rude uses organ language and actually gets tired and then has a legitimate excuse to retire from the conversation. There are people who are chronically physically tired because of lack of interest in life. We have at the moment a woman patient who is paralysed in both legs, because she "cannot stand up to life." Her paralysis says more effectively than words, "I can't go on and what is more I am not going to go on."

Effort syndrome. We have seen that when emotion such as anxiety produces visceral changes such as palpitation, the anxiety may then be concentrated on the heart or lungs. On this account the patient is concerned about making any effort in case he brings on the symptoms. He then becomes over-susceptible to fatigue and effort, and this together with the emotion aroused gives the clinical picture of "disordered action of the heart" (of the first World War), and "Effort syndrome" (of the second World War), in which even slight effort produces sweating, heart symptoms and breathlessness. These conditions are brought to light particularly in wars, and we rarely see them in civil life: not that they do not exist then, but these persons in civil life take on quiet jobs like gardening where they can take their time. One of our patients was a municipal scavenger because "he could rest when he liked!" When drafted into the Army they are quite incapable of making the grade, and after a few weeks they are sent to hospital where they remain for some months during which frequent examinations of the heart or lungs make them more preoccupied with their symptoms and they are discharged in a worse state than when they entered, having wasted their time, cost the country a year's maintenance and occupied a valuable bed in hospital. Sweating of the palms of the hand, the soles of the feet and in the axilla should therefore be suspect of a psychosomatic state. But in "effort syndrone" as in several other psychosomatic disorders we have reason to suspect a constitutional predisposition which makes this the symptom of choice, and we question the opinion of those who regard it always as purely psychological.

Hypochondria. This may throw some light upon the hypochondriac, who is preoccupied with his heart, liver or bowels. He claims that his symptoms are organic and nothing will convince him to the contrary. They are in fact somatic, and it is extremely annoying to him to be told constantly that his symptoms are imaginary. This makes him exaggerate them the more to make his point. His symptoms are somatic, but not organic; they are psychological, but not imaginary. But the patient cannot be expected to know that any more than the physician unacquainted with psychosomatic disorders, and it is not surprising if he exaggerates them into a fear of cancer and such-like.

CHAPTER VII

TRAUMATIC NEUROSIS

TRAUMATIC neurosis provides us with a disorder so obvious in its origin, so simple in its formation, mechanism, psychopathology and treatment, that it will be a convenient starting point to our study of the more complex psychoneuroses.

A traumatic neurosis is one which results from accident or shock. It is a condition in which the *precipitating factor, usually of an objective nature, is the most important factor in the production of the disorder.* This does not mean that there are not predisposing factors; indeed we find that there almost invariably are. But the predisposing factors may be of such little significance that many of these individuals have passed for normal and have always previously regarded themselves as normal: and the treatment of the precipitating cause, such as the experience of being blown up, may be enough to cure them.

Traumatic neurosis usually takes the form of hysteria, whether conversion hysteria, anxiety hysteria, or an attack of hysterics such as we have witnessed in a Quartermaster on the bridge of a minesweeper wrecked in a storm.

We shall deal with a case of traumatic hysteria in some detail because there must be thousands of people who continue to suffer quite unnecessarily from headaches, pains, depression and other symptoms due to car accidents, which are comparatively easily cured by the abreaction method. General practitioners may be called upon to treat such cases where expert advice is unobtainable.

A typical case is that of a Highland officer who came for treatment three years after he was blown up in Norway, suffering from headache, anxiety, depression, terrifying dreams and fatigue. He had fought a rear-guard action as cover to our retreating troops until he successfully brought his men to the coast where he was promised transport but met with disappointment when he found there was none. There he was blown up by a shell, and lay unconscious; when he regained consciousness he found his hands and face in flames from burning petrol and suffered excruciating pain. He was taken off in a destroyer which was continually bombed, and ultimately arrived in Scotland in a state of severe shock, and was treated in hospital for six months for his wounds and burns. He returned to duty, was given responsible work, and not for three years after did he come for treatment for his present symptoms He had lost his memory for the whole experience from being blown up to his arrival in Scotland, where he became aware of feeling intense cold, shock and severe pain. In a series of analyses he gradually remembered every detail of being blown up, even the flash and noise of the shell, the sensation of being carried through the air, the burning of his hands and face, lying there thinking he was dead, praying that it might be over quickly, and then being brought to by the severity of the pain to find himself on fire, getting up and staggering away till he got help. All of these experiences he vividly relived during analysis, sometimes rolling on the floor in agony as he had on the beach. After each episode he would take some minutes to recover and then he would usually feel a sense of relief, "just as when you have an abscess pricked," to use his words. Sometimes, however, he would feel worse between treatments which indicated that he was in, but not yet through, a particularly painful part of the experience, which he would shrink from remembering even though he did not know what it was. On two occasions the anaesthetic Pentothal was used successfully to release the block.

This case illustrates the following facts, characteristic of most traumatic cases, most of which are familiar to the expert, but they are perhaps worth recording for those who may be called upon to treat these conditions when no expert help is available.

(a) *The precipitating cause* was of an objective nature, and was the determining factor in the breakdown, since he had never before had a nervous breakdown and had always passed for normal in that respect.

(b) *The physical shock* was important because it rendered the patient temporarily incapable of adjusting himself to the situation: the blow made him bewildered, helpless and incapable of proper readjustment. The physical explosion which knocked him out also had the effect of throwing him off his guard; taken unawares, he temporarily lost his morale. By the time he had recovered from the shock and pulled himself together it was too late; in those few minutes the damage was done. The physical shock is therefore of importance in these traumatic cases, and justifies us in the use of the term "shell-shock" for such cases.

The term "shell-shock" was discarded after the war of 1914–18 because it came to be used synonymously with neurosis in general, and of many soldiers who had never been near a shell: and also because it suggested that the physical shock alone produced the disorder. But we have been told so frequently that the war neuroses are no different from those of civil life, that we may fail to do justice to the importance of the physical shock itself as a precipitating factor in the production of the breakdown. The objectivity of the experience, the suddenness of the experience as well as its severity justifies us in distinguishing these cases of traumatic hysteria from the ordinary type of hysteria. The physical shock is not merely an excuse for breaking down; it is a causative factor in the breakdown.

(c) *The emotional conflict.* But the fact that these conditions supervene on a shock does not mean that this is the only factor in the production of the disorder: indeed that is proved not to be the case, for many a man recovers from such accidents with no after effects. Drunken men who fall and get concussed do not suffer from neurosis: and there is the curious fact that those subjected to electric shock treatment do not suffer from subsequent neurosis, although if such treatment is wrongly applied to the psychoneurosis, it may make the patient worse. It is the reaction of the patient to the shock which determines the neurosis, and that depends largely on his previous personality. The person who suffers traumatic hysteria is always one who already has emotional problems, of which he may be unaware, whether of the present or of the past. In the soldier the most common present conflict is between the fear aroused by the danger and the sense of duty: what the soldier fears more than death itself is that he should prove a coward; he fears most his own fear.

Traumatic cases in civil life, especially car, cycle or industrial accidents, follow the same pattern as this war-shock case. Neurosis in such cases does not occur unless the traumatic experience is associated with mental conflicts of a personal or domestic nature, predisposing the individual to breakdown.

(d) *Contributing emotional factors* in this case were the resentment and disappointment that the promised transport was not there. Such contributing factors play an important part in traumatic neurosis, and we often find that a sense of grievance against the Army, suppressed anger of the ordinary soldier against the Sergeant, anxiety about those at home who may be subjected to raids, concern about his business, worry about wives subject to the blandishments of our gallant allies, and such-like conditions undermine the morale of the soldier, so that he becomes an easy victim to the final blow. Discontent in one's work is a common contributing factor in industrial neurosis.

(e) *Predisposing factors.* Although the precipitating factor, physical and emotional, may be considered the most important in traumatic cases, this case illustrates the fact that we find predisposing causes in most cases of traumatic neuroses, although these might never of themselves have caused a breakdown. This officer had in childhood and youth always been told by his mother that he would be a failure as compared with his favoured brother; at school he was poor at games, and only average in his work; so that when he became a regular soldier he had determined that in soldiering at least he would make good, as indeed he had both before and during the war. The loss of morale due to his being blown up filled him with the old sense of failure. It was this moral issue and not the explosion or the burns which was the most distressing feature and therefore the most repressed of this experience.[1]

(f) *The super-ego.* This officer's sense of duty and morale were of a high order and this is typical of most of those suffering from traumatic hysteria. They are not the funks, the cowards, the weaklings, but often those who have a *strong devotion to moral and social demands*. It is the *repression* of their fear which does the damage. That is why these war neuroses are more frequently met with in N.C.O.'s and officers, people of responsibility, than men in the ranks, for they must maintain a high standard of courage before their men. Their breakdown is occasioned by the strain of having to live up to a higher standard of courage. It is this sense of duty and high morale which distinguishes the psychoneurotic from the coward and the funk. Owing to their devotion to duty neurotics often make excellent soldiers (and hard-working conscientious civilians), as long as they are not subject to excessive strain, and to reject them on the grounds of their predisposition would be to lose many a valued officer and man: indeed it is frequently the nervous and highly strung man who receives the decorations for bravery.[2]

Nevertheless, the courage in these cases is not a natural courage, but usually an over-compensation for some old fear or feeling of inadequacy, which the patient has repressed. He covers up his sense of inferiority by assuming a courageous attitude

[1] The importance of the predisposing emotional factor was illustrated in another case said to be due to an explosion in a gun-pit. This occurred when the officer was due for a court martial for a mistake that cost the lives of two of our men. This meant particular disgrace because his older brother had always scorned him, but when he had joined up and his brother had not, he felt he could crow over his brother and return from the war crowned with glory. Instead he was threatened with dismissal and disgrace. The explosion in the gun-pit was not the cause of the neurosis, it was the excuse which enabled him to return home as the broken hero instead of being in disgrace. The ground is always prepared even in traumatic neuroses.

[2] The author had three V.C.'s to treat after the first World War.

beyond the ordinary, and compensates for the feeling of fear by acts of daring. For this reason such people are more predisposed to break down than the naturally courageous man, and it should be the duty of the regimental medical officer (the factory, or school doctor in civil life), to recognize these people when they are near breaking point, and to order them the rest which they are themselves reluctant to take, and thus save a breakdown. As it is this sense of duty which distinguishes such a man from the coward, it is this over-compensation to the feeling of inadequacy which distinguishes him from the man who is *naturally* courageous, whether constitutionally or by proper conditioning in childhood, though outwardly they look very much alike.

(g) In traumatic neuroses *there is always repression and dissociation*. In every case of traumatic hysteria part of the experience has been forgotten (in spite of the patient's claim that he remembers everything). It is this dissociated part which perpetuates the trouble, even if it is only the moment of the crash; and it is this part which often reproduces itself in dreams which is its attempt to reach consciousness. Dreams by reproducing the traumatic experience are nature's attempt to bring repressed and forgotten experiences to consciousness and therefore to solve them; indeed we have known cases where the dream has brought the whole experience back to memory, and the patient has been spontaneously cured. But for the purposes of cure the recovery of the *whole* experience is necessary. If only part of the experience is recovered the unrecovered part acts as a foreign body which perpetuates the wound; and though the patient remembers some of the experience, even this part may be rapidly forgotten again unless the whole is reproduced. Patients often forget what they recovered in the previous analysis.

(h) *The symptom* may be regarded *mechanistically* as the emergence of fear that had been kept repressed, reproductions of the buried and now forgotten experience; hence the headaches, restlessness, sleeplessness, and depression. Or it may be regarded *purposively* as a means of escape from an intolerable situation, or more accurately from an intolerable mental problem.

(i) *The function of the symptom* is; therefore, to assert the rights of the natural self with its fears against the exaggerated demands made upon it by the super-ego with its moral and social demands and excessive sense of duty. Its purpose is to enable the patient to escape from an intolerable situation, moral as well as physical, yet without surrendering his prestige. It does this by a compromise, that instead of running away, the patient develops an illness, which serves the same purpose of getting him out of the war without losing face. It satisfies both the natural self and the moral ego but at the expense of an illness, which however is more tolerable than disgrace.

(j) *The period of meditation.* The emergence of these symptoms did not take place at once, nor as long as he was physically ill with the burns, but only six months later. The "period of meditation" represents the time required for the transformation of the physical and emotional shock into a neurotic symptom. This delay so often noted between the actual trauma and the onset of neurotic symptoms, gave rise in the first World War to the saying, "You never see shell-shock in the front line," a saying not wholly true, but true enough to call attention to an undoubted fact. People suffer from "railway spine" or other symptoms days and even weeks after an accident, which naturally gives rise to the suspicion that they are malingering, an after-thought to get compensation, which may or may not be the case.

This delay in reaction probably may be explained in various ways. (i) We keep going as long as we are actually confronted with the crisis, but when we relax, as the soldier behind the lines, the suppressed emotion emerges and creates an active conflict. So the mother anxiously nursing her sick child breaks down only after the crisis is over. (ii) Secondly, after it is all over the patient at a distance from the traumatic experience tends to dwell upon it in imagination and in doing so exaggerates the awful horrors of what *might* have been which is far worse than the actuality, and of what might happen next time. We often noted in the London blitz that people got a sense of relief, not to say exhilaration, immediately after a bomb had burst, as though to say "It wasn't so bad after all!" not so bad as the anticipation. (iii) In this case, as in many trau-matic hysterias, the onset of the neurotic symptoms coincided with recovery from the physical illness. The symptom was, therefore, a delayed reaction. This is because as long as he was ill with the burns, the moral problem did not arise; but as soon as he got well, and the reason for being out of the line was no longer operative, the dread of returning to the Hell from which he has only just escaped was reactivated, and the symptoms developed. This corresponds to the saying in the first World War that "the wounded man never got shell-shock," since he required no other excuse for being out of it. This not infrequently happens in civilian patients who suffer from the "after-effects" of illness and operation which are often of a hysteric nature, implying a continued desire for the care, attention and freedom of responsibility experienced in the illness.

(*k*) *Prophylactic first-aid.* These facts are important for preventive treatment. Taken before he has time to think it over, that is to say during the "period of meditation," and dealing with his fear before it can be transformed into a symptom, many a man can quickly be returned to duty. In the first World War airmen found that the simplest cure after a crash was to send the pilot up again immediately. It is simply a case of reconditioning one's fear *while it is accessible.* Once his fear has been repressed and fixed to a particular symptom it becomes inaccessible to reconditioning and requires more radical treatment. In the second World War far more first-aid treatment was given near the front, with gratifying results. So in civilian life brooding over our grievances and harbouring our resentments tend to make us neurotic: getting them off our chest helps us to readjust ourselves to them. The wise industrialist deals with such grievances and restlessness, even before they have found expressions in deputations, still less in strikes.

(*l*) *Treatment.* For the treatment of these traumatic disorders the abreaction method (the release of repressed emotion of fear) is most effective; and very commonly dealing with the traumatic experience alone without going back to predisposing factors is often enough to "cure" these symptoms and return such patients to civil life.

(*m*) The method we normally use in traumatic cases for the recovery of memories is that of free association and sometimes hypnotism. But the use of narco-analysis[1] with Evipan or Pentothal given slowly by intravenous injection has largely superseded hypnosis, and is most valuable as an adjunct to free association when resistances are particularly strong.[2] In the case of this officer we used it on two occasions, in one of which there was reproduced surprisingly the sensation of pleasure at being dead and therefore out of it all! In the second the feeling of collapse as he fell to the ground with momentary loss of courage when he gave up, an experience so alien and distasteful to his pride in being a courageous man.

But narco-analysis should be used only as an occasional aid to the breaking down of resistance and not a substitute for free

---

[1] Horsley: *Narco-Analysis.*

[2] In our experience the more slowly the drug is given, the longer the patient takes to come out and therefore the longer time is given for talking. We take about five minutes to give 6–8 c.c.

association. For it has its limitations. For instance, in the case of this officer, when, under Pentothal, he came to the point of "dying" he kept saying, "I can never think of that; it is too awful! I know I ought but I can't!" whereas under ordinary free association he did face it and recovered the memory, probably because he gave his more willing co-operation than when he was doped. Not only so but whilst narco-analysis is of value in releasing repressed emotions, it frequently cannot deal with the more subtle super-ego and moral sense which has kept them repressed. Sometimes the release of these emotions alone sweeps away the false super-ego and the patient no longer pretends that he is a superman who knows no fear. But if only the emotions are liberated and the super-ego remains, the patient is in a worse state of distress, so that some patients treated by narco-analysis alone have become permanently worse.

(*n*) In traumatic neurosis the abreaction of the forgotten experiences whether by hypnoanalysis, free association, or drug narcosis is enough to bring about a cure. This "cure" may be permanent in so far as the patient has not again to return to the same conditions. In the first World War it was a good rule that once a man was diagnosed "shell-shock" he was not sent back to the line. This officer was a case in point; he was "cured," returned to a responsible job and after three months wrote saying he was 100 per cent fit. Later he had the misfortune to be a few yards from an exploding bomb and had to go sick again: but he quickly recovered and is now doing a full day's work in a civilian job.

(*o*) But in some cases even of traumatic hysteria, the symptoms do not yield unless the predisposing causes in childhood are dealt with, as is usually the case in non-traumatic hysteria.

Non-traumatic hysteria

The ordinary cases of hysteria met with in civilian life differ in some respects from traumatic hysteria in the fact that they are not connected with physical shocks which as we have seen are of some effect in producing the condition: the precipitating cause is usually of little significance as compared with the predisposing causes; and they are not primarily due to present-day objective conditions which in many cases are ideal, but to emotional conflicts within the patient's own personality which come to a head irrespective of circumstances. Thus a person will break down on the slightest provocation and under conditions of the most trifling nature. It may have been environmental conditions in childhood which produced the complex; it is now the complex which makes it impossible for the patient to cope with his environment.

Further consideration of these more complicated cases we leave to the next chapter.

Note on concussion

The complete recovery of the whole experience in these traumatic patients who are said to suffer from concussion, raises questions of considerable importance with regard to the nature of concussion. Whatever theory of concussion we hold, it is usually assumed that the brain is temporarily put out of action, perhaps from pressure, perhaps from disturbance of the molecules of the brain, as distinct from "contusion" in which there is a definite injury, so that in either case the brain does not function and consciousness is lost. This theory of concussion cannot be maintained if it can be shown that in these conditions of supposed concussion from shock, the functions of the brain are not completely put out of action, although consciousness may be greatly impaired: for the recovery of the memory in every detail proves that consciousness must have been present throughout. In the case of this officer we were able to revive the whole experience in detail, even to the noise of the explosion, the hot blast of the air, the feeling of every bone in the body being bruised, of being whirled in the air, and the thought that he is actually dead (a very common experience in these cases), all of which proves that the brain is *not* put out of action, although the patient lies completely inert, is apparently unconscious, suffering from "concussion," and remembers nothing of the experience afterwards, until it is recovered in analysis.

To say with one writer that what we can recover is due to psychological amnesia, what we cannot is due to concussion, is to beg the question, for it makes the diagnosis of concussion in any given case depend on the skill of the analyst in recovering the memory! On several occasions this patient stated "that is where I became unconscious: I can remember no more," and yet in free association or under Pentothal he was able to recover these experiences in every detail.

In the war of 1914–18 we made special investigation of this problem and were able to recover the complete memory in every such case treated over a period of eighteen months (over 100 cases). An apparent exception was that of a man who had a severe fracture of the skull, an obvious case of contusion. Another interesting "control" is that if in the process of recovering the buried memory of the experience the patient has an operation under an anaesthetic (which actually does put the brain cells out of action), the recovery of the memory ceases, and we have been quite unable to get any response. If the patient had been making it up, he would have continued to "tell the tale." But in any case the violence of the patient's recovery of fears and actions leaves no doubt that what he is recovering and reproducing is an actual experience. These facts, which we observed in the first World War, we have confirmed in this war, as well as in many accident cases with "concussion" during the intervening years. In such cases there are, we understand, changes noted in the electro-encephalograph, but that does not imply any necessary loss of consciousness. What we suggest, in view of the recovery of these memories, is that what is usually called concussion is physiological shock plus amnesia, and that the amnesia is recoverable.

This question is of more than academic interest, for the recovery of the whole memory usually brings about cure, and is necessary to cure, and if we assume that the memory cannot be recovered, the patient remains uncured, as thousands unfortunately do.

CHAPTER VIII

HYSTERIA

HYSTERIA has always been in disrepute. It is stigmatized as "just nerves," "only hysteria," "all imagination," and as next door to malingering. There is, however, no such disease as "only hysteria," any more than there is a disease of "only pneumonia." Hysteria is a serious disorder, definite in its pathology and often disastrous in its consequences, leading to life-long incapacity and misery. It may be a disorder of the imagination, it is certainly not an imaginary disease: in any case imagination is the most potent factor in the world, upon which all invention and all progress in science and industry depend, all instruments of construction and all weapons of destruction are devised, and must be treated as a reality, not dismissed as illusory.[1]

The ill-repute into which hysteria has fallen is chiefly a relic of the days when it was associated with the "Humours," the "Vapours," and the "Migrims," which were regarded with contempt. But a consideration of these disorders suggests that far from being imaginary, they were not even psychogenetic, but chiefly disorders of physical origin. The following quotation from Purcell[2] describing such an attack makes this clear. He describes the patients as suffering from

"a heaviness up their breast; a grumbling in their belly; they belch up, and sometimes vomit, sour, sharp and bitter humours; they have a difficulty in breathing; and think they feel something that comes up into their throat which is ready to choke them . . . perceive a swimming in their heads, a dimness comes over their eyes, they turn pale, are scarce able to stand, their pulse is weak, they shut their eyes and remain senseless for some time; after little by little their pulse returns, their face regains its natural colour; their body grows hot as before; they open their eyes, sigh and by degrees come to themselves."

Such an attack bears little resemblance to what we should call hysteria, and most of us should recognize in such symptoms an attack of bio-chemical origin.

[1] "And she seems such a *nice* girl!" was the remark just made by the matron of a nursing home to the author, when told that a girl's paralysis was hysteric.
[2] *Treatise on Vapours or Hysteria Fits*, 1702.

It is interesting to note that Sydenham stated that, "Venice treacle alone, if continued for a good space of time, is perchance the most effectual remedy in this disease"—an anticipation of the treatment of "acidosis" and hypoglycaenia by glucose. Similarly, the "migrims" and headaches of the Victorian ladies, which were usually regarded as hysterical, would now be recognized in many cases as due to eye-strain from doing fine needlework with an uncorrected astigmatism. That neurotic symptoms followed on this failure in diagnosis is only to be expected, but that was not the fault of the patient. Purcell himself more correctly ascribed these disorders to a physiological cause, namely, to the "humours" of the body.

The modern psychopathologist is therefore justified in disclaiming responsibility for these "humours, vapours, migrims and hysterics" of the past century and in handing them back to the physician, paying due credit to those early physicians who, like Purcell, recognized, even if they did not understand, the physical nature of these disorders, and consequently did not treat them with a scorn, which arose from a failure in diagnosis.

But the bad reputation into which hysteria has fallen is also due to the fact that the neurotic is one whose personality has failed in meeting the responsibilities of life. But there are reasons for this failure, for which he is no more responsible than the man who fails in life because of endocrine disorder, or chronic tuberculosis contracted at birth; for hysteria is mostly due to predisposing causes in early childhood over which he has no control.

Biologically considered, hysteria is a failure in adaptation to the objective demands of life. When an animal is in a situation of danger, its first reaction, as we have seen, is in the autonomic nervous system and viscera, preparatory to action; and if the situation is such that it can neither attack nor escape, its first reaction is by exaggerated movements of the viscera, which we have studied in the psychosomatic disorders. But it may react in various other ways, expressive of its helplessness. Being frustrated, it utters a *cry of distress,* or gets into a state of panic in which it rushes about wildly and apparently without aim, though, as with a rat in a cage, this wild dashing about may at any moment achieve an accidental release and way of escape. In extreme cases this ends in *hysterical convulsions* and fits, in which there is complete inco-ordination of movement and inability to cope with the situation, so that the energy produced for the occasion expends itself in degraded and purposeless movements.[1] These reactions may be observed and experimentally induced in the animal as a result of frustration.

As a case in point we may mention the experiments of Prof. R. F. Maier, of Michigan, who introduced four rats to a piece of apparatus in which there were two cards, one of which was white with a black circle on it, the other black with a white circle. When the rats jumped at the first it revealed food behind it; when at the second they just bumped their noses. The rats soon learnt to jump at the first card, after which the cards were changed and rechanged, which so confused the rats that they refused to jump at all. Then one of the cards was removed, upon which the rats "jumped out of the apparatus, ran round in circles for a while, then stopped and exhibited convulsions, and *finally fell into comas, their eyes expressionless and glassy.*" Such experiments seem to indicate that in animals nervous breakdowns can be brought on "by the necessity of responding to a situation in which no mode of behaviour is available."

In other cases the animal may get into a state of stark fear in which it is immobile, rooted to the spot, *paralysed with fear.* This immobility is the normal reaction of animals like the "stick insect" which remains stock still when subjected to light. This immobility serves the biological purpose of avoiding detection, whereas a screaming animal, whilst giving warning to other animals, will attract the attention of the enemy, and an escaping animal will invite pursuit, as we find when we run from a barking dog.

All these reactions have their uses, for when one cannot escape, it is best to remain stock still, and when crying is of no avail it is best to be mute so as to avoid detection. This is illustrated in children with night terrors who are speechless with dread, for crying out would only call the attention of the bogies and other evil beings to them.

Hysteria follows the same pattern as the biological response, and serves much the same purpose. It is the result of frustration, and is an expression of helplessness, of dependence, of failure in adaptation. The hysteric symptom is a disability, originally the result of fear, but now designed to serve the same biological end of escaping from an intolerable situation.

Psychologically considered, therefore, the hysteric is one who

---

[1] Sherrington, *Integrative Action*, p. 117, says: "If there resulted a compromise between two reflexes . . . the compound would be an action . . . adapted to neither and useless for the purpose of the other."

when faced with the difficulties of life, shrinks from its responsibilities, shuns rather than faces its difficulties, avoids rather than meets the danger, retreats to safety and security. The hysteric is the herbivorous animal depending for its safety on flight, whilst the obsessional is the carnivorous animal, which depends on aggressiveness and attack. Confronted with a situation of danger, the hysteric gets into a panic, cries out for help, falls into a faint, gets a fit, becomes paralysed with fear, or avoids the danger by getting blind or deaf.

Transition from biological to psychological reactions. But hysteria goes a stage further than these biological reactions amongst animals. (*a*) Amongst human beings, possessed as they are of a sense of pity, *this physical helplessness and disability makes a mute appeal for help* and calls forth sympathy; it calls the attention of others to its state of helplessness and need[1] The paralysis which was at first a normal reflex response to danger is now used as an appeal to others for sympathy. (*b*) But it then goes even further, for the illnesses which call for sympathy are then *created with the object of gaining sympathy*. Thus the symptom which was originally the *result* of the biological response to an objective situation, has now acquired a *purpose*. This is the state of things in most cases of conversion hysteria. When this resort to illness is consciously and deliberately done, we call it *malingering*; when unconsciously it is a *neurosis*. Malingering is resorted to when the ordinary appeals for sympathy and help would have no effect; when pretending illness is the only way of achieving our ends. Conversion hysteria occurs when one will not allow *oneself* to run away, to be afraid or ask for sympathy. Indeed one is not aware that one is afraid, wants sympathy or desires to escape. (*c*) In hysteria, therefore, *the inhibition comes from within*, not from without: it is not that we cannot escape, but we will not. (*d*) Not only so but in hysteria the *stimulus* of fear is not the objective difficulties and dangers, but subjective conflicts and difficulties. The "intolerable situations" that the hysteric cannot face are usually within himself. These fears are not only fears *for* ourselves for our safety and security; but they are fears *of* ourselves, of impulses and forbidden desires within ourselves, the consequences of which we fear. It is not so much the bombs but our own fear that we cannot cope

---

[1] The crying out of an adult animal is of little service to itself; indeed, like the cry of the rabbit when caught in a trap it calls the attention of the fox who devours it. But it gives warning (not intentionally of course) of danger to others. It is one of those reactions which are detrimental to the individual himself, but of value to the race. The cry of the young human, however, does call for the protection of the parent.

with. (e) But curiously enough, though these problems are now subjective, *they give rise to the same physical symptoms* as though the situation were an objective one, the panic, the paralysis, and the cry of distress. The organism reacts similarly to subjective as to objective situations.

There are three main types of hysteria. In the first place, there are those conditions better known to a former generation as *Hysterics*, which consist of outbursts of uncontrolled emotion, often of weeping and laughter. In the second place, there is *Anxiety Hysteria*, the main characteristic of which is a morbid fear of harm to oneself. This may be localized, such as fear of open spaces, fear of darkness, of heights, of illness, of death, and fear of being afraid, which are the phobias; or generalized anxiety of everything.

The third and most characteristic form of hysteria is *Conversion Hysteria*, in which the failure to meet the demands of life ends in breakdown in the central nervous system, whether afferent as in pain, or of efferent functions as in paralysis. It was so named by Freud because a mental conflict was "converted" into a physical symptom. These are to be distinguished from psychosomatic disorders which are the direct *result* of emotional disturbances, though both are somatic.

These three types of hysteria differ so widely in their manifestations and symptoms that at first sight it is difficult to understand why they are all grouped under the same name. Those suffering from conversion hysteria, for instance, present a marked contrast to patients suffering from hysterics, for whilst the latter are characterized by unrestrained emotion, those suffering from conversion hysteria are often peculiarly unemotional, controlled, and show very little sign of any psychic abnormality, their emotional conflict having been transformed into the physical symptom.

It is this apparent lack of emotion which has given to the conversion hysteric the label of "la belle indifference." Apart from their physical disabilities these patients are often happy, well adapted to life, and sexually well adjusted. In our cases of war neuroses, the patient with the paralysed arm or leg was often extroverted, hobbling along with his friends, the life and soul of the party: he had found a solution of his problem in his physical disability. The anxiety hysteric on the other hand presents a very different picture, for he has not found such a solution, so that his days are filled with apprehension, and his nights with terrifying dreams. The truth is that in conversion hysteria there is the same emotion but it is repressed and converted into a physical symptom: whereas in hysterics it bursts out as uncontrollable emotion. But beneath the apparent indifference of the conversion hysteric there is often a pool of apprehension which at any moment may burst forth into hysterics or turn into an anxiety state. Indeed it frequently does so during analysis, as in a recent case in which a patient suffering from paralysis of both legs, when cured of the paralysis, began to suffer from anxiety, sleeplessness and nightmares, and then from uncontrollable hysterical laughter every evening, the compulsive expression of his sense of freedom. We must then regard the different types of hysteria, as indeed the different types of psychoneuroses, not as disease entities, but rather as varied reactions to a situation which are interchangeable, or may exist simultaneously. But though differing in form, *the essential feature of all these types of hysteria is that of helplessness and dependence*, incapacity to meet the demands of life, and a retreat from life.

HYSTERICS

Hysterics consists of outbursts of uncontrolled emotion such as grief, panic, rage, fear, self-pity, or attacks of weeping alternating with laughter and other states of emotional instability. Such outbursts are more apt to occur in people of a constitutionally highly emotional temperament, and also in those who have never learnt to control their emotions. An obvious illustration of the former is found in the emotional disturbances which affect some women at the menstrual periods, at which time they are often "temperamental," unstable, irrational and liable to outbursts of unreasonable jealousy, hate or craving for affection. Such physiologically induced hysterics are to be distinguished from the psychological types due to lack of discipline and self-control, as in the case of the woman so spoilt that she cannot brook the slightest frustration without bursting into tears, the man who bursts into uncontrolled rage when he misses his train, or the woman who is thrown into a paroxysm of grief because her pet kitten has died.

Some get into hysterics because their sensuous or sexual feelings are excessively stimulated beyond their control, like the girls we recently saw being whirled round in a merry-go-round at a fair, who were thrown into a typical state of hysterics, with alternating weeping and laughter, till rescued by the gallant young attendants whose services a wise directorate had retained for that purpose. A doctor from a South American city tells us that he has to spend the night after a ball attending hysterical females whose sexual feelings have been over-stimulated and left unsatisfied.

Hysterical outbursts *usually follow a period of suppression*, when emotions strongly aroused are held in check until they cannot be held any longer. When the moment of release comes the pent-up emotions burst forth with great violence and unrestraint. Such a case was that of Bismarck, who is said to have had a typical attack of hysterics, weeping and laughing, when, after a day of strain and expectancy, news was brought to him of his victory over the Austrian forces.

This suppression may explain why hysterical attacks so often take the form of the alternation of weeping and laughter. During the period of strain there is suppression both of grief at the possible disappointment, and joy at its possible success: but when the tension is relaxed, whatever the result, both the suppressed emotions surge up and overwhelm us, so we weep and laugh at once or alternately. A patient was stuck half-way down a cliff, unable to go up or down. But when she was safely hauled to the top, instead of showing signs of happiness at her rescue, she lay down and sobbed hysterically which expressed the pent-up horror to which she had not previously been able to give expression.

Another instance of hysterics is that of a person receiving tragic news who laughs instead of expressing grief. It is akin to "sardonic laughter," which is laughter without mirth, in a situation calling for chagrin. This may be because the grief is so unbearable that it has to be suppressed, and can only emerge as its opposite: the real reaction may come later. But we have known cases where it has not come out at all and has led to insanity.

A clinical example is that of a young married woman (usually of a controlled nature) who suffered from attacks of sobbing working up to screaming. Her husband was serving in Malay and informed her that he was going by troop plane to Australia on a certain day. The day after, she read that the plane had crashed. The shock was terrible, but she kept herself under control arguing that if he had been killed, the War Office would have informed her. Three weeks later, when she had received word from her husband that he was safe since he had not travelled by that plane, she started attacks of weeping and screaming, obviously the outburst of her previously suppressed emotion. So we have the curious circumstances in such cases that the hysterical emotion bursts out when there is no longer any occasion for it; and that the emotion expressed is the opposite of what is called for.

An interesting phenomenon of hysterics is mass hysteria found in girls' schools. Freud[1] has possibly given the correct explanation

_____
[1] *Group Psychology*, p. 64.

of these: one girl has hysteria because of an emotional crisis, e.g. receiving a letter from someone she loves which arouses her jealousy and all the others identify themselves with her and get hysterics out of envy, because they would like similar secret love affairs. But a more important factor is surely that being cooped up in schools in which their love life has no outlet most girls have pent-up feelings which in such situations are easily touched off by suggestion from the other girl's hysterics.

Hysterical outbursts also differ from ordinary emotion in that they are entirely *undirected* and useless whereas ordinary emotions like rage or fear, however exaggerated, are usually directed towards a definite end. Hysterics serve no useful purpose except that of relief of pent-up feelings: sometimes it is difficult to diagnose what emotion the screaming female is supposed to be expressing, self-will, self-pity, anger or despair.

The *hysterical fit* goes a step further in the degradation of the emotions. In the fit there has been such a complete breakdown that the energy produced to cope with the situation expends itself in completely unco-ordinated movements (as in the case of the rats) in which no specific emotion can be differentiated, such as spasms, convulsions, spastic contractions sometimes producing the *arc de cercle* (since the extension muscles of the body in the back are stronger than the flexors of the body in the abdomen), and ending in flaccidity and coma. Hysterical fits were very common in the two World Wars, and were usually reproductions of experiences at the front, the emotion of which had been repressed.

The treatment of hysterical attacks follows an understanding of their nature. As hysterics are outbursts of uncontrollable emotion, they depend on the relative inability of the inhibitory forces in the personality to control strongly aroused but suppressed emotions. They may arise therefore when the suppressed emotion is excessive (as with Bismarck), or when the inhibitions are poorly developed (as in the undisciplined). Recognizing this, "hysterics" may be treated in either of three ways: by allowing the emotion to expend itself ("let her have a good cry!"); or to allay the emotion by quietening treatment (by suggestion for instance); or by firm handling, to provide the individual with the needed self-control to pull himself together until the crisis is past. All these are employed in everyday life, and all are effective. But whilst this may be sound treatment for "hysterics," it is of no use in the more complicated cases of conversion hysteria, in which the repressing forces are already too strong, and the emotions completely repressed and unconscious.

CONVERSION HYSTERIA

Conversion hysteria is the most typical form of hysteria, and exemplifies the psychopathology and mechanism of the psychoneuroses in general. We shall therefore give a case illustrating these various points (the reactions being in italics).

Mrs. B., a married woman, suffered from intense physical fatigue associated with an acute pain in the back: she also had an obsessional fear of injuring her children. She herself recognized there was something abnormal in her symptoms because she was able to play two rounds of golf without fatigue or pain, whereas if she wheeled out her children in the pram for half an hour she became exhausted and suffered this pain. Yet she was a most devoted mother; in fact, as she had previously been an infant welfare worker, who, when married, prided herself on being a perfect mother, her condition was the more unaccountable. Her father was a crofter in the north of Scotland earning a hard living and was none too good-tempered. She was the eldest, and for a time the favoured child, but the birth of another child not only made her jealous and resentful, but laid new responsibilities upon her to help in the home. She felt deprived of that affection to which she was accustomed, and craved it the more. One day as a child of three, she was standing on the kitchen table when her mother came in, and in her craving for affection she tried to fling her arms round her. Her busy mother was irritated and brushed her aside with the result that she fell on the floor and hurt her back, for which she got some temporary attention. But her feelings were hurt more than her back. She felt *resentment*, decided she would never ask for affection again, abandoned the idea of getting love from her mother. But this made her lonely and depressed and full of *self-pity*. But to remain so was unbearable so she repressed her resentment and self-pity and assumed an *independent attitude of mind*. But to regain her mother's approval she helped about the house and started to look after the baby, and developed her *super-ego*. So she was restored to the inner circle under different terms. When she was twelve her mother died, and the responsibilities which she had undertaken were greatly increased, to keep house for her father, yet she welcomed the self-importance of it. She was often wearied to death with the task, but having adopted this stern standard of helpfulness she refused to ask for sympathy and grimly continued, in spite of the fatigue. Later the opportunity came to go to College, where she did well, and ultimately she went into child welfare work, in which she attained a high position. When the opportunity came to marry, she abandoned her career to devote herself to her children, and in view of her ideals in child welfare work, determined to be the *perfect mother* (her super-ego once more). But in time she found the rôle of mother, however perfect, did not bring her the glamour she had received in her public work, nor did she get any compensation by way of affection from her husband, who was a busy man also in an important position. But of course she could not admit failure, nor allow herself to entertain any regrets, which she immediately repressed as being unworthy of her noble ideal. But her repressed craving for love as well as the repressed resentment were reactivated by these conditions, though still unconsciously, with the result that a violent conflict was precipitated between her determination to do her duty, and the old repressed craving for love and self-pity, to say nothing of the feelings of resentment, now directed against her husband.

It was at this point that the neurosis was precipitated: she developed *fatigue and a severe pain in the back*, which in fact was a reproduction of the identical pain which she had suffered when she had been rebuffed by her mother, under similar emotional circumstances. But what is of striking interest is the fact that apart from this conversion hysteria, she also suffered from an *obsessional compulsion*, namely a fear that she might leave the gas turned on in her child's bedroom so that the child would suffocate to death. She had constantly to return to make sure she had turned it off. In fact in one case she went in to do so, found the gas turned off and unwittingly left it turned on! This was a curious expression of her unconscious wish to get rid "accidentally" of the child who now stood in the way of her career. The hysteria represented her repressed need of love and dependence, the obsession her repressed aggressiveness.

The mechanism of conversion hysteria is clearly exemplified in this case. We have here the double repression which we find in all the psychoneuroses. Firstly, there is the exaggerated craving for love, in this case fostered by her being the favoured child for three years. This was followed by its deprivation and repression from the rebuff, and the reaction of disappointment, rage, bitterness, self-pity, depression and a sense of grievance took its place. If the process had stopped at this stage these reactions might have persisted as reaction character traits and the patient might have continued all her life, as many do, to have moods of self-pity, resentment and sense of grievance. But commonly this attitude cannot be maintained because the child cannot bear the continued pain of humiliation, loneliness and disappointment; its self-pity only results in despair, its anger in isolation; its sense of grievance effects nothing, its depression is unendurable, its rage futile. In any case such a child must have the love of the mother for its protective security. So the reaction is abandoned and repressed in favour of a third stage, namely the formation of an ego ideal, designed to secure social approval, in this case an attitude of helpfulness, a sense of duty, of responsibility, by means of which she hopes to ingratiate herself with those from whom she demands affection, and be restored to love. Finally, the symptom is occasioned by the emergence of these repressed elements, which refuse to be repressed any longer. These mechanisms apply to other forms of neurosis as well as to hysteria.

Because of this double repression, in all the psychoneuroses as distinct from most character traits there is an endo-psychic conflict between two or more elements, *both* of which are repressed in favour of an ego ideal, the adoption of standards of behaviour more in conformity with social demands. Another case will make this clear.

A girl of three was jealous of her younger and prettier sister, who was petted by the father: when they were alone she gave her a "sock on the jaw" for which she was reproved by her grieved father; so she decided to be independent, not to want "sloppy" love any more. But this attitude led to another scene because in her sulkiness she refused to see visitors, for which she was punished. She felt so lonely that ultimately she decided she must be a good, sweet and obedient little girl, but combined this with her aggressiveness by imposing these ideals on her sister and so developed a *self-righteous bossiness*, which she maintained as her ego ideal. In this she found she could get outlet for her assertiveness and at the same time get approval by self-righteousness and priggishness. She carried this attitude into school life and bossed over her school-fellows, which met with the approval of her teachers in whose eyes she was a valued leader and a good example. But it made her unpopular with the girls, and the basic need for their love was too much for her and she broke down.

It is necessary to recognize the double or even more complicated repression in the psychoneurosis proper, for otherwise we shall fail to analyse out all the elements of the conflict, and so fail to effect a complete cure. Partial analysis may break up the symptom into its component parts and cure the patient of his symptom, but leave him with the morbid character traits of which his symptom is composed; we may cure his paralysis, but leave him with self-pity or craving for attention; we may cure his phobia, but leave him with a sense of depression; we may cure him of his pain, but leave him with feelings of anxiety; and we may relieve his anxiety and leave him aggressive and resentful. In such a case there is some justification for the patient's complaint that analysis "only makes him feel worse." Such character traits are the components of which the symptom is formed and from which his symptom is in some part intended to relieve him, and into which the symptom may be broken by analysis. So that whilst the symptom may disappear, it gives place to morbid character traits which now become the main symptoms, and require to be further investigated and treated.

Psychopathology of Conversion Hysteria

(I) *Biologically* considered conversion hysteria is fundamentally due to a *sense of insecurity*, resulting in a failure in adaptation to the external world; therefore those functions which serve our adaptation to the external world, the functions of the central nervous system, especially of movement and sensation, become disordered.

Psychologically considered conversion hysteria is fundamentally a morbid reaction to the feeling of deprivation of love.

The typical hysteric reaction may be seen in any large nursery: the child who feels left out and unloved, who is not getting the attention he wants, says "I have a pain in my tummy," "I have got a sore toe," "I feel tired," by means of which he hopes to regain the sympathy and attention he has lost. This is an early manifestation of *conversion hysteria*. Whereas another child feeling the loss of affection becomes frightened and cries out from his bedroom "Oh! Oh! I'm frightened! Come to me quickly!" as a means to compel his mother to come to be with him. This is the prototype of *anxiety hysteria*. Unless these situations are properly dealt with these reactions may develop into chronic hysterias of adult life. The right means are not always obvious: to deny attention in such cases is to increase the desire and so perpetuate the neurotic reaction; to give all the attention demanded encourages the child to continue using the same methods of getting attention. What should the harassed parent do?

This craving for love is well exemplified in our case. It was at the moment of deprivation of love in childhood, when she fell from the table, that her pain in the back first appeared. It was then an organic symptom, but as the patient admitted, it was the mental hurt, the rebuff to her feelings, not the physical pain which concerned her. Nevertheless the physical pain and injury got her the attention, at least temporarily. When later she experienced the deprivation of love from her husband there was a reproduction of this pain. The injury had secured for her the mother's love; why should it not succeed with the husband? So she revives it all unconsciously.

A child who was denied affection from her mother, got attention only when she had a sore throat. The conscious desire for love was thereafter repressed, but at a later age when she had a disappointment in love and craved for affection, she fell back on the "sore throat" and developed "aphonia."

(II) *In conversion hysteria the love craving is always exaggerated.* As we have seen, the feeling of deprivation of love is characteristic of all the psychoneuroses, the obsessions, the sex perversions as well as hysteria. The difference is that in conversion hysteria the love craving has always been previously exaggerated in childhood, whether by encouragement or by frustration, and that is why the specific reaction of the hysteric to the craving for love is one of helplessness, dependence and self-pity, whereas the reaction of the obsessions is that of anger, and in the sex perversions a resort to sexual gratification. Each depends on what was previously exaggerated.

This exaggerated craving for protective love is everywhere apparent in hysteria. The *precipitating cause* of the hysteria is often of such a nature; terrifying experiences as in traumatic cases (soldiers in battle have been known to shout out for their mothers), a disappointment in a love affair, the loss of a husband's affection, an illness which arouses the desire for sympathy, or responsibilities in life which the patient finds too hard to bear—any situation in fact in which there is the feeling of inadequacy to face life, and a need for help. The exaggerated craving for love is also obvious in the *symptom* which is an appeal for sympathy. If any further doubt exists upon this point this is immediately dispelled during the course of *analysis* itself, when the patient is reviving the experiences which produced the symptoms: he often gives way to surges of self-pity and the need for affection. A patient, a good unselfish daughter, who devoted her life to her parents, and "could never let them down," suffered from persistent hysterical headaches. In the course of analysis she surprised herself by suddenly breaking out in a tirade against her mother, complaining that she has never had a chance, that her mother has imposed on her all her life, that she has been unjustly treated, that fate has been cruel to her, and finished with a hysterical outburst of sobbing and self-pity, dried her eyes and said, "There! I feel better now." This case is typical of what happens in the analysis of most conversion hysterics: the self-pity no longer repressed surges up in its overt form instead of being disguised as an hysterical pain. The basic need for love also accounts for the fact that the *transference* in hysteria is usually a positive love transference to the physician, not a negative hate transference.

(III) *The origin of this exaggerated craving for sympathy* and affection in the hysteric is interesting as it may come about from either of two opposite sets of circumstances. (*a*) It may come from a child being spoilt and pampered and given an *excess of love* in the first place, so that it has an excessive expectation of affection and is correspondingly rebuffed if it feels deprived of love. (*b*) In other cases the exaggerated craving for love comes when the child has from the beginning felt *deprived of love* so that it craves it the more. The first usually produces a conversion hysteria, the latter an anxiety hysteria such as fear of loneliness.

(*a*) The biological function of love is to give protection and security to the child so that he may grow up able to face the demands of life. If he is given an excessive amount of love, and by "excessive" we mean *beyond the needs and demands of life*, instead of encouraging biological adaptation to life, it tends to incapacitate him from meeting these demands. If the child, therefore, is pampered, if it is protected where there is no danger, guarded when there is no threat, adored till it feels so wonderful that he comes to despise even those who adore him, rendered incompetent by having everything done for him, or so overwhelmed with sensuous coddling, instead of encouraging biological adaptation to life this "excess of love" renders him both incapable of meeting the responsibilities of life, and over-sensitive to its rebuffs. If such a child is then deprived of affection, or feels denied it, he falls victim to the first severe onslaught of objective difficulty, and takes refuge in hysteric reactions whether as a biological expression of helplessness or as a means of regaining the care and sympathy he has lost.

The circumstances, therefore, that are most commonly found in the early life of the *conversion hysteric* are those in which the child is pampered, made to feel important and then snubbed: where he is an only child for two or three years and then has to surrender his privileged place to another; where the youngest child is kept a baby by his parents but scorned by the older children; where the only boy is the pet in a family of girls; where the girl who is the favourite of her father, but arouses the jealousy of the mother and *vice versa*; where the child is brought up by grandparents who dote on him to gratify their lost parental opportunities, or by a widowed mother, or a mother disappointed in the love of her husband, who are apt unwittingly to gratify their sex cravings, as well as their affection, by doting on and fondling the child. Such situations fail to fulfil the biological functions of love, which are to render the child fit to face the responsibilities of life; they paralyse volition.

(*b*) But the exaggerated craving for love may also come about because of its *original deprivation*, which is usually the case in anxiety hysteria.

The circumstances, therefore, which lead to *anxiety hysteria* are those in which a child suffers from some primal fear in early childhood, such as from illness, from suffocation, over-anxiety of the parents, loss of a mother, or cruel treatment at the hands of a nurse or mother. Such a child from the beginning develops an attitude of fear towards life, and clings with all the more tenacity for the protection and security of which he feels himself, and indeed has been, denied. The choice of symptom in these cases, whether conversion hysteria or anxiety hysteria, is therefore largely determined by the different circumstances of their early experiences, which naturally call for the different reactions. Both the conversion and the anxiety hysteric are helpless and want sympathy and care, the one because he has received too much "love," and the other because he has not received enough. The conversion hysteric, therefore, welcomes the illness which brings him sympathy; the anxiety hysteric dreads it, since he has experienced its terrors in early childhood.

These circumstances account for the fact that we find the essential conflict in conversion hysteria to take place about the age of $2\frac{1}{2}$ or 3 when there has been time and opportunity for the sentiments of love to be more completely developed and even exaggerated, whereas in anxiety hysteria the fear is developed at a more primitive level, usually in the first year of life, before a personal attachment has been formed, at which age most of the phobias are found in analysis to originate. The older child of 3 also has the intelligence to make use of a pain to get sympathy; the infant has not, although it may find that it does get sympathy, and so reproduces it later for that purpose. These circumstances also account for certain other distinctions between conversion and anxiety hysteria.

In conversion hysteria a strong *personal* attachment to one or another parent has been formed, and hence its symptom takes the form of an appeal for sympathy and pity by means of a physical illness such as paralysis or pain, whereas in anxiety hysteria the fears originate in infancy before a personal attachment has been formed, and take on an *impersonal* form; it is therefore characterized by stark fear and panic, as in the fear of darkness, of animals, agoraphobia or isolation. It is this exaggeration of personal affection which seems to be at the base of the Freudian view that conversion hysteria occurs at an "Oedipus level," that is, at the stage of personal relationship. Freud explains this relationship as a sexual one, the girl having incestuous desires towards the father and the boy towards his mother. No doubt these sexual relationships often occur (though in our experience usually originating in the attraction of the opposite parent to the child rather than the reverse). But the essential feature in hysteria is not the sex relationship, but a love relationship based on the child's need for protection and security. That is why the symptom takes the form of an illness, a disability which is an appropriate and effective means of escaping from life and securing attention and sympathy, but is not an appropriate expression of sexual gratification.

In many cases there is a combination of both exaggeration and denial of love producing a double attachment to the mother. To these is sometimes added a third, namely a sexual attachment due to her fondling. All of these may combine to render the child completely dependent and mother-bound, so that such a child, petted, spoilt, pampered, afraid and sexually attached is hopelessly incompetent to meet the demands of life, and later suffers from phobias or is compelled to resort to illness as an escape from the responsibility for which he has been totally unfitted. Where the sexual motive is predominant he may also suffer from sexual impotence which represents both his sexual fixation to his mother and fear of the responsibilities of marriage. Some such cases are extremely difficult to cure because the patient so clings to infantile dependence that he has no incentive to get well when he will have to face life, and we may with some justification regard such a patient as a "hopeless neurotic." But with the co-operation of the patient no case should be "hopeless."

(IV) In conversion hysteria *the exaggerated craving for affection is always followed by its repression.* The exaggerated craving alone does not produce a neurosis, though it may predispose to it. A child given a great amount of affection under favourable conditions responds with affection, and later transfers this devotion to a husband, or wife and child. Even an excess of foolish devotion such as we have described rarely has a bad effect upon the otherwise healthy child except to make him revolt against this pampering and assert his independence; whereupon his over-devoted parents accuse him of ingratitude. The ordinary child tires of a hot-house existence. The pampered child may become selfish, self-centred, self-willed, incapable of taking responsibility, monopolize the attention of the parents, and develop other undesirable characteristics, but these are character traits and tend to be modified in the process of time and in the painful school of life. Similarly, many children have illnesses in infancy, traumatic births or ill-treatment giving rise to fear, and so have an exag-

gerated craving for protective love; but this alone does not produce anxiety hysteria. For if circumstances are favourable, they
later find that life is not as bad as they were led to believe. They
were conditioned to fear by infantile experience; they are reconditioned by favourable conditions to self-confidence. Nor indeed
does the *deprivation* alone produce a neurosis. The child who feels
deprived of affection may seek it elsewhere, or get it where it can.
The crucial point comes when the child turns its back on love
and says, "I don't want anyone's love!" and falls into self-pity,
resentment and depression. This is true repression, for it is by
the child itself, and the child denies that it any longer wants love.
It is definitely abnormal because it sets up a perpetual duality in
the personality: the child wants love but denies that it wants it.
That is why in our formula we state not merely that it is the
deprivation of love but the repressed craving for love which
produces the neurosis.

The reason for this repression of love is the disappointment
in not getting it as in Mrs. B's case. Nothing is so painful to a
child as to continue wanting affection and to be perpetually
denied it; and so to avoid the pain, disappointment and humiliation it says, "I can do without it! I don't want anyone's love."

(V) *Reactions to the repression of the love.* The first reactions are
resentment, self-pity, depression and anxiety.

Self-pity. The child who is denied the love of others indulges
in self-love: nobody feels sorry for him, so he feels sorry for
himself. It takes this form of self-pity since the love craving has
previously been over-developed, and must find an outlet somehow.
One patient referred to his childhood in these terms. "I used to
get attention all to myself: but now I must do something to get it.
So I stay behind when they all go out to enjoy themselves, and
feel lonely and sorry for myself." It is a curious phenomenon,
this self-pity; for why should a person enjoy dwelling upon the
sadness of his lot? Why should he wallow in his misery and
brood over his misfortunes? Why should he even bring misfortunes and pain upon himself that he may pity himself? It is not
primarily masochistic, as some would have us believe, for in most
cases the sexual element does not enter into it at all. The reason is
that in self-pity he is playing a double rôle: he is not only giving
himself sympathy, but he is getting sympathy—from himself; and
of the two the latter is what gives the greater satisfaction. There is
no one else to pity him so he pities himself: his main gratification
is not in pitying himself but in *being pitied by himself*. He may
even develop a headache, so that he may give himself good cause

for self-pity, and what was the result of the self-pity is then taken by the patient to be the reason for it. Ultimately he becomes the victim of it, and the headache which he welcomed as a means of self-pity, becomes his master from which he would give anything to be released. But an added reason for bringing illness or even death on himself is to make others sorry and so pay them out.

A boy has a sore eye, but he deliberately goes into the wind to make it worse. "Nobody," he says, "cares if I lose my sight or not: women can give in and go to bed if they like, but not me! I have to keep going till I drop dead." In this case we see the suppression of the love craving in favour of self-pity, but also the transition from a hysterical character trait of self-pity to a true conversion hysteria taking the form of a sore eye, from which he later suffered.

Resentment, though more characteristic of the obsessions, is also common in hysteria, and is often associated with hurt pride. This is to be expected of the child who has previously been pampered and spoilt, who expects everything and therefore feels jealousy and hate, sometimes towards the mother, sometimes towards the baby, when it loses this attention. Thus whilst some hysterics are characterized by complete self-pity others are domineering and use their symptoms to get their own way—the "resistive hysterics." They are almost obsessional in their demands for love and attention. They are indeed a mixture of hysteric and obsessional, but we call them hysteric because it is by means of their helplessness that they get their own way and tyrannize over others.

These reactions of self-pity and resentment may remain and persist throughout life. There are those who go through life full of self-pity, wanting sympathy and attention, always dependent on others, demanding preferential treatment, always leaving it to others to tidy up for them, late for appointments, sorry for themselves, nursing grievances, always complaining of "bad luck," easily discouraged.

(VI) But so far these are only reaction character traits, and though abnormal, do not constitute a psychoneurosis. To be transformed into a neuroses *these reaction traits also must themselves be repressed*. The child cannot for ever live in a state of self-pity or resentment against those on whom it depends; for he still needs love although he denies it. Jealousy and hate of the baby only bring upon him more punishment and disapproval which he cannot bear: loneliness and isolation give poor comfort, and self-pity is poor substitute for the love he needs. His resentment also gets him nowhere, except that he loses more love. Therefore he is compelled to repress these reactions in favour of a line of conduct more compatible both with biological needs and social demands. Hence the formation of the super-ego or ego ideal.

(VII) *The super-ego*, as we have said, in its broadest sense is the adoption and incorporation into the personality of the standards, aims and modes of behaviour of those round about. The super-ego, it is to be observed, is the result of the intolerable conflict, not as is sometimes assumed in psychological writings, the repressing force: it is the product, not at first the agent of repression. Once formed, however, it perpetuates the repression and assumes the rôle of repressing agency, keeping down both the resentment, self-pity and craving for sympathy and love. So the super-ego becomes the devil in the piece, and stands as the barrier to the patient's spontaneous recovery. The result of this double repression, first of the craving for love, and, secondly, of the reaction of self-pity or resentment, is the adoption of an attitude of mind that consciously wants no love, feels no resentment or self-pity and is only anxious to be helpful, brave, self-sacrificing and efficient.

The popular view of the hysteric as one who demands attention, is full of self-pity and craves for sympathy, is therefore true, but only provided we recognize the very important fact that it is not a conscious, but repressed and unconscious need for sympathy. If therefore we accuse the woman with a hysterical headache or pain in the back of trying to get sympathy and notice, she will stoutly deny it, and rightly maintain that on the contrary, far from seeking sympathy, whenever she gets a headache she goes to her room so as not to worry other people, and carries on with her duties in spite of the pain. If we charge a war-shock paralysed man with wanting to get out of the war he indignantly replies that far from being the case the one thing he desires is to be back fighting with his pals in the front line; his only reason for not going back, he will tell you, is that his paralysed hand incapacitates him from holding a gun. The men who suffered from war neuroses were not the funks or the slackers; they were men of responsibility and courage whose very breakdown was largely occasioned by the strain of having to live up to so high a standard of courage. Some soldiers are cowards; others are like frightened animals; still others are malingerers: but the true conversion hysteric, who suffers from paralysed legs or pain, far from consciously craving for sympathy, refuses to accept it. "I hate," said the lady with a paralysed hand, "that anyone should know that there is anything wrong with my hand." "I went on reading," said the half-blind girl, "long after I was unfit"; and used to take work home from the office and worked late to conceal the fact. Mrs. B. stuck to her job despite the added hardships of the constant fatigue and pain in the back.

Whilst therefore the craving for sympathy is the common characteristic of the conversion hysteric as such, his *character* is usually the opposite; he is consciously one who shoulders responsibilities; who is out to do his duty, to face life courageously, helpful to others, carrying on with his work even in face of this illness and pain, and suffers in silence. The physician therefore who tells a hysteric that he is "only wanting sympathy" is not only wasting his time but acting ignorantly and unjustly. In saying that the hysteric has a craving for sympathy, popular opinion is right; in assuming that he consciously seeks it, popular opinion is wrong; and in denying him that sympathy it is perpetuating his disorder.

It is this fact of *unconscious motivation* which, as we have indicated, differentiates a hysterical symptom from malingering. In both there is a desire to escape because the difficulties of life are too great, but in malingering the shirking is deliberate, whereas in conversion hysteria the desire is latent but repressed by the sense of duty, and that is why it emerges in the substitute form of a pain or paralysis.

So we must clearly distinguish these hysteric *character traits* like self-pity, and hysteric *symptoms* like paralysis, from the *character* of the conversion hysteric, for he is one who represses all these tendencies and adopts an attitude of self-sufficiency, dutifulness and helpfulness.[1]

From the practical point of view *the function of the super-ego* is, first, to keep the goodwill of those around upon whom depends our life and happiness; it is based on a need for security. The secondary function of the super-ego is therefore to keep guard against our own impulses, self-pity, aggressiveness and sex which threaten disapproval and danger, and keep them repressed. The further function of the super-ego is to give some expression to the repressed impulses in an approved form.

The nature of the super-ego will therefore be determined partly by the circumstances of the moment (the child subjected to danger is compelled to adopt an attitude of self-sufficiency),

---

[1] It is this repression of his emotions and feelings which leads Janet to speak of "la belle indifference" of the hysteric person. Freud, on the other hand, speaks of the "mental hypersensitiveness" so common in hysteria which leads him to "react to the least suggestion of depreciation as to a deadly insult." The difference is to be explained by the fact that Freud refers to the underlying hysteric nature; Janet to the attitude adopted.

partly by the nature of the moral standards demanded by the
parents with whom the child identifies himself (whether the
parent wishes the child to be good, hard-working, sociable, or
independent); but also by the nature of the repressed impulses.
If it is resentment or aggressiveness which is repressed, the super-
ego is likely to be one of ingratiation and submissiveness, whereas
if fear is repressed the super-ego is more likely to be one of
courage. The sex pervert, on the other hand, having to repress
sensuous tendencies, is commonly ascetic or aesthetic.

In conversion hysteria it is the personal love motive which is
dominant; therefore the super-ego whilst repressing these tendencies takes on a form which disguises yet gratifies this need. The
super-ego of the conversion hysteric is often one of helpfulness,
unselfishness, devotion, or even one of charm: but if the love
motive is more deeply repressed, the super-ego may appear in the
form of a sense of stern duty or self-sacrifice which is also socially
approved.

In the anxiety hysteric, on the other hand, in whom the repressed tendency is that of primal fear and dread, the super-ego
is usually one of self-sufficiency, success, bravado, power and
achievement all designed to keep the primal fears at bay, and to
give security by personal prowess. The conversion hysteric is one
who, because of his early conditions, relies on others; the anxiety
hysteric tries to rely on himself.

Thus *the super-ego is a compromise* satisfying social demands yet
giving expression to the basic repressed needs. The super-ego of
being "helpful," for instance, is socially approved yet gives some
outlet both to the need for affection and to the aggressiveness.
Mrs. B. is a case in point; if being helpful did not give her all the
love she wanted, at least she got approval; if it did not give outlet
to all her rage and resentment it nevertheless gave her the sense of
self-importance. The super-ego gratifies both, while it completely
satisfies neither side of the conflict. We see then that whilst these
tendencies are repressed, a considerable amount is released to be
sublimated in the super-ego. *The super-ego consists of that part of
the forbidden tendencies which has escaped repression and been
sublimated: whereas the symptom, as we shall see, is that part which
has remained repressed and therefore must emerge in abnormal form.*

The development of a neurosis therefore depends upon how
much of the forbidden impulses is left repressed, and how much
is successfully utilized in the formation of the super-ego and finds
expression in socially useful channels: upon this does the success
of the super-ego depend. The greater the proportion that is thus

utilized or sublimated, the less liable will the patient be to have a breakdown. That is why most of us, although we all have repressions and complexes, manage to carry on satisfactorily without any marked neurosis. But when the emotions are strongly developed and deeply repressed not only is there less available for the use of the personality but such a condition is almost certain to end in psychoneurosis of a mild or severe form.

In the psychoneuroses *the super-ego is always exaggerated*; for it is at such pains to hide the forbidden desires and impulses that it goes to the opposite extreme of ingratiation to hide hostility, of toughness to hide effeminancy, of hardness to hide sentimentality, of piety to hide evil desires and of helpfulness to hide antagonism. So to repress the sexual we must be ascetic or aesthetic, to repress the aggression we must be excessively gentle, to repress the sense of dependence we must put on a bold face and be tough. In psychological language the super-ego is always an *over-*compensation.

For the same reason the *super-ego in the psychoneuroses is always abnormal*. It is not that we pretend to be judges of what are objectively true ideals and what are false; nor does the psychologist as such pretend to be the arbiter of what objective standards are right and wrong. But we have our own standards of judgment, and the very fact that the patient suffers from a neurosis proves that there is a repression, and this means that his super-ego is maintained at the expense of keeping tendencies repressed which ought never to have been repressed and ought to have been given free expression and utilized for the purpose of the personality as a whole. The super-ego has obviously failed in its true function which is that of harmonizing and directing the impulses of the personality towards a common end, and so making the personality function as a complete whole. Therefore, if a person has a neurotic breakdown, if he has an obsession however mild, if he has sex aberrations or a tic, it proves that *however objectively right his ideal may be, it is not right for him*; for the rightness of an ideal, judged in terms of mental health, depends upon its power of direction and harmonization, and the presence of the symptom proves that this has not been effected.

In contrast with such a super-ego, a true ego ideal is not a compromise but a directing power; it does not repress tendencies in our nature, it controls and directs them. It sacrifices nothing but makes use of everything; so that we have a strong will and healthy character. Such an ideal is not at variance with reason, which selects the ideal most conducive to these ends; it is not at variance with morality, indeed it gives support to morality, for to be mentally healthy we need to give scope to our social as well as to our more individualistic tendencies, and this makes us considerate of others.

The following illustrations will further illustrate the foregoing points both of mechanism and psychopathology.

The girl who suffered from hysterical blindness had, as the youngest child, received both love and attention till her older brother got delicate and ill, when he began to get the attention; she then took the attitude that she didn't want the love; *he* was a baby and had to be coddled, while *she* was capable and efficient. She ultimately became a most efficient secretary to the head of a firm till the demands of love asserted themselves and her revolt against the task and standards she had adopted produced blindness.

A boy furious at the loss of affection when another child came was severely punished, decided "that gets you nowhere," and repressing both love and rage assumed an attitude of independence, of not wanting anyone, of self-sufficiency. Even then he had outbursts of aggressiveness which were punished; and he found that there was something missing in his self-sufficiency; so he repressed all feeling and became "docile and harmless." By this means he gained peace; but later came complaining of tiredness and lack of energy, which is not surprising as he had repressed all incentive to act. This instance shows how one may develop two super-egos, the one being of self-sufficiency, and the other of being docile and harmless. A super-ego, therefore, may itself be repressed, a fact of particular importance in the obsessions.

Another instance of the foregoing characteristics of the super-ego is that of a patient jealous of her younger pretty sister: she reacted by engaging in sex practices as a solace and was discovered by her father who scolded her as nasty and dirty, and finished off by saying she wasn't his little girl any more, and he would have nothing more to do with her. She was terribly distressed and cried wildly that she would never do it again. "It was simply awful, and I felt wild and wanted to do something violent and crash through the window. But it's no use. I'll have to be good. I must convince Daddy that I'm not like that; that I am a nice little girl and so be happy and secure. I've been an absolute fool to have anything to do with sex. I must just be exactly what Daddy wants me to be. Then I behaved so meticulously that nobody could *imagine* that I had such feelings." She later suffered violent blushing at the thought or mention of sex.

It is a point which we commend to the study of the moralists and also to those who consider social adaptation the main criterion of normality, that a person may be of excellent character but psychologically unhealthy, the very excellence of whose character is morbid. That is why in discussing the standard of mental health, we found that even people of unexceptionable character broke down.

(VIII) *The precipitating causes of the breakdown* (which claim the attention of the social psychologist as well as the psychopathologist), may be (*a*) whatever arouses the latent repressed tendencies of the ego into activity, or (*b*) on the other hand, whatever brings about the weakening or breakdown of the super-ego so that it can no longer keep these tendencies in check. Commonly it is both factors in combination; for whatever weakens the super-ego encourages the emergence of the repressed impulses, and whenever the impulses are aroused they threaten and weaken the super-ego.

(*a*) The precipitation may take place from the *arousal of the repressed emotions* which refuse to be repressed any longer, and overthrow the super-ego. In conversion hysteria it is primarily the arousal of the repressed love or self-pity which gives to the hysteric his characteristic symptom. To such conditions we have already referred (p. 196). But the precipitating cause may be the arousal of the secondary repressed tendencies, like resentment, sex or a sense of guilt which are also capable of upsetting the balance of the personality. In the case of Mrs. B. it was the waning of her husband's affection which aroused her latent craving for love; she was disillusioned in the romance of love. But also her resentment was aroused at having to abandon her career and being confined to domestic duties for which she got no credit or attention. She revolted against having to be the good wife and perfect mother, and this precipitated her breakdown.

(*b*) This process of disintegration is encouraged by the weakening of the super-ego. As we have mentioned, the super-ego is always false because it can maintain itself only at the expense of repressing these tendencies. For a time it may do so successfully so that the personality is able to carry on with the objective conditions of life. But assailed from within by the repressed impulses and from without by adverse circumstances it cannot maintain its exaggerated standards and breaks down. Adler's dictum is right, that all psychoneuroses are due to false ideals. The breakdown is the overthrow of fictitious ideals.

The reason for the breakdown of the super-ego is that it fails in its original purpose, which in hysteria was to gain attention and approval. Mrs. B. got no credit for wheeling her own children out, as she had for her welfare work. The "willing horse" found that she was being imposed upon by her brothers and sisters who took her good nature for granted and expected her to "fag" their tennis balls, and to stay at home with their mother while they enjoyed themselves. Another child who felt deprived of affection found that she got great credit for being clever, adopted this as her ego ideal and became a teacher. As long as she won prizes at school and scholarships at college all went well. But when she became a teacher she got no credit for being clever as it was expected of her, and little praise from the headmistress; indeed she was not particularly liked for it, for while people admire cleverness in children, they dislike it in adults, especially when it is obviously intended to win applause. So it failed to give her the love for which she really craved. Her super-ego having failed of its purpose she developed a severe pain in the abdomen, which was a means of getting attention more effectively and was less troublesome than being clever: it also excused her from teaching.

In other cases the failure of the super-ego is because, being exaggerated, *it is impossible of attainment.* The over-ambition of one man, like the ultra-goodness and over-conscientiousness of another, the over-ambition of a third, and the devotion to duty of a fourth, may all be designed to maintain the integrity of the individual and may all be temporarily or even permanently successful; but psychologically regarded, they are pathological attempts to solve the problem and are liable to failure. They are too much for us, we cannot keep it up, we become weary in well-doing and break down.

The first effects of this threat from the impulses of the ego is to stimulate the super-ego to further effort; so the patient works harder, is spurred on to even greater ambition and achievement, is more anxious to live up to his ideals of helpfulness or goodness, more earnest in his moral endeavour. This anxious endeavour and strain, often accompanied by sleeplessness, is commonly the prelude to a nervous breakdown, which is naturally regarded as due to overwork, whereas in reality the overwork is due to the latent anxiety resulting from the mental conflict. Throughout this period of incubation, such a personality is perpetually in a state of tension because of the necessity of keeping these forbidden tendencies repressed, but at any moment he may be thrown off his balance, in which case the repressed emotions surge up to precipitate the symptom. The term "unbalanced" is therefore rightly used of these conditions of mind, since the balance between the ego and the super-ego, the repressing forces and the repressed forces, which has been maintained for so long, has now been disturbed; and by "breakdown" we mean the breakdown of the

standards of life by which the personality has so far been inte-
grated and kept itself going; in brief, the breakdown of the super-
ego.

In some cases, as we have seen, the lack of balance is such that
it requires but the most trifling experience to tip the balance
and produce a breakdown, so that some people break down for
apparently no reason. Many men during the war maintained their
integrity as long as they were in a quiet occupation, but the mere
fact of joining the Army, living in unaccustomed surroundings
and amongst strangers was sufficient to break them down. On the
other hand, where the balance is well maintained it requires a
severe shock as in traumatic hysteria or a series of misfortunes to
break this down. This balance of the personality depends on the
development of a well-co-ordinated personality in childhood.

(IX) *The symptom.* The emergence of the symptom may be
interpreted either (a) mechanistically or (b) teleologically and
purposively.

(a) *Mechanistically, the symptom is the emergence into conscious
activity of the repressed dynamic tendencies and impulses* which
cannot be kept repressed any longer. These impulses themselves
may surge up, and the individual who up till now was carrying out
his responsibilities and duties in life may suddenly have outbursts of bad temper, complain bitterly of his conditions in life,
of being imposed on by others, of having to slave at his work. He
then recovers himself and apologizes for his behaviour, as his
super-ego begins to function again. In other cases the rebellion is
complete and permanent, as with some adolescents. But when in
spite of the arousal of the repressed impulses, the super-ego
refuses to give way even for a moment, the only means whereby
those impulses can express themselves is by a neurotic symptom
which is a perverted form of these same impulses.

(b) According to the *teleological or purposive* idea the symptom
works towards some end, or achieves some purpose for the individual. Indeed the original biological responses serve a purpose,
the crying out to get help, the paralysis of "shamming death" as
a means of escape. The purposive idea explains the symptom and
its manifold forms better than the purely mechanistic view.

This purposive idea is expressed by Freud in the term "wish
fulfilment"; but to say, as some do, that "every hysterical symptom
is wished" is to put the matter too crudely—no one desires to
have a headache as such, nor wishes to be paralysed, nor is there
a "wish to be ill" as such. But it is true to say that every symptom
represents a wish; it may be a wish to escape from responsibility,

to get out of a difficulty, to solve a moral problem, to get sympathy and attention; and as the symptoms, unpleasant as they are in themselves, are the only means permitted to gratify these desires they are suffered for the sake of achieving these ends.

It is interesting to find that this conception of "wish fulfilment," as well as the analytic method, which has in recent years been so strongly urged by Freud, was long since anticipated by Purcell. The following quotation from Purcell's *Treatise on Vapours* (p. 155) is worth preserving:

"For upon diligent search and enquiry you will almost always find that those who are troubled with vapours have some deep passion or concern . . . wherefore the physician ought to consider attentively what may be the cause of her concern, which having found out, he must with the aid of her friends and relatives *facilitate to her the means of obtaining what she desires.* . . . An ancient gentlewoman used to lye for two months together in violent fits . . . all the remedies she had taken for two years and a half were inefficient but the doctor had no sooner *found out what it was that troubled her and put her into the way of obtaining what she so passionately desired,* that all the violent symptoms were abated to a miracle."

It is a pity the nature of the "passionate desire" is not stated, but the treatment is truly modern and analytic, and how much wiser than that advocated by some physicians at the present day who, recognizing that the patient wants sympathy, instruct the relatives that on no account must they give her any, thereby perpetuating her trouble!

The purpose of the symptom. (i) First and foremost the *hysterical symptom represents a repressed craving for sympathy.* There is no better way of securing sympathy than by being ill. *Illness is the royal road to sympathy.* When once the symptom is formed the patient projects his self-pity upon it: he is sorry for himself because he has a pain and he demands sympathy for his blindness. But the pain is the result of the self-pity, not its cause. *The hysteric is not one who wants sympathy because he is ill: he is ill because he wants sympathy.* Every case of conversion hysteria demonstrates the same fact.

(ii) *The hysteric symptom represents an escape from responsibility:* there is no better excuse for escaping from responsibility than by being ill. After a severe accident with a fractured skull a patient says:

"If anybody says anything to me, I've always that pain in my head to fall back upon if they make me do things. I can do what I like. They are beginning to forget my accident now—still there is always the scar. I would cry and say the pain in my head is hurting. My brothers would call me a cry baby—but I would go to my father and he would be very angry with them."

The soldier in the stress of battle seizes upon some symptom as a means of escape—his sense of duty forbids him to run away, so he escapes by an illness. As we have seen, those who were severely wounded did not as a rule get shell-shock (the slightly wounded more so); they did not require to develop a neurosis as a means of escape because they had one ready at hand in their wounds. It is the same with anxiety hysteria: the business man's fear of travelling is designed to release him from responsibilities which he forces himself to assume, but cannot bring himself to abandon. The woman's phobia of leaving home is to avoid the danger of falling into sexual temptations which the moral super-ego she has adopted will not entertain.

Other forms of disability carry out this same desire to escape from responsibility; in particular the sensory disabilities of blindness, deafness, anaesthesia, and amnesia (loss of memory) are means of blotting out the painful experiences of the objective world, and blind us to the horrors of life. They make us anaesthetic so that we feel nothing. A patient who was blown up in a battleship became completely anaesthetic over the skin of his whole body. Even such symptoms as feeling of inferiority, shyness, blushing or stammering may be an unconscious means of avoiding social life, and therefore avoiding the inevitable comparisons. We not only avoid society because we blush; we blush because we feel inferior in society and in order to avoid society.

(iii) The symptom is also *an excuse for possible failure*, and therefore helps to retain a false phantasy of one's superiority.

At one time the author was called upon to treat two Oxford students, a man and a woman, both of whom had suffered from hysterical blindness. The man was so brilliant that he had been offered a Fellowship before he took "Greats"; the woman before her finals had already been appointed to a lectureship in another University. How dreadful if after all they got only a second-class honours instead of a first! Better to escape from the possibility of such failure by an illness, while the going was good; that at least would give an excuse for failure, and so maintain their prestige. So the man became stone blind before the examination and was unable to sit; he failed to get a degree and lost his Fellowship. The girl got blind during the examination in her best paper, but by the help of a medical certificate was granted a second class. Her worst fears were fulfilled, but now she had the excuse of blindness. In each case the fear of failure from an excessively high standard was stronger than the desire for success, but each retained the inner gratification that they *would* have got a first if they had not had this trouble. So phantasy triumphed over reality.

(iv) The further purpose of the symptom is *to relieve the patient from an intolerable mental conflict.* A physical pain is far easier to bear than mental pain; the begetting of a paralysis not only delivers the soldier from the dangers of the front line, it solves the distressing conflict between his fear and duty. That is why a patient often gets worse during analysis because the mental conflict from which he tried to escape by illness needs to be revived in order to be solved.

A patient in analysis said, "I would rather go on having physical attacks than for all my mind to be churned up." A child in a violent conflict between rebellion and fear, feels that "everybody hated me and made me feel miserable and depressed and nasty because I was rebellious. If I said I wasn't well and felt tired, I wouldn't need to decide one way or the other. I wouldn't need to be good, and people would not hate me because they would say I couldn't help it." A man who had what for years had been diagnosed as epileptic fits revealed in analysis that as a boy he had a hard life not only because of the bullying of an older brother, but because "whilst my mother taught me Latin, my father thrashed me for not knowing it! The trouble," he concludes, "is in having a will at all. By unconsciousness and oblivion, as in the fits, I get out of having to exercise my will and yet without giving in to my desires." His fits were cured when the cause was revealed.

(v) The super-ego may play an important part in the motivation of a symptom, so that a pain or paralysis may be a form of *self-punishment* for forbidden impulses. Or the function of the symptom may be by appealing for sympathy to avert the consequences of the guilt. Thus a child may feign illness to turn the wrath of the parent into pity and so avert the punishment of his sin. It serves the same function as an obsessional propitiatory act, with which it is closely allied.

(vi) But the hysterical symptom is not merely an escape but a revolt, giving expression to the resentment that is so often present in conversion hysteria. It is *a revolt against the demands of life, and especially the intolerable demands which the super-ego makes upon him.* When the super-ego refuses to allow us to give up the task, the ego rebels and produces the symptom to make it impossible to carry out the demands. That was a further motive in the Oxford girl just mentioned. It was found in analysis that she had had a very unhappy childhood because of brawls between her parents. Her only hope of winning love and attention was by cleverness at school. This drove her on from one success to another; failure in this meant the loss of everything. But her need for affection in adult life asserted itself in other ways. She revolted against a loveless career, a reason for wanting failure: so she revolted against the unnatural demands placed upon her by getting blind and so refusing to pass the exam. Her symptom served the three purposes: to get the sympathy she had always craved; to escape from a too great responsibility; and an excuse for the failure which she unconsciously desired. The problem was solved both psychologically and objectively, for she is now married *and* is a lecturer in the University.

A girl who had a paralysed hand had been petted and adored by the older sister; the arrival of a boy cousin then claimed the sister's attention; the patient insisted on playing with them, was repelled, made an onslaught on the boy, and generally made herself so objectionable that she was separated from the others and put into the hands of an old nurse. Her loneliness and misery made her come to terms with them; it was a mistake to want all this love and attention, henceforth she must be docile, do their bidding, fetch their errands and generally became the door mat. She gained their approval at the expense of her individuality. But it brought her no love and her revolt took the form of the paralysed hand which was not only designed to get sympathy without asking for it, but to excuse her doing these jobs which she had imposed on herself.

Mrs. B. had voluntarily assumed the responsibility of a wife and a home, and set out to be the perfect mother, the original motive being to get approval and feel self-important. She could, therefore, not openly revolt against a standard of life she had placed on herself and refuse to be so devoted to her children, for this meant abandoning all that she stood for, and losing her prestige by which alone she now got attention. So her refusal expressed itself in illness. Another alternative was to get rid of her children, and so return to her old public work. This could be done by unconsciously leaving the gas turned on, which in fact she proceeded to do, and for which she therefore developed a phobia.

Whilst the symptom is the revolt of the repressed tendencies against the super-ego, it does not abolish it. The symptom of pain or paralysis may incapacitate the patient but he refuses to give way and often carries on in spite of it. He now gets the worst of both worlds for *the symptom remains side by side with the super-*

ego, and even if the symptom entirely incapacitates him, he protests that he "ought" to be doing this or that, although in fact he is not doing so, no longer wants to do so, and is no longer capable of doing so. But he blames the disability, the pain and tiredness for his failure to live to its demands, So the super-ego persists in maintaining its futile existence. As we have seen, the girl partially blind struggled on with her tasks in spite of the handicap. So that, although the symptom is designed to deliver us from the excessive tasks and responsibilities we lay on ourselves, it does not in fact necessarily do so: and we are in far worse state than before.

But it is this very fact that gives us the hope of cure, for when the patient realizes that the symptom is no longer fulfilling its original purpose, he sees that there is no point in it, and is prepared to abandon it. It is no use having a headache to get sympathy when it brings him none. If on the other hand the symptom is successful in getting sympathy, as in so many cases of chronic hysteria, the patient may prefer to retain it; and if his paralysis secures him a pension for life which relieves him of the responsibilities of life from which he has always shrunk, what incentive is there to get well?

Indeed to give a hysteric patient sympathy and to deny him sympathy equally perpetuates the symptom: for to deny the sympathy reproduces the conditions which originally caused the symptoms; and to give him all the sympathy he wants makes him hold to a symptom which serves its purpose so effectively. The discovery and abolition of the causes are the only effective forms of cure. But we should err on the side of sympathy.

A case which illustrates both the motive of the symptom and the motive of cure, is the following:

A patient who suffered from headache and fatigue was made as a child to feel useless and a failure by his father, a distinguished artist, but determined to be as great a success as his father. "But the strain was too great for me and I could not keep up with it; yet I refused to admit my failure. All this strain gave me a headache, but it was a headache I welcomed; and I welcomed it because it gave me a moment of blessed relief when I could let go the strain. I have been preoccupied all my life in getting notice for being tired because of the overwhelming burden I have to carry! If I could get better—what things I could not do! —only this frightful tiredness overwhelms me. I always have to have physical illness to fall back upon. Nowadays the headache produces an additional anxiety that I cannot do my job, but at the same time, excuses me from it. But I am coming to see that obviously if I can do my work with the strain and headache, as I can, I am all the more capable of doing it without the strain!" The motives for the symptom and the revolt against the excessive standards, the escape from responsibility, the excuse for failure, and the means of cure are all here illustrated.

(X) *The symptom in hysteria as in every form of psychoneurosis is a compromise* between two opposite tendencies, *both* of which are repressed, and the super-ego. To illustrate:

A child has a furious row with her father, in which he threatens her and locks her up. She feels sick with the struggle. "I realize I cannot get my way, and so I say 'Daddy, I feel so ill;' because as I am sick I needn't say I'm sorry." So she can obtain her father's sympathy, and yet remain defiant. By her sickness also she makes him feel that he was responsible for her sickness, and it pays him out. But further, once formed, this symptom, originally designed to get sympathy, is utilized by the super-ego as a means of punishment for wanting sympathy—as though she says to herself, "That is what you get for wanting sympathy!" The compromise is further illustrated in the following case of a young man suffering from hysterical weakness in the knees. In childhood this boy failing to get the attention he wanted from his mother, struck her. His father came in and threatened him, and he was torn between fear and defiance. "When one is afraid," he says in free association, "the impulse is to run, but when I was confronted with my father I couldn't run. But if I was defiant and said, 'Very well, then, beat me!' he would have thrashed me worse. So there is the conflict: I want to run away, but the weakness in my knees prevented me running away: so by that means I express my defiance without being openly defiant. But I also get weak in the knees because I want to arouse my father's pity: it is a way of throwing myself on his mercy—just as a child whimpers before it is punished." By the symptom therefore he satisfies both the repressed defiance, and his repressed self-pity, but without yielding the pride of his super-ego.

(XI) *The symptom and the super-ego.* But if the super-ego is a compromise between the conflicting elements, how does it differ from the super-ego which is also a compromise between them. The *super-ego* of Mrs. B. was to look after her children, and be the perfect mother, thereby to gain approval, but also to assert her self-importance. Her *symptom* of pain in the back was also a compromise between the same general impulses, satisfying her self-pity and also her resentment against having to carry out these duties. The main difference between them is that *the super-ego is that part of the conflicting tendencies which has escaped repression and been sublimated;* whereas *the symptom is the emergence of that part of the conflicting tendencies which has remained repressed.*

The health of the personality depends on the relative quantity of each of these. In complete mental health all our potentialities are utilized and none is repressed. In neurosis a considerable part has been repressed and demanding expression can only appear as a symptom. From the point of view of function, the distinction is that the super-ego is turned towards the outer world, designed to enable us to carry on in life, to adapt ourselves to life and to the people around; whereas the symptom does the very reverse; it incapacitates us from facing life by making us ill. The super-ego is an acceptance of life, the symptom is an escape from life; the super-ego goes forward to face life, the symptom is a regression back to the security of infantile life. It is not surprising therefore that people ordinarily regard the super-ego, with its standards of duty, of responsibility, of unselfishness, as normal, right and approved, and the symptom as abnormal and disapproved; and it is to be treated of the symptom that the patient comes to the physician, for this he regards as abnormal, and very rarely to be cured of his super-ego, for this he accepts as right.

But in fact both these conceptions require correction. In the first place, the super-ego, whilst biologically and socially right, and enabling the child to meet his present obligations, is psychologically abnormal, as we have seen, in that it keeps repressed emotions and tendencies which ought never to be repressed. It is falsely motivated, it is over-compensated, it is exaggerated in its demands, and it places so heavy a burden of responsibility upon the personality that the latter breaks down under it.

On the other hand, though the symptom is obviously abnormal, it is an attempt, though a poor attempt, to regain normality, since it represents the emergence of impulses and tendencies which ought never to have been repressed. *The symptom may therefore be regarded as an attempt of the personality to restore itself to health.* The urge to completeness is fundamental in human nature. In every psychoneurosis the personality is functionally incomplete because of the repression of tendencies which should never have been repressed, but should have been utilized for the purpose of the personality as a whole. The super-ego perpetuates this morbid state by denying expression to these impulses. The natural self after all has its rights over the demands of society: and if these demands are too severe, and if the repressed impulses have been denied their normal outlet because of the false standards, the natural self can only maintain its individuality by revolt. The symptom is the attempt of the repressed part of one's personality to express itself as a function of the personality and so complete it. The hysteric who denies himself love is doing violence to his own nature, and his hysteric pain is an attempt to regain what he has denied himself and what he needs. That it does so crudely and pathologically is not the fault of the natural self but of the powers which deny it expression. The story of Pygmalion, in which the stone statue comes to life, bears on this theme of the coming to life of emotions and impulses which have been petrified. Such emotions are needed for the fulfilment of the personality; the symptom an attempt to make it whole. The symptom, like a high temperature, is a sign that there is something wrong with the organism; but like the temperature it is also an attempt at cure.

The function of analytic treatment is clear; it is to liberate these repressed tendencies so that they may express themselves, and develop in a form in which they would have developed if they had never been repressed.

In treatment, therefore, the psycho-physician does not regard the symptom as something to be got rid of, but as containing a source of potential energy to be released. He ranges himself, as it were, on the side of the symptom, and seeks to release the emotional tendencies bound up in it for their fuller development. By this means he not only gets rid of the symptom which is the perverted form these impulses take when they are repressed, but restores the personality to wholeness and completeness.

(XII) *The specific symptom.* A significant feature about hysteria is the multitude of forms taken by the symptom; to it has therefore been ascribed the term "protean," many-headed. In conversion hysteria the symptoms are mostly physical and affect the functions of the central nervous system. But what is it that determines the choice of symptom? Why does one patient develop a headache, another an abdominal pain, one neuritic pains in the limbs, another pain in menstruation, pain in digesting, pain in the heart, difficulty in swallowing or breathing: or how is it that one has paralysis, or weakness or tiredness of the limbs, while another develops vomiting and another loss of sensation in the skin, blindness, loss of taste, deafness. "The frequency of hysteria is no less remarkable than the multiplicity of the shapes it puts on. Few of the maladies of miserable mortality are not irritated by it," said Thomas Sydenham, as far back as 1670. Minor forms of it are far more common than the text-books would have us believe. Why the specific symptom?

(a) A great deal is made in the text-books about "medical suggestion" as the cause of a particular symptom, the question

"Have you got any pain there?" producing the pain for the next visit. We have in fact found this very rare. The malingerer is more liable to take such a hint than the hysteric.

Moreover, such a suggestion, even from a doctor, would not have any effect unless the patient is already suggestible; without such a state of mind the suggestion of the symptom would fall on stony ground. Why then, it may be asked, should a patient be prone to accept such a suggestion? It is because the symptom serves some purpose, fulfils some need of the individual. It is because the patient is already wanting to be relieved of responsibility and to get sympathy that he welcomes the suggestion of illness. It is not the suggestion but his proneness to suggestibility which is the important factor. Given such a predisposition, suggestions from any source, doctor, advertisements, sympathetic friends, previous illness or any other are capable of precipitating a particular symptom.

(b) More potent than medical suggestion is suggestion due to *identification*, which is a prolific cause of the choice of symptom. An instance of this was that of a girl who had nursed a paralysed mother for months, and when the mother died, herself developed a hysterical paralysis which put her to bed.

(c) The most common cause of all determining the choice of symptom is an *organic illness*; the hysteric symptom often starts with an operation, an attack of indigestion, influenza, neuritis, an accident. The organic condition itself passes, but the pain, paralysis, or sickness *persists as a neurotic symptom*. This accounts for the fact, so often pointed out, that *hysteric symptoms simulate any form of organic disease*, which sometimes makes the diagnosis difficult. If therefore we have an anaesthesia of the "glove" variety we may diagnose it as hysterical because it does not follow any known nerve distribution. But we cannot argue the converse—that if the patient has an anaesthesia which *does* follow the nerve distribution, it is organic for it may be a hysterical reproduction of a previous organic lesion which it therefore exactly simulates. A man who had lumbago when he heard he had lost his job simulated it later in every detail. Conditions of neurotic origin are therefore treated as organic by the general physician probably more frequently than organic conditions are treated as functional by the medical psychologist.

(i) There are several forms of organic suggestion. In some cases the symptom is due to *accidental association* in which the organic disorder happens to coincide with an acute mental conflict and is seized upon to serve the purpose of the conflict.

There was the case of the girl who had buzzing noises in her head with a feeling of giddiness and fainting; these were the sensations she experienced when she had a motor-cycle accident, in which she fell on her head and was knocked "unconscious," the buzzing sound being the noise of the racing engine, which she heard during her state of "unconsciousness." Traumatic cases such as war neurosis furnish many such instances, a soldier suffered from a pain in the chest, which originated in the fact that he happened to have pleurisy at the time he was blown up. The pleurisy had nothing to do with the conflict but was utilized as a means of escape from the conflict. In this respect our experience agrees with that of Freud who regards such an endopsychic conflict as the essential cause of the symptom, as against the French authors (Babinski, Roussy and Lermitte) who regard the disorder as being merely the result of suggestion.

(ii) An important group of this type are the "after-effects" of illness or operations.

An interesting case was that of a girl who had a severe operation on the back of her neck. After the wound had healed she continued to have an acute pain in the neck, which was assumed to be due to a nerve ending being involved in the scar tissue. The pain, however, proved to be of an entirely hysterical kind associated with the following emotional shock. In the operation some of the muscles of her neck had to be severed so that she was unable to support her head properly. When a relief nurse was dressing her wound she accidentally let her head fall back, which gave the patient a horrible jerk, and she thought her neck was broken. This pain persisted as a hysteric symptom and was entirely cured when the cause of it was discovered, and the repressed emotion of fear released.

The same applies to the so-called "after-effects" of ordinary illnesses. Fatigue after illness is usually physical, but in many cases it is the precipitation of a wish to remain ill which has seized upon this opportunity to express itself.

In one case a woman patient slept for eighteen hours a day for seven years. The reason was found to be that when she had an infant with pyloric stenosis she had very little sleep for some months; and this prolonged sleep was to make up for lost sleep and to prepare for future emergencies. The discovery of this explanation and her readjustment to the situation cured her.

The importance of these hysteric "after-effects" of illness was impressed on us during the war of 1914-18 when many patients were sent to the Neurological Hospitals suffering from so-called "after-effects" of a virulent type of influenza. Finding them on our hands, we investigated these conditions by the same methods already employed with the "shell-shock" patients, and discovered that many of these so-called "after-effects"—headaches, tiredness, indigestion—were really psychoneurotic and were cured by psychotherapy.

One such soldier patient suffered from headaches and depression, the supposed organic "after-effects" of influenza. These symptoms, however, proved to be the result not of any toxic condition but of an emotional shock, for he had been put into the "Death Ward" to die with other hopeless patients, and naturally fell into a state of dread and despair, which perpetuated the headache. The psychogenetic nature of his disorder was confirmed by the cure of his symptoms by the abre-action method.

Such cases suggest that possibly many after-effects following surgical operations as well as other illnesses may have the same psychological origin, this explanation of the after-effects of surgical operations being one that we find the surgeons are not unwilling to accept! It can readily be understood that if a patient already has a hysteric disposition, she will welcome an illness or an operation in which she is given the care and attention she has so long craved, but which she would not permit herself, and she would naturally be reluctant to leave this oasis of rest. Sometimes such patients invite illness in a more positive fashion. In one case a young woman completely fabricated an appendicitis which she therefore had operated on. (Asked what the removed appendix was like, the surgeon merely replied that she was as well without it!) This may be conscious malingering, but the malingering was done by a hysteric personality and for hysterical motives, as is so often the case. It raises the question whether healthy personalities ever malinger. Or should we distinguish a class of "hysterical malingerers" from the coward or shirker?

(iii) In many cases there is a real organic illness present, but this is greatly exaggerated in order to escape responsibility. Such is the "skrimshanker" as distinct from the pure "malingerer," for the latter consciously pretends to have an illness which he has not. In the case of the "skrimshanker" the symptoms are organic but greatly accentuated by a hysteric motive.

(iv) In a few cases, the origin of the specific symptom is not illness but purely normal physiological functions like movement of the bowels, throbbing of the heart, of which we are usually unconscious, to which the morbid emotion becomes attached. An old lady during the war was listening for the German planes one night during an air raid; as she listened she could hear its throbbing—and she went on hearing the throbbing after the war, for it was the pulsation of her own circulation in the ear to which she had now become over-attentive.

In the case of such visceral disturbances the symptoms are greatly accentuated by a hysteric motive.

(v) Amongst the most common organic disorders utilized as an hysteria are the allergies and the *psychosomatic conditions*. A psychosomatic indigestion, headache or palpitation is the direct effect of an emotion; but these symptoms may then be utilized like an organic illness, as a means of getting sympathy and escaping responsibility. So the psychosomatic symptom which was the result of the emotion is then used to satisfy the emotion by being transformed into a hysteric symptom, as we have seen. A patient may get asthma from an allergen like dust, and he may utilize this symptom, or hay fever, or migraine, as a means of getting sympathy and avoiding responsibility. But the fact that a patient utilizes his symptoms for hysteric purposes does not mean that these conditions are wholly psychogenetic. The fact that a patient gets an attack of asthma from an artificial rose, does not prove that his asthma is purely hysteric, still less that all asthma is psychogenetic, as we have seen. The same applies to some cases of mild schizophrenia: the psychogenetic factor may be cured, the basic constitutional factor remains. The so-called "cure" of a schizophrenic by psychological means does not imply that schizophrenia is psychogenetic; nor does the fact that schizophrenia has a constitutional basis mean that psychological treatment is to be excluded in any particular case. We have seen (p. 165) that the psychological factor may be merely the precipitating cause of an attack; we now see that the organic illness may be used purposively to develop a hysteria.

(vi) In other cases the patient has no present illness or other excuse by means of which he can stage his hysteria, so that he must borrow an illness from the past. That is why infantile experiences which originally got sympathy are so often revived as hysteric symptoms. This corresponds to the saying of Freud that "the hysteric suffers from reminiscences."

The girl who was semi-blind, for instance, informed us that she had never had trouble with her eyes before; but her mother corrected that by saying that at the age of four (at the time she was jealous of her brother and was feeling left out) she had measles with complications in her eyes and had to be carefully nursed in a dark room. She had previously been given sympathy for bad eyes; why not again? The

professional man with the abdominal pain had, as a boy, starved himself
in the fit of sulks and depression in which he had been thrown by his
mother's unkindness. He then got the pain as a result of over-eating
hot buttered scones, and got his mother's attention. Later in life when
he felt left out and had no other illness to fall back upon, he revived
this old symptom to call attention to himself.

An interesting case was that of a man who had very severe headaches lasting a few days, which came from a bad injury to his skull,
fractured at birth with forceps, leaving a bad scar in his forehead.
The headaches were naturally regarded as organic and due to injury;
but in analysis the patient revived all the terrible sensations and fears
at birth, which left him with such a dread of life that he resorted to the
original headache whenever life was too hard for him.

(vii) *Occupational psychoneuroses* are those in which there is a
disability of a function employed in the patient's specific occupation. It always arises where there is a loathing for work which one
is nevertheless compelled to do. The occupation disorder is a
means of escape from the situation by the production of a symptom
which makes it impossible to continue the disagreeable task.
Typical occupational psychoneuroses are clergyman's throat,
writer's cramp, telephone girl's deafness, telegraphist's cramp,
musician's neuritis, and not the least important, soldier's "shell-
shock."

An instance was that of a missionary who having translated the whole
Bible into an obscure native language was compelled by the publishers
to copy it all out in large and legible handwriting, and had to spend
eight hours a day for two years doing this. It was not surprising that
after eighteen months of this boredom he developed writer's cramp.
It was a task he must achieve or else his ten years of previous work
would go for nothing, but the weary task made him cry out in revolt,
to which his paralysis gave expression. Resort to his left hand simply
meant that this also was immediately paralysed, indicating that it was
his soul that revolted, not his hand.

Another instance of such an occupational neurosis is that of the girl
violinist who developed neuritis of the arm which prevented her
playing. This was a revolt against having to take up a career paid for by
her uncle on the condition that she put marriage out of the question.
The claims of love expressed themselves by obstructing her career.

The fact that these symptoms have to do with the functions
employed in the specific work suggests that they are due to physiological strain such as neuromuscular fatigue in writing, or the use
of the larynx in speaking. That may be in some cases, for most
clergymen use their voices badly; but if that were the only cause,

rest would put it right. Sometimes even in neurotic cases it cures temporarily in that it gives the patient some relief from the mental strain under which he is working. But it is apt to return when he returns to work. That neuromuscular fatigue is not the explanation is proved by the fact already mentioned that if in writer's cramp the patient begins to use his left hand instead of the right, he gets cramp in the left hand also, which indicates that the cause is central, and not a peripheral fatigue of the localized muscles.

The symptom chosen is necessarily one which specifically incapacitates the individual from performing a function from which he unconsciously wishes to escape. That is why the symptom takes the form of a disability to perform the particular function used in one's work. It would be useless from the point of view of escape for the telephone girl or clergyman to get a paralysed foot which would not prevent them continuing with their work.

Occupational neuroses always imply a hysteric personality, but they differ somewhat from most cases of conversion hysteria, in that (a) the symptom has to do with a disability to perform a *specific task* concerned with the uncongenial occupation; (b) that the urge may come not so much from a false super-ego as from *uncongenial circumstances*. Change of conditions will therefore sometimes cure them.

(viii) As we have indicated, the choice of symptom may also be derived from the original specific *biological reaction*. An animal in a state of danger and unable to escape, becomes paralysed with fear: soldiers under bombardment, if prevented from escape either by objective circumstances or more often because of inner inhibitions also become paralysed. Similarly, the woman with illicit but repressed sexual desires develops a paralysis which is a representation of the physiological rigidity accompanying a wished-for orgasm. Again, pain is a signal of danger, of something wrong which calls for action; in hysteria also, pain is used and indeed designed to call the attention of others to our distress, even though this is moral distress. When we are wounded we suffer pain: so when we are mentally "wounded" by a friend's disloyalty, or "hurt" by their behaviour, but do not wish to admit it, we revert to physical pain as a vivid expression of it. In all these cases, however, the symptom cannot be interpreted as a simple biological reaction, though derived from it: it is utilized by the personality to give expression to internal moral problems. So the primitive biological responses of panic, of the cry of distress, and of paralysis, find their counterparts in anxiety hysteria, hysterics and conversion hysterias respectively, but their motivations may be far more complex than a mere biological response.

(ix) The hysteric symptom may be chosen as a *symbolic expression* of the conflict. The subject of symbolism we have dealt with under the psychosomatic disorders, the main point of difference being that whilst these disorders are only expressive of the suppressed emotion, the hysteric symptom is also purposive and this perpetuates what would otherwise be a passing psychosomatic disturbance. Many disorders of the central nervous system are of this order.

The substitution of a physical fatigue for a mental fatigue, a physical pain from an intolerable mental pain, are not merely symbolic, but serve the purpose of side-tracking the attention from the real mental pain. Voluntary functions are sometimes used for the same purpose. We recall the case of the woman with a hysterical torticollis in which the permanent turning of her head to the side symbolized a turning away from the unpleasant experiences of life and so actively avoiding them. In a case of spasmodic blinking the idea was the same, shutting her eyes to the unpleasant. In another case the patient's unhappy life made her "shut herself in," with all her feelings, and this symbolized itself in chronic constipation in which everything was "held up."

(x) *Hysterical anaesthesias* are means of avoiding the unpleasant experiences of life. They are often simple inhibitions of sensory functions such as psychic blindness. There were many cases of this in the war; one of a patient whilst gazing at an enemy aeroplane coming overhead became blind, another became totally blind at sea as he watched an enemy submarine which they were chasing and which might let go a torpedo at any moment. The patient who became completely *anaesthetic* to touch and pain all over his skin got the nickname of "Pin-cushion," the symptom representing a refusal to feel anything. There were during the war a number of cases of *psychic deafness*, a means of shutting out the painful objective world of bombs and gun-fire.

Complete *loss of memory* is another indication of this avoidance of life, so that the patient desiring to forget the painful experiences of the past, may make doubly sure by forgetting his whole past life, even his name, identity and occupation. *Fugue states* are of this nature, an escape from an intolerable situation with loss of memory. Another form which this takes is *clinical regression*, in which the patient sinks back into childhood, lives and behaves like a child, in complete oblivion of all the responsibilities of life.

Another means of escaping life is to *become unconscious*, so as to obliterate everything from one's mind. Hence the forms of hysterical stupor such as we often meet with in war cases, quite apart from "concussion." They are sometimes diagnosed as narcolepsy. Conditions of *trance* are in the same category, an escape from life.

Drug addiction like alcoholism often serves the same purpose as hysterical symptoms, being a means of escape from life which is too difficult or distressing, whether objective life, or subjective problems. This remains true even if we regard it as a regression to an infantile state (to the oral state in alcoholism). In "drunkenness" the desire to escape and the means of escape are usually conscious, so that a man deliberately gets drunk in order to forget. But the cause of the drinking may be unconscious, so that the alcoholism may be compulsive and involuntary. Such is the "alcoholic," as distinct from the drunkard. But alcohol also serves to release repressed emotions and is a form of abreaction, which may partly account for its popularity all the world over; it is so far a therapeutic agency.

NOTES ON THE ESSENTIAL NATURE OF HYSTERIA

Hysteria, suggestibility and dependence. The hysteric as such, a. we have stated, is one who shrinks from responsibilty. craves for sympathy, and feels inadequate to face life. His main characteristic may therefore be summed up in the word "dependence."

Dependence is characteristic of all forms of hysteria: the conversion hysteric becomes paralysed when he is called upon to face danger, blind when he cannot bear to look at life, sick and helpless when he must have care and attention. In anxiety hysteria it takes the form of fear of life, fear of being alone, fear of everything. In hysterics he throws up his arms in helpless surrender to his emotion without aim or purpose. It is his dependence which makes the hysteric, like the child, crave for protective love and sympathy.

Evidence of this dependent attitude in the hysteric is not far to seek. The symptom itself is evidence enough; the hysteric symptom is a retreat from life, an escape from responsibility, a refuge from difficulties, a demonstration that the patient is incapable and needs help. Moreover the hysteric symptom itself is always a disability taking the form of a paralysis pain, inadequacy, weakness, fatigue or fear. It incapacitates him for life, makes it impossible for him to carry on; it is an act of surrender, a gesture of failure. In other cases the symptom is a manifest craving for sympathy, a mute appeal for pity by means of illness.

Dependence as a phase in human nature has been too much neglected as against sex and aggression. But it is of the greatest importance in child life, in social life and in all the neuroses, especially hysteria. It is also on account of the need for help and protection that these impulses to sex or aggression have to be repressed. But even this feeling of dependence which is the essence of suggestibility, appears to be based on a still more deep-seated stereotropic tendency, the tendency of an organism to keep in close contact with another body, like the starfish to the rock, the baby to its mother. It is primarily for safety and security that men and beasts join together in herds. Hysteria is a morbid manifestation of this basic need in human life.

Several other stigmata have been described by various authors as the essential feature of hysteria; such as suggestibility, dissociation, or histrionic personality.

Suggestibility has been regarded by some as the main characteristic of hysteria. Janet holds that "the first stigma of hysteria is suggestibility." Babinski has made suggestion the criterion of his "Hysteria or Pithiatism," i.e. curable by suggestion (p. 40). He defines hysteria (p. 17) as "a pathological state manifested by disorders which it is possible to reproduce exactly by suggestion in certain subjects, and can be made to disappear by the influence of persuasion alone." Hurst "On the special senses" says that hysterical symptoms are "Symptoms which result from suggestion and are curable by psychotherapy." Inasmuch as suggestibility is a characteristic of every human being, we theoretically agree with Hurst that "there is nobody who may not develop hysteria, if the provocation is sufficiently great," and with Kahn[1] when he says that "Hysteric reactions are potentially present in every man." But the fact remains that everybody does not develop hysterical symptoms even under the greatest provocation such as that of war: nor does the type of neurotic disorder depend on provocation alone, but also on the previous experiences and complexes of the patient, which makes him fall victim to the slightest provocation.

We agree as to the importance of suggestibility in hysteria. But none of these authors have explained the reason for the excessive suggestibility: indeed it is a question they have apparently not troubled to ask themselves. It is not enough to say that the hysteric patient is characterized by suggestibility; we must know what is and what causes this suggestibility. *Suggestibility is psychic dependence,* which makes us accept without question the moods and ideas of others. It is a state of mental passivity and receptivity which accepts the opinions of others without question. It implies this temporary abolition of criticism and the surrender of individual judgment, and operates particularly in these conditions, such as in a crowd and under emotional states whether fear, sex or love, which encourage dependence and the surrender of our will.

Suggestibility is probably a function of the granular layer of the cortex of the brain (which is concerned with sensory receptivity), the supra-granular or pyramidal layer (which is concerned with reason and volition) being temporarily in abeyance.[2]

[1] *Psychopathic Personality*, p. 385.
[2] Wilson: *Proceedings of the Royal Society of Medicine*, February 4, 1927.

Suggestibility is a development of the feeling of dependence. The physical dependency characteristic of infancy develops naturally at about the age of two and a half or three into suggestibility, which serves the natural function of keeping the child close to the mother, so that it may imitate her, identify itself with her, and so learn to prepare for life. This dependency and suggestibility naturally develop into the "gang spirit" which lead adolescents to surrender their wills to their leaders and implicitly obey them. Later this dependency naturally develops into social life the basis of which is *inter*-dependence on one another, making us suggestible to the moods and opinions of others. Trotter has shown,[1] that suggestibility to others and to the crowd is one of the most marked features of social life.

Suggestibility itself is therefore a normal attribute of life, the basis of sympathy, of mutual understanding, of common feeling, of corporate action, and of mutual help. Without suggestibility social life would be impossible. It is most highly developed in the higher animals which have the longer childhood, that is to say the longer period of dependence. Therefore it is those species of animals which have the longest childhood which are the most sociable.

This tendency is exaggerated in some people, either temperamentally and constitutionally, or because of over-development in early childhood. It is mainly exaggerated when the child feels deprived of protective love, for this induces an excessive dependence on others. It is morbidly manifested in timidity, in subjection, in cringing, ingratiation, over-suggestibility and other morbid characteristics, as well as in hysteria It is this dependence which determines that the hysteric is so open to the suggestion of illness: without it the suggestion of illness would have no more effect than it does on the rest of us. Conversion hysteria is a condition in which this dependence is first over-developed as a craving for love and sympathy, and then repressed, but later emerges in the symptom. In Anxiety Hysteria the dependence is due to the primal fear in infancy.

Hypnosis and hysteria. The over-suggestibility of the hysteric is demonstrated by the well-known fact that hysterics are most easily hypnotized, for dependence and passivity are the features of hypnotism as they are of hysteria. Freud has said that the difference between hysteria and obsessions lies in one relating to sexual passivity and the other to sexual activity.[2] We agree with this except that this dependency is not necessarily sexual, but a basic biological disposition.

So closely allied are hypnosis and hysteria, that some have been led to the view that hypnosis is only a form of hysteria, and is only found in hysterics. Charcot, for instance, whilst recognizing the heightened suggestibility of the hysteric, and especially the fact that he can be easily hypnotized, maintained that hypnosis was closely associated with *hystero-epilepsy*. This conclusion was based on two fallacies, first that Charcot apparently only used so-called hystero-epileptics for his

[1] *The Instincts of the Herd.*　　　　[2] *Collected Papers*, vol. 1, p. 156.

experiments, and it was therefore not difficult to "prove" a fictitious connection: and secondly, many of the phenomena he observed in these patients and regarded as characteristic of hypnotism were of his own doing, the result of his own suggestions. It is said that patients in fact knew beforehand what was expected of them! Hence the phases of his *Grande hypnotism*. It would, however, be true to say that *both hysteria and hypnotism are characterized by dependence and suggestibility*. In so far as anyone is dependent he is suggestible, but in hypnosis that dependence reaches so marked a degree that the subject is almost completely dominated by the hypnotizer, and so identified with him that the commands of the hypnotizer are implicitly obeyed and acted upon as though they were his own.

People in a crowd subject their personalities in dependence to the crowd, and are therefore suggestible, by virtue of their identification with it. But anything which tends to abolish criticism tends to suggestibility, one of the most important of which is the emotional state of the individual, for emotion tends to check thought, reason and criticism.

Dependence to authority makes a person surrender his individuality and suggestible. Fear puts a person into a state of subjection and therefore ready to follow any lead however foolish, an example of which is those statesmen who install fear into their people so that they will follow them implicitly. Being in love endows the lover with the most god-like qualities.

The histrionic and dramatic characteristics of the hysteric, which some accept as the sign of hysteria, arise partly from his excess of pent-up emotion as in the patient with hysterics, but partly from his desire to make an impression on others: he must exaggerate his needs, he must dramatize his symptom to get the attention he craves. But it cannot be taken as a primary criterion of hysteria for many people are dramatic without being hysteric and many are hysteric without being histrionic, especially the conversion hysteric with "la belle indifference."

Dissociation or splitting of the personality has been taken to be the characteristic feature of hysteria, for instance by Janet,[1] according to whom "Hysteria is a form of mental depression characterized by the retraction of the field of personal consciousness and a tendency to the dissociation and emancipation of the system of ideas and functions that constitute personality." Therefore he includes somnambulism and fugue states under hysteria.

Janet has shown that the splitting of the personality may be due to a variety of causes, constitutional, emotional, or physical like fatigue— anything in fact which leads to the "lowering of psychological tension." This differs from Freud's view that dissociation is due to active repression, this repression being due to the painfulness of the experience, or its incompatibility with the personality as a whole. These views are not exclusive, and in our experience both types of dissociation take place. There seems no doubt, and the war has given many instances of

[1] Janet, *Hysteria*, p. 332.

the fact, that dissociation can occur through physical weakness, exhaustion and disease, with confusion and loss of memory, in which case the treatment is physical rest and rehabilitation and encouragement, not psychological analysis. Dissociation in fact may simply be the disintegration of the personality which fails to hold together as a synthesis and this failure, with the resulting dissociation, may come about either because there is constitutionally lacking the energy to hold the personality together because of physical causes like fatigue, as Janet says, or because the stress of psychological conflicts may be so great that it results in repression of one part of the personality, with consequent dissociation, as Freud says.

Dissociation as such cannot be regarded as the stigma of hysteria.

There is obvious dissociation in conversion hysteria, but that is true of all the psychoneuroses; for where there is repression, there is dissociation. The phobia or the tune ringing in the head is just as dissociated as a hysteric pain; the obsessional compulsion to do a certain act is as autonomous as the hysteric's inability to use his arm. It is merely that in hysteria the dissociated symptom being physical is more apparent.

Hysteria and schizophrenia. Because it is assumed that dissociation is the stigma of hysteria, and because dissociation is a marked feature of schizophrenia as the name implies, some have assumed that schizophrenia and hysteria are related. There are some resemblances, but more differences. There is dissociation in both, there is the inability to face life in both: there may be patches of anaesthesia, and paralysis in both. But in the schizophrenic the basic cause of the failure to face life is his *constitutional* inability, whereas in the hysteric it is primarily due to early conditions in life and is psychogenic. In symptomatology the hysteric is extraverted whereas the schizophrenic is introverted; the hysteric turns to others for affection, the schizophrenic turns into himself: the hysteric wants affection, the schizophrenic wants none. The schizophrenic has given up the struggle of life, he does not even put up a fight, nor does he feel called upon, like the hysteric, to find an excuse for giving in. The hysteric struggles on in spite of his symptom, retains a purpose in life, and often a very determined purpose, whereas the schizophrenic has none. The hysteric, conversion or anxiety, has deep emotions, the schizophrenic is characterized by apathy and is unemotional. "La belle indifférence" of the hysteric is only apparent, as we have seen, due to the suppression of his emotion; the apathy of the schizoid is real and due to the constitutional lack of emotion not to its repression. The supposed superficial resemblance between the two must therefore not deceive us into identifiying them.

Other factors than dependency may, however, obtrude and give their tone to different clinical types of hysteria.

We have observed that whilst the hysteric is characterized by dependence, the obsessional is characterized by aggressiveness, and the sex pervert by sensuousness. But that is not to say that these other elements do not play a part in each case. The three main types of neuroses, we have said, are like the three primary colours, of which there may be many mixtures. In hysteria other factors than dependence may give their tone to different types of hysteria according to the amount of dependence, aggressiveness and sensuousness entering into the composition of each case.

The purely dependent type provides us with the *"pathetic hysteric"* who is full of self-pity for his pains and disabilities, who is always ill but bears up bravely, always lets you know he is ill but never asks you for your sympathy. He may weep with pain (being careful that you get to know), yet push you away if you offer sympathy. On the other hand, there is the aggressive or *"resistive hysteric"* who exploits his illness to get his own way, and tyrannizes over the whole household. Adler emphasizes the fact that the hysteric uses his symptom to gain power over others.

But aggressiveness is not the primal factor in hysterical subjects. They must have what they want, but what they want is to be cared for.

The sexual factor also plays an important part in hysteria. The woman who constantly collapsed with paralysis in front of her doctor's house did so to get a physical examination and gratify her sexuality. The sensuous hysteric may use his pain not only as self-punishment but as a means of masochistic self-gratification. The original meaning of hysteria may have a sexual significance, the womb wandering about the body, seeking for satisfaction. There is no doubt that in the condition which we have called hysterics, there is often sexual arousal and frustration, producing restlessness, emotionalism, weeping, depression, rage and sleeplessness. But sexuality may also produce anxiety states from the overplus of frustrated libido, and often psychosomatic disorders like headaches and ovarian pains. Plato in the *Timæus* recognized this as a clinical entity: "The matrix is an animal which longs to generate children. When it remains barren for a long time after puberty it finds it difficult to bear, it feels wrath, it goes about the whole body, closing the issues for the air, stopping the respiration, putting the body into extreme dangers, and occasioning various diseases, until desire and love, bringing man and woman together, make a fruit and gather it as from a tree."

Freud regards sex as the essential feature in hysteria. His dictum that "in a normal sexual life there is no neurosis" is not difficult to maintain if we start off with the premise as he does, that the Oedipus complex is universal. It is true that the hysteric is sometimes abnormal in his sexual life, but in point of fact we find those suffering from conversion hysteria surprisingly free from sexual abnormality, and they make no complaint on that score, whether man or woman. Indeed, it is curious to find that patients suffering from so much arrest of emotional development can be so sexually normal and adult. Wives who have conversion symptoms usually find normal pleasure in sex relations with their husbands; what they complain of is not lack of sexuality but lack of affection: it is their love life, not their sex life, which is starved; it is their need for security not their need for sensuous pleasure which manifests itself in their symptoms. The hysteric symptoms take the form of an illness and disability, designed to secure the care and sympathy of others, not as a rule to satisfy sexual desires. But if the sexual element dominates over the dependent element, as it does in masochism, we regard the condition as a sex perversion, and not hysteria. Patients suffering from anxiety hysteria, on the other hand, are often impotent or frigid since fear naturally inhibits sex. These facts were amply demonstrated in the cases of war neurosis in the two World Wars.

If we may then summarize the various characteristics of hysteria: hysteria is an exaggerated condition of dependence and suggestibility derived mainly from the feeling of deprivation of love. This produces an abnormal craving for affection and sympathy, and a shrinking from life and responsibility. This abnormal craving for affection becomes repressed, and produces a dissociation of the personality. This craving for love aroused by later conditions is unable to restrain itself any longer and emerges, now as hysterics, anxiety hysteria or conversion hysteria, all of which are biological reactions expressive of inadequacy to face life, but are then used as means of evading the responsibilities of life and securing the attention and sympathy of those on whom the individual depends.

CHAPTER IX

ANXIETY STATES

ANXIETY is a morbid condition of fear. Its forms are varied, and as numerous as the sands on the seashore; for there is nothing on earth or in the heavens, nor in the mind of man, which may not be the object of morbid fear. In the form of "worry" it is one of the most common distractions of daily life, from which few people are fortunate enough to escape.

We use the term anxiety state to cover all forms of morbid anxiety, whether neurotic or otherwise.

Fear is a normal constituent of life. Biologically it sharpens our perception, makes us alert to detect danger; it releases energy necessary to cope with the situation and is a spur to action. The need to cope with the dangers and difficulties of life makes man courageous, determined, self-controlled, and so develops qualities of character. It is primarily fear which makes men band themselves together in social communities for mutual protection against the common danger, and thus becomes a basis of communal life. Being a member of society, man must pay regard to its demands; and the desire for the goodwill of his fellows, born in the first place of the need for security, encourages social and moral qualities, and leads to consideration of others, politeness and cultural pursuits. Fear, in the broadest sense, may therefore be said to be one of the basic factors in social, ethical and cultural life.

But fear may paralyse as well as act as an incentive to action; instead of being a spur, it may fill our minds with such morbid dread that we cannot act at all and are reduced to dithering incompetence; instead of making us alert it confuses us. Fear of starvation may urge us to work hard, but fear of losing our job may make us inefficient. Fear of consequences may make us deceitful or cowardly; it is fear which makes the child lie and the adult secretive; fear of the past may darken our future, fear of the future may fill our present with apprehension and dread. Fear is as much a cause of war as is aggressiveness, for agressiveness often arises from fear. The fear of hell which the Church inculcated in past ages may have helped to make men moral, but undoubtedly cast a gloom over the whole of life, and probably produced more unhappiness than the hope of heaven ever produced of happiness.

Fear may stir men to bravery, but it may also transform the courageous man into the hopeless neurotic, afraid of his own shadow. The fear that binds us into communities may be turned into the fear of breaking the laws and taboos of society, and produce an obsession.

One of the main problems of "social security" is how to secure freedom from want so as to rid ourselves of the fear which paralyses, without getting rid of the fear which is an incentive to action and a spur to endeavour.

Fear and anxiety are constituents of many behaviour disorders and of most psychoneuroses. They are the dominant symptom in anxiety neuroses such as a phobia of travelling in trains, or a morbid fear of contamination which makes a woman live in bed for the rest of her life covered with sterilized gauze. They are present in many cases of conversion hysteria, especially traumatic hysteria, which is an escape from fear. Sex perversions are often resorted to as a solace from fear, as we may observe in the child; and obsessional acts are propitiations to avert the fear of consequences of our forbidden impulses.

It is not surprising that many consider that *fear is the basic factor in psychopathology.*

But fear is due to lack of security and protective love which is the *cause of most abnormal reactions.*

Fear is also the most common cause of repression for it is for fear of consequences that a child is compelled to repress its hate, its jealousy or its sex pleasure, so that these impulses being repressed are transformed into morbid character traits or psychoneuroses. So varied are the forms, so tragic may be the consequences of fear and anxiety, that it is of the greatest importance to pay regard to this, one of the most compelling forces in human nature, not only for an understanding of the psychoneuroses, but for social psychiatry and human behaviour in general.

THE NATURE OF ANXIETY

To understand the nature of anxiety we must see its relation to other mental processes.

Impulse. We have seen that when the organism is confronted with a critical situation it prepares for action by the activation of the autonomic nervous system, releases energy for the emergency, and discharges this energy in voluntary mobility as an impulse. Such impulses are directed towards the adaptation of the organism to the particular condition of the environment which calls it forth;

fear reactions, if the situation is one of danger; pugnacity if the individual is thwarted or attacked; sex if aroused by the appropriate stimulus; tenderness in the presence of a helpless offspring. The expression of this energy in a specific direction we call an "impulse." The word impulse may be used either of energy itself, so that a man may say he had an impulse to fight, though he did not actually do so; or, preferably, of the actual discharge of energy itself as in attack. Ordinarily the production of energy should be commensurate with the demands of the situation, in which case we may speak of it as a *simple impulse*: we are hungry, reach out for food, eat and are satisfied; we see a car coming towards us, anticipate danger, and step out of the way; a man accuses us, we have a perfect reply and so keep calm. There is in all this little or no excitement, emotion or feeling, for the impulse is one in which the response is exactly commensurate with the demand of the occasion.

Excitement. But prior to the discharge of energy as an impulse, the whole organism, body and mind, may work itself up into a state of tension which we commonly call *excitement* or excitability. This excitement is irrespective of the emotion it subserves: so we speak of being sexually excited, or of nervous excitement when we are afraid, and we tell a man "not to be excited" when he is getting angry. Excitement as such is relatively undifferentiated. But as the excitement increases and becomes more intense, the energy tends to assume a more specific form, and discharges itself as an impulse to bring about a desired end, such as an impulse to run, to answer back, or to plead for mercy, as we have seen.

Feeling. Sometimes the stimulus may be so slight and the excitement of so mild a nature that it is not strong enough to produce a response in the form of an impulse, but merely affects our viscera and arouses changes in the heart and other organs, which we only sense or feel. *The consciousness of these bodily changes we call "feeling" or "affect."* They may not be sufficient to arouse us to action, but only to "affect" us with feelings of pleasure or displeasure, comfort or discomfort: or they may be more specifically related to certain emotions, such as a feeling of annoyance in the case of anger, of apprehension in the case of fear, or of sentimentality in the case of love, for sentimentality is love without action. If these affective states tend to persist we call them "moods," such as an irritable mood or a depressed mood. A mood is a persisting feeling devoid of action. Feelings then primarily arise from consciousness of changes in the organism, which affect us; and we therefore suggest that James's definition of an emotion as "the sensation of our bodily changes" is really a more appropriate definition of feeling than of emotion; for an emotion, as the word implies, is better used of an active conative process like rage, and not merely of a "sensation," as we shall see.[1]

One characteristic of feeling as distinct from the special senses or from cognitive processes is its *vagueness*, which is to be expected since it arises from changes in the autonomic nervous functions. So much is this the case that when any emotion or cognitive process is vague, we are apt to speak of it as a feeling; so we speak of a feeling of uncertainty, of hope, of confidence, or familiarity, and we say, "I have a feeling I know that person," or "I have a funny feeling in my head," when it is something undefined. Another characteristic of feeling is its *wide distribution*, which is also to be accounted for by the fact that it is associated with the autonomic nervous system, whose ramifications are widespread throughout the whole body which is "affected"; so we feel "all over" in love, are "full" of despair, and the feeling is not confined to any one part, as in the case of the special senses like sight. It is very difficult to localize a feeling of apprehension or of uncertainty.

Feelings then may exist when the stimulus affects us but is too weak to produce any conative activity or impulse, as we have instanced above. But if feelings are the consciousness or awareness of our bodily changes, they will also accompany the most ardent passions of rage and fear, for when the organism is aroused to great excitement violent changes take place in the viscera, the sensations of which arouse in us the strongest feelings, as in the case of dread.

Feelings themselves may, because of the physical tension, *become a stimulus and impetus to action*, first as excitement, and then, as the tension increases, as an impulse. Thus consciousness of bodily discomfort aids the original biological urge to change our position. The discomfort of hunger is an incentive to make us seek food, annoyance urges us to remove the irritation, danger makes us apprehensive, and apprehension discharges itself as an impulse to flight. Pleasant feelings are also a stimulus to action, encouraging us to strive for what gives us pleasure. But even

---

[1] We do not fear because we run away (as James says): the stimulus of danger produces the biological urge to flight, which is associated with violent visceral changes preparatory to action. These changes produce feelings of apprehension, and the energy produced finally discharges itself in flight, which tends rather to ease the tension of fear than produce it. *The feeling is associated with the visceral changes, not with the flight.* On the whole, therefore, the balance is in favour of the popular view that we run away because we fear.

pleasant feelings may become unpleasant if too intensive or too prolonged, a provision of nature which is an encouragement to constant change of action, and guards us against taking an excess of what may be otherwise desirable; for we may have too much even of a good thing. We get fed up with delicacies, bored with a surfeit of sex; we long for rest, but continuous inactivity makes us restless; in winter we long to bask in the sun, but in summer a few days of heat makes us feel oppressive and welcome the cool shade. So nature keeps us always on the move; she tempts with pleasures and then makes the pleasure nauseating, and thus provokes us to seek for something new. Thus both pleasant and unpleasant feelings act as a perpetual incentive to action.

Emotion. A simple impulse discharges itself in action as an impulse: we see a car coming and we step out of the way. But suppose, for any reason, we cannot escape so easily from the situation of danger (when for instance the car is suddenly upon us), then the energy produced cannot find immediate discharge and is temporarily dammed up within the organism, throwing it into a state of great excitement and tension, until it discharges itself in action, and we leap to safety! *This condition of accumulation of energy prior to discharge we call an emotion,* such as an emotion of fear or anger.[1]

Such an accumulation of energy is of biological value in that it makes the discharge more urgent and compulsive, giving the impulse greater driving force, just as the head of water above a weir makes the surge of water all the more powerful. That is why when any impulse is checked it becomes the stronger: for the accumulation of energy has the effect of sweeping away all obstacles to the full expression of the impulse for the attainment of its ends. Popular opinion has always therefore regarded emotion as a driving force—"fear impelled me," "rage gave him super-human strength." Emotion is what moves us, as the name implies.[2]

[1] The term "affect," used in psychology as synonymous with "feeling," is now used in psychopathology to describe these conative-affective experiences, but there is no reason why we should not retain the original term "emotion" to express these experiences in spite of the fact that the term emotion has received so many meanings and definitions at the hands of psychologists.

[2] This view of emotion as signifying the accumulation of energy before discharge not only agrees with the popular view of emotion as a driving force, but it is not inconsistent with the view of McDougall (*Outline*, p. 322) who defines emotion as the sum of the physiological effects when an instinctive impulse is brought into play. Nor is it altogether inconsistent with the view of those psychologists who hold that our emotions only occur when our impulse is being thwarted (J. Drever, *Instincts in Man*). But we cannot agree with Claparède, who goes so far as to say that "fear is only experienced when flight is *impossible*" (*Feelings and Emotions*, p. 126).

Normal emotion is aroused by an appropriate stimulus, and although temporarily held up, ultimately discharges itself in purposive action.

Anxiety. But suppose the danger is upon us and action is impossible, these energies, unable to discharge themselves in voluntary action, discharge themselves in violent trembling, palpitation, difficult breathing and other psychosomatic disorders aleady discussed, and also violent mental changes of *anxiety and dread.*

Anxiety is frustrated fear: it arises from the state of tension when we can do nothing to meet the situation, when escape is impossible. It differs from the normal *emotion* of fear which though temporarily held up, ultimately discharges itself in purposive action.

Some psychologists, like Hart, regard fear as being aroused by objective stimuli, whereas anxiety is stimulated from some internal cause. This is hardly satisfactory, for surely we can be in a state of anxiety when awaiting the crash of a bomb, or when being driven at seventy miles an hour along a busy highway. Also we may have a real fear of our impulses from within. *The difference between fear and anxiety lies not in the nature of the stimulus but in the effectiveness or otherwise of the discharge*; in fear the discharge in purposive activity is normal and effective, in anxiety the discharge is frustrated and expends itself in useless and purposeless movements of panic and in a dread that paralyses and renders us inefficient to cope with the situation.

Strictly speaking *anxiety is specific to fear,* and implies a threat to our personality whether from within ourselves or from without. There is no specific term to describe the corresponding experience when anger and sex are thwarted, so that we often use the term anxiety of these also, as when we are "anxious" to get our own back. There is, however, some justification for this usage, for the thwarting of any of our impulses is a threat to our personality, and any threat is associated with fear. When we say we are "anxious to do well," our anxiety is lest we do badly. So we may suffer from "anxiety states" as we can from psychosomatic disorders from the frustration of *any* emotion. On the other hand, these impulses of rage and sex may themselves be the object of fear when they threaten the aims of the personality as a whole. This as we shall see is the basic problem in obsessional anxiety.

A condition often closely related and so confused with anxiety is that of *depression*: but they are different experiences. For in anxiety there is still the effort to achieve, to overcome the frustration;

whereas depression comes when we have given up hope and cease to make any effort.

All anxiety is abnormal; for in any given situation of danger we ought to be able to produce exactly the requisite amount of energy and to discharge it in purposive action as a simple impulse. But this is a counsel of perfection, for it is natural to have "anxiety" before we hear the result of an examination, receive news of a friend being operated on, contemplate proposing to a girl, take our first aeroplane flight, or await the reply to a rude letter we have written. Such anxiety may not be normal, in that it is a waste of energy, but it is very natural! Indeed, the "anxiety" experienced, say before making a speech or running a 100 yards race, is generally regarded as a good sign, for at least it indicates a surplus of energy and therefore the preparedness of the organism for action, like a steamer letting off the pressure of steam before it leaves the quay-side: it may be a waste of steam, but it is also a sign of preparedness. In any case the anxiety in these instances may be regarded as normal in so far as the energy is later discharged in action, and disappears as soon as we run the race, or have proposed to the girl; or it may give place to depression! But where it cannot be so discharged it becomes chronic and definitely abnormal.

Whilst, therefore, we may regard a certain amount of anxiety as natural, if it is exaggerated it acts as a hindrance instead of a help, so that we may be so anxious that we are unable to make the speech or concentrate on the examination at all; we may make a bad start in the race or fumble in proposing to the girl. Anxiety may also distort our actions and make us, for instance, too aggressive in our interview to cover our sense of inferiority.

This conception of anxiety as thwarted fear helps us to understand why, when we have a crash in an aeroplane, a fall from a horse, an accident driving a car, it is better immediately to go up again, to mount the horse or to drive the car, for this gives outlet to the accumulated emotion in purposive action. Indeed, *to do anything* is better than to do nothing, as long as the pent-up energy discharges itself in voluntary mobility. In a state of crisis, individual or national, an accident in the street or the invasion of a foe, people therefore clamour for "somebody to do something," it does not matter what, since any action even if useless helps to relieve their anxiety. A harassed woman in the London blitz remarked, "If I were an airman and could *do* something about it, I should not be suffering so!" The man who runs away, shows his anger, or expresses his guilt, even in words alone (as in the confessional, or by getting it off his chest to a friend, or in analysis), has a sense of relief of mind as well as of his psychosomatic symptoms, because the energy has found outlet and the organism is restored to equilibrium.

Anxiety tends to be *chronic*; it persists more than normal fear, for when the emotion of fear has discharged itself in action the organism is restored to equilibrium and the fear ceases to exist. Anxiety, on the other hand, failing to find proper discharge for the energy, tends to become chronic and subject to the principle of perseveration, the tendency to revert back to an unsolved problem. This is what we mean by worry. It is still more chronic when the cause of the fear is something within ourselves, and especially if that is unknown, as in neurotic anxiety.

We conclude, then, that whilst the emotion of fear is normal in that it is directed towards an end and may be biologically healthy, anxiety must be regarded as abnormal expressing itself in dread and purposeless movements.

CLINICAL TYPES OF ANXIETY

Clinical types of anxiety vary from the almost normal type we have just described as experienced before an examination, to the most complicated forms of anxiety, such as we find in obsessional guilt.

(a) Ordinary Objective Anxiety

Ordinary objective anxiety is the condition in which there is an *adequate objective danger, but inadequacy of response,* because of the impossibility of escape: it is the anxiety of ordinary life. This is the kind of anxiety we experience when in the trenches, at "action stations" in a ship, when we are cut off by the tide, stuck half way up a cliff, facing financial ruin, or in the presence of dangerous illness in someone we love. The stimulus is objective; the fear is justified; but it is true anxiety since the fear has to be held in check without opportunity for discharge. The fears of infancy are typically of this nature for in a state of dread the infant can do nothing about it. Therefore the first year of life is the typical age for the origin of anxiety states, which are reproduced in later phobias. Most anxiety hysteria like agoraphobia originates at this early age.

(b) Ordinary Conditioned Anxiety

Ordinary conditioned anxiety differs from ordinary objective anxiety in that the response is occasioned not only by the present stimulus but by *reinforcement from earlier experiences*, and therefore exaggerated; such is a fear of a barking dog, of water, or of the dark. The present situation is insufficient to account for its excess; the individual is already predisposed.

Ordinary conditioned anxiety may be specific or generalized.

(i) *Specific conditioned anxieties* are those in which the fear has become attached to some special object or situation, like the fear of water from having fallen into a river in childhood, fear of suffocation from having a pillow over the face in infancy, or fear of doctors from an early operation. The actual stimulus of danger may be slight, the mere sight of water being sufficient to cause a panic. They are abnormal in that they have little relation to present danger, and they are exaggerated because the fear of the past becomes added to the slight fear occasioned by the present situation. We cannot cope adequately with them, since the main source of the fear is unknown, and the fear is therefore transformed into anxiety.

Conditioned fears often arise because of the tendency of a child to universalize its experiences, or rather to fail to discriminate between danger stimuli. If a stranger terrifies a child, a child may thereafter be terrified of all strangers: if one feels guilty, then the sight of all policemen makes one self-conscious. This no doubt has its value as a biological precaution, for since one stranger can harm one, others may do the same. But it means that we are subject to terror on many occasions when it is quite unjustified, so that the man once blown up, leaps under his bed every time a door bangs, and feels foolish.

Specific fears of childhood usually pass away, just as all conditioned reflexes pass away unless they are reinforced. But if they are reinforced they may become chronic—so the man who was suffocated in infancy may get over this, but may have it reinforced by being shut up in a tunnel. Thus we find that many attacks of claustrophobia relate back to long-forgotten experiences, such as suffocation at birth.

(ii) Generalized conditioned anxiety constitutes a "nervous disposition." A child who is subjected to constant illness or operations, to a disordered house, quarrels amongst parents, or any generalized cause of insecurity may develop an anxiety towards life; he sees danger at every corner, feels apprehensive at every new situation, shrinks from every new task and grows up with a nervous disposition.

The treatment of conditioned fears and anxieties is by *reconditioning*; so a child may be cured of a fear of the dark by someone sleeping with him to give him the sense of assurance; whereas to try to toughen him may only reinforce his fears. In other cases morbid fears may be cured by *explanation*, as in the case of the boy who as a small child was terrified of all noises. This was derived from his grandmother who had a fear of thunderstorms and made him so by suggestion. This became a great humiliation to him before other children. An explanation of this origin of his fear was sufficient to cure him, for on hearing it he remarked, "Oh! I see it was Granny who was the fool, not me!" He was later employed dropping depth charges at sea. Generalized anxiety may also be favourably treated by *suggestion*, which brings confidence to the despairing and courage to the fearful. Suggestion may also be used to break the morbid association between the fear and its object in specific phobias.

(c) Ordinary Subjective Anxiety

Ordinary subjective anxiety is that in which *the source of danger is from within*, threats from our impulses and desires, but of which we are quite conscious. There are dangers from within as well as from without: a man may fear not only shells and explosions, illness or losing his job, but his own temper. These are threats of which he is aware, arising from his aggressiveness and from the consequences of his sexual passions: there lurks danger in his tendency to lethargy and indolence. He may be afraid of being rude, or of making a fool of himself. A man breaks down, not only when he is betrayed by circumstances, but when he becomes a traitor to himself: he dreads those sinister evil forces within himself which sap his strength and cause his courage to run away like water. These threats to our personality, to our social, moral or spiritual self, may be as real as threats to our physical organism. A man may fear for the loss of his honour more than death; he may indeed take his own life so as to avoid the disgrace of cowardice, as many have done on the field of battle, or disgrace of bankruptcy, or dishonouring his family. We first identify ourselves with an ideal standard, and then fear those impulses which threaten its integrity. In the broadest issue fear arises from the sense of annihilation, of obliteration of the self, and this may apply as much to our moral self as to our physical self.

These dangers from within are very liable to produce anxiety because of the impossibility of escape from ourselves: moreover the inhibiting forces preventing the expression of these emotions are also within ourselves; the whole conflict is subjective.

Ordinary subjective anxiety is distinguished from neurotic

anxiety in that *the source of the danger is recognized*. A man may be perfectly aware of his temptation to be a coward, or to take the easy path in business which threatens his moral integrity, or of his temper which will lead him to humiliation, or his self-importance which leaves him open to ridicule. Not only in these cases is the threat to the integrity of his personality a conscious one, but he is justified in being afraid, that is why we call it *ordinary* anxiety: yet inasmuch as the cause of the fear arises from within ourselves we call it *subjective*; and since we can find no escape from it, it is true *anxiety*. Hence the term "ordinary subjective anxiety."[1]

(d) Neurotic Anxiety

Popular psychology ascribes most abnormal fears to objective situations of the types we have mentioned, as the sole cause of phobias. But if such fears of falling, of the dark, of suffocation persist, we have strong reasons to suspect that they are not as simple as they appear, but represent a more deep-seated subjective fear which has been projected on to this objective danger, as analysis so often proves. The fear of dogs may be on account of having been bitten by a dog; but it may also symbolize fear of an angry father. But to go further, the father may not be angry, and the fear may come only from a sense of guilt which is deserving of such anger. Phobias are often objective fears regarded as the consequences of forbidden desires, and the night terrors of children are commonly of this type—moral fears.

Neurotic anxiety is a form of anxiety state in which the cause of the fear is not only subjective, but *repressed and unconscious*. The term "neurotic" is sometimes used of all morbid anxiety such as a conditioned fear of water. But we prefer to use the term "neurotic" and "anxiety neurosis" in the sense of all conditions of morbid

---

[1] Freud dividing the functions of the personality into the Id (our primitive self), the Ego (that part which faces reality) and the Super-ego (our moral self), has stated that fear is always on the part of the Ego, whose fear is derived from three quarters, fear from the external world, from the Id and from the Super-ego. But surely Freud is confusing the "Ego" as meaning the personality as a whole, and the "Ego" in the more limited sense in which he has defined it. It is true that the personality as a whole (the Ego in that sense) does have fears from these three quarters: for fear and anxiety may arise from any threat to our personality. But any of the three functions of the personality may be "afraid" of the others. The Super-ego, or moral self, can fear the impulses of the Id, as well as external circumstances which threaten its integrity; the Id, or primitive impulses can fear the Super-ego and the Ego, which threaten to annihilate it, and frustrate its desires: and the Ego (in the Freudian sense representing the reality principle) may fear the impulses of the Id like aggressiveness, which may get it into danger, or the demands of the Super-ego which threaten it, as a man's sense of honour may endanger his life in battle.

anxiety which are the result of repression and dissociation, the objects of which are unknown and unconscious.[1]

Because of the hidden nature of these fears we cannot cope with them adequately, so that the fear turns into anxiety. Because they are repressed they are *dissociated*; because dissociated they are *beyond the control of the will*; and because the true object of fear is unknown they often *project themselves* on to other objects of fear, and manifest themselves in abnormal forms as phobias. These are the characteristics of a psychoneurosis proper—repression, dissociation, and unconscious motivation of the symptom.

Anxiety Hysteria is one form of anxiety neurosis: it is a clinical term which has not been clearly defined, but we shall use it of those forms of neurotic anxiety in which *fear of harm to ourselves* is the main motive, such as claustrophobia, fear of suffocation, agoraphobia or fear of open spaces, fear of isolation, of loneliness, of the dark, of illness or of death, or a vague generalized fear of nothing in particular which is liable to develop into a fear of everything in general.

But such phobias may be derived from two sources: some of them are of a purely hysteric type merely due to the revival of some repressed fear; some are of an obsessional type, the fear of the consequences of our forbidden desires.[2]

Anxiety hysteria is therefore of two types: (i) *Hysterical Anxiety* is that in which the anxiety is a reproduction or *revival of a repressed dread* in childhood. (ii) *Obsessional Anxiety is a fear of a forbidden impulse in ourselves*, especially sex or aggression. The latter is characterized by self-will and assertiveness, and therefore takes on a compulsive form; for every time the self-willed impulse is activated there is also aroused the fear of consequences. In both of them the fear of harm to oneself is the dominant motive. (iii) But apart from these there are phobias which take the form

[1] The present-day use of the term "anxiety neurosis" differs from Freud's original conception of anxiety neurosis which is physiological and largely quantitative, due to the excess of production of libido over discharge, as in "coitus interruptus." We are encouraged in the more *general* use of the term by the statement of Ernest Jones (*Psychoanalysis*, p. 506) who says that "there is no difference of principle between the conceptions of anxiety neurosis and anxiety hysteria. . . . The anxiety neurosis may thus be regarded as a single type or a syndrome of anxiety hysteria."

[2] As regards the distinction between Hysterical and Obsessional anxiety, Freud (*Introd. Lectures*, p. 334) says, "We group all these phobias under anxiety hysteria, that is, we regard them as closely allied to the well-known disorder called conversion hysteria." But he does not say what the connection is, nor does he appear to admit the distinction between the hysterical and the obsessional type of phobia. Indeed he says that what used to be regarded as obsessional are now to be regarded as anxiety hysteria. E. Jones, on the other hand (*Papers*, p. 476), speaks of "obsessive phobias" as distinct from anxiety hysteria. In this we concur.

of *fear of harm to others*, such as fear of poisoning, of strangling, of stabbing in which the aggressive element is more apparent. These for want of a better term we shall call *Compulsive or obsessional aggressions.* (iv) The term *Sex obsessions* we shall use of those conditions like the fear of raping in which the forbidden sex element appears in the phobia and which differ, as we shall see, from ordinary sex perversions in being compulsive and repulsive not desired. They are like the obsessional aggressions but the forbidden desire which emerges into consciousness in the symptom is sexual not aggressive.

All these neurotic types we shall deal with in later chapters.

OTHER MORBID AFFECTIVE STATES

We have so far dealt with fear and anxiety. But there are many other affective states like depression, shame, disgust, humiliation, self-consciousness, guilt, and a feeling of inferiority which play precisely the same rôle as fear in the production of morbid states. Such feelings may frustrate our whole personality and ruin our happiness, as those suffering from shyness, self-consciousness and an inferiority complex can testify. A man may be overwhelmed with symptoms of shame, or depression, as he may with a phobia. Such morbid emotions may be simple and objective such as depression due to objective conditions, which is justified, but about which we can do nothing: or they may be ordinary and subjective like the shame at our own conscious folly; they may be conditioned like the inferiority complex derived from conditions in childhood, which is constantly revived; or they may be neurotic.

These affective states may, like fear, be the *agents of repression*, for a feeling of shame may be just as effective as fear in repressing sex; and a feeling of inferiority may make us repress our assertiveness. But these affective states may, like fear, be themselves repressed and give rise to opposite *abnormal reaction traits*, the repression of the feeling of inferiority, for instance, making us bumptious, or the repression of the feeling of aggressiveness making us ingratiating. Or if repressed, they may produce *psychosomatic disorders*, such as neurotic blushing due to a repressed feeling of shame, or sweating due to repressed guilt. But the repressed shame or depression may themselves emerge, as fear does, in the form of a *psychoneurotic symptom*, as a feeling of inferiority or a morbid depression, when there appears no justification, cause or reason for the feelings.

Thus, as with fear, these neurotic affective states may be of the hysteric type, the *mere revival* of some old repressed feelings of shame, guilt or depression. On the other hand, these morbid emotions may be of an obsessional kind, being *the consequence of some forbidden desire* of which we are unconscious, but which persists and therefore produces a chronic obsessional sense of disgrace, shame, guilt or disgust with oneself which seem entirely unreasonable because the cause is unknown. The aggressive child is humiliated, the showing-off child, if snubbed, made to feel ashamed, the sexual child disgusting, so that later it both fears these tendencies and feels the sense of humiliation, depression or shame whenever the feelings are aroused even though it may not be aware of what they are. With these we shall deal later.

The Mental Hygiene of these affective states of fear, depression and the rest follows as a consequence of this psychopathology. In so far as anxiety originates in early childhood from *objective causes* of fear, whether from birth, illness, lack of protection, unkindness, jealousy of parents, brothers and sisters, or from operations such as circumcision and adenoids, these objective causes should as far as possible be avoided; but if they are inevitable, the greatest care should be taken to give the child affection and love so that it may have the sense of security. The same applies to depression, self-consciousness, exaggerated shame and guilt or a feeling of inferiority, the causes of which should be avoided. Yet these are the very punishments and threats so often inflicted on the child by the parent.

It is the function of the parent to give the child reassurance not fear, to adapt the child to life so that he feels confident to meet its demands and responsibilities, not to make him feel inferior and ashamed of himself. To force the child to face life's objective problems too soon is to exact too much, so that he shrinks before it in fear. To inflict upon a child moral demands which he cannot live up to and which in fact the parent does not live up to, is inviting trouble since it compels the child to repress his natural self, thereby producing a conflict within the personality, and possibly a subsequent obsessional neurosis.

The function of education is the establishment of such aims and moral standards as will utilize and direct these emotional tendencies, so that they are at the service of the personality, and the child goes into life full of confidence in himself and for that very reason willing and able to conform to life and co-operate in a social community. This is a task requiring the greatest skill, intelligence, and common sense in the parent: yet that is what is demanded of every parent! Those parents can best give effect to it who are themselves healthy-minded.

CHAPTER X

ANXIETY HYSTERIA

ANXIETY hysteria is characterized by morbid fear of harm to oneself, typical examples of which are agoraphobia, claustrophobia, fear of illness, of operations, of accidents, of loneliness, of separation, which are the reproduction of repressed primal fears in infancy.

It is of two main types, hysterical and obsessional. Hysterical anxiety is the emergence of suppressed and repressed fears; obsessional anxiety is the fear of the consequences of forbidden impulses. Both are characterized by fear of harm to oneself, both are derived from infantile objective fears, and both may take precisely the same form. It is the former which clinically most commonly goes by the name of anxiety hysteria.

Hysterical anxiety, with which we deal in this chapter, may be divided into three groups: (a) In the first type, morbid fear is used in precisely the same way, and for precisely the same purpose, as a conversion hysteria, namely as a means of getting notice and attention. (b) Secondly, there is the type in which the illness is unconsciously desired, as is conversion hysteria, but it is feared because of its dreaded consequences. So we develop a fear of the illness we desire, instead of developing the disability itself. (c) In the third type there is a primal fear in infancy which has been repressed by an attitude of independence and self-sufficiency, but which emerges in its original form as a fear of loneliness, separation or suffocation.

We observe a *transition from conversion to anxiety hysteria.*

(a) The first form of chronic hysterical anxiety is that in which fear or anxiety is used, precisely in the same way as a conversion hysteria paralysis or blindness may be used, as an unconscious means of getting attention and sympathy, or as a means of escape from responsibility. One child gets attention by developing a pain in the back; another child by developing a fear. We have heard a child, after being put to bed, call out for her mother to come to her, and when her persistence was of no avail shout, "Oh! Oh! Come! I'm afraid!" She was using fear as a means of getting the attention she wanted, in this case deliberately. But then comes the time when the process becomes unconscious and automatic, and the child becomes victim of its own fears. In other cases children use fear, as they may use conversion hysteria, as a means of getting the sensuous comfort and sexual gratification from being petted.

A patient suffering from anxiety neurosis revives its infantile causes. "I have that anxiety because I can't call out and I can't call attention to myself. The only way I can call attention to myself is by being anxious. If I forget to be afraid, and so remind people of my existence, I should be forgotten. If I am left in your waiting room now for a quarter of an hour, I should be forgotten if I didn't get into a panic and so call attention to myself. I don't howl because I'll be slapped if I do. To be anxious is the only thing I can do not to die, not to be annihilated. If I allow that anxiety to go out of my head I sink into nothingness: I should be passive and restful, which would be very nice, but I should die."

Which of these an individual adopts, whether the conversion symptom or anxiety, depends partly on circumstances, but partly on which is found to be the most effective in getting what is wanted.

Where the process is conscious and deliberate it is malingering, as in this case. If the mother yields it encourages the child in later life to resort to anxiety hysterics whenever she does not get what she wants, and this becomes a habitual response to any difficulty in life. If on the other hand the mother does not come, further developments may take place. One child realizing that the game is up goes to sleep. But in another child the assumed fear turns into a real one, for she argues, "Suppose I am *really* ill, and mother does not come!" She then becomes the victim of the panic she has herself induced. At first voluntarily evoked, the fear becomes a monster, and she becomes terrified of the creature she has created. In such a case the child is terrified of her own voice and stops crying, but lies in bed in a state of abject dread, whilst the mother congratulates herself on the success of her firm treatment. In fact she is laying up a possible neurosis for her child, but whether the neurosis actually develops depends on later factors.

(b) Thus a second type of hysterical anxiety is that in which the patient, like the conversion hysteric, wants to develop an illness to get sympathy, but fears it; and this for two reasons. (i) In the first place he wishes to be ill, but owing to the fact that he has already had an illness in early childhood, he dreads its recurrence. So he fears the illness which he wishes and he wishes the illness which he fears; thus he develops a phobia of illness, a fear of his wish.

A simple case in which the anxiety hysteria represented a repressed wish was that of a girl of sixteen who like her mother had a fear of illness. In infancy she felt neglected because she was healthy and her older brother an invalid. She tried crying to get attention, which was no use. Then she tried being ill as it was that which won attention for her brother, and this succeeded; until one time she pretended it and her father seeing that she was putting it on, insisted on taking her mother out. Then the girl felt that suppose she was really ill and needed her mother, her mother might refuse to stay! She could no longer rely on her mother: so she gave up the desire to be ill, said she wanted no one's sympathy, and assumed an attitude of independence and self-sufficiency. But at puberty when there is the natural tendency in a girl to be dependent and to want to be loved, a conflict arose between the old independent self-sufficiency and this desire for love which reawakened the original repressed desire for love in early childhood. She would not *say* she wanted affection from her parents because she had already eschewed it in favour of independence; she could not *be* ill because she already feared illness: so the symptom which emerged was the fear of illness. This was at once a means of getting attention like any conversion hysteria, but was also a genuine fear of the illness she wished. The precipitation of the fear was the sight of other girls being ill in the Sanatorium with measles. This aroused in her both the desire to be ill to get the same care and attention for which she longed, but also the dread of this wish.

(ii) The second reason why the patient does not develop an actual illness like the conversion hysteric is that whilst he has a wish to be ill to escape responsibility he has built up a sense of power and self-sufficiency in the way already described, and this power psychology will not permit him to develop an actual illness, as the conversion hysteric does. An illness is a disability, an incapacity, a threat to his power, and contradicts all that he now stands for. Therefore whilst the conversion hysteric being a more dependent type develops an illness, the anxiety hysteric only fears it, because it is a threat to his power.

(c) In the third type there is a primal fear in infancy which is repressed in favour of an attitude of independence and self-sufficiency which becomes the dominant characteristic of the patient: there is no one else to protect him, therefore he must protect himself, there is no one whom he can trust, therefore he must rely on himself and be self-sufficient. He therefore represses his fear and assumes an attitude of bravado and self-sufficiency which is assumed *as a barrier against the fear to keep the fears at bay*.

But the time comes when these barriers against fear break

down, and the fears emerge in the form in which they were originally experienced in infancy, such as the dread of loneliness.

This reaction may take place at a very early age, even in the first
year of life, as an automatic self-preservative measure; for *fear and
assertiveness are both native responses to a situation of danger.*
Thereafter he must succeed, he must make money, for money
means security, he must reach the top of his profession, he must
always keep up to the scratch, must never fail. Perpetual achievement is necessary to reassure him against inadequacy, to bolster
his self-confidence.

Self-assertiveness now becomes the dominant feature of his
character. Such men and women become hard-working, efficient,
energetic, successful, ambitious, reliable and conscientious, but
always with strain and anxiety because of the underlying fear.
Indeed it is this anxiety which drives them on to greater and
greater efforts. The early dread which such a man has repressed
then gets transferred to his work, so that he is anxious about his
success and is never satisfied with what he has done; he is tense,
he never rests, can never relax, and even his recreations he takes
too seriously. Everything he does is by an effort, lacking spontaneity. Because of this urge it is usually the successful man who
gets anxiety hysteria, rarely the dud. Yet the very oppressiveness of
the demands his super-ego is making on him accentuates the wish
to be ill and to be cared for. He has laid on himself burdens
grievous to be borne; he must be successful, he must work
day and night to prove his power and to keep the fears at bay.
But the task is too great, he becomes weary, he longs to lay it
all down, to sink into a state of lethargy, he yearns for Nirvana.
So whilst there is a drive urging him forward to achievement,
there is also a strong pull drawing him towards this lethargy and
indolence. Like Ulysses' companions he finds the indolent land of
the lotus-eaters far more enticing and pleasant than the arduous
journeys of life. But he dreads these tendencies, for to give in
would mean the abandonment of all he has stood for; he cannot,
he must not give way to these temptations to ease, he must fight
all the harder, put forward still more strenuous efforts, until he
suffers the inevitable breakdown in which anxiety, sleeplessness,
restlessness and fear play the predominant rôle. These breakdowns
so common to the successful business man, are said to be due to
overwork: *the overwork is in fact due to his over-anxiety.*[1]

[1] The voyages of Ulysses appears to be a saga of the voyage of man's soul
through life. The land of the lotus-eaters represents the phase of lethargy and
passivity in which we are in earliest infancy, and even before birth. This passes

In practically all these cases of neurotic anxiety, whether hysterical or obsessional, we have found an original objective dread in infancy. The infant, deprived of its sense of security and helpless to do anything to cope with the situation, is thrown into a state of anxiety and dread. It is precisely this appalling state of dread, so overwhelming and so terrifying, which is reproduced in later attacks of anxiety.

It is useless to tell such a man to relax, for he feels that if he lets go he will go to pieces altogether, and be overwhelmed by the fears he has dreaded all his life. These people as employers are severe with others, but are hardest on themselves, driving themselves to impossible tasks which they overdo in an attempt to evade fear. They say they never demand of others what they do not demand of themselves, without realizing that they have no right to demand it either of themselves or of others. All his life such a man is a slave-driver, fighting against a fear which he has repressed and of which he is now quite unconscious. Then comes some blow to his sense of power which precipitates the breakdown. He experiences some set-back to his success, some threat or failure, some illness, an operation, a slight car accident, and down comes his castle of cards; the barriers against fear are broken down and his fears surge up to produce a nervous breakdown.

An instance is that of a professional man who after a trying interview developed claustrophobia. He had been delicate and sickly, suffering from rickets as a child, and had very little affection from a mother who was cold, and a father whose only ambition was for the puny son to become an international football player! Failing help elsewhere he must be self-sufficient, repressed his feeling of inadequacy, his one motto being "I must get on!" Strained, over-conscientious, in a continuous state of tension, always aiming at efficiency and yet constantly criticized by his father as a failure, things proved too much for him and he broke down, not because he was inefficient or failed in his work, but the task he had put on himself was too great. The precipitation came when he had spent an afternoon standing up to partners senior to himself who were trying to make him do something detrimental to

to the reign of Circe, the mother who casts her sensuous spell on us in infancy and makes "beasts" of us in our abandonment to these pleasures. Polyphemus represents the giant of the father whom the child in the aggressive phase may defy, but at the risk of his life, as Polyphemus though blinded threw the rock at the defiant Ulysses and his companions and nearly wrecked them. The sirens represent a more adult type of sexuality, maidens who lure us on to destruction. Ulysses himself stands for the guiding and directing principle in our personality, the super-ego who is urging us on to face life and its difficulties, and delivering us from its dangers until we reach the end of the voyages of life and find our true home.

his professional honour. He stood out successfully, but all through the struggle he felt the oppression of the situation and felt "I must get out!" which he projected on to the closeness of the atmosphere. Going down into the Tube, after the strain was over, he was suddenly possessed with this panic, the fear of being shut in, partly a reminiscence of an infantile fear, but partly symbolic of the fear of frustration of his personality. He was always in a hurry and naturally got palpitation; and this brought the old dread, he was getting ill with heart disease, and he might die at any moment, or perhaps worse, faint and make a fool of himself. The barriers of self-sufficiency and power broke down and precipitated the claustrophobia. This was a reproduction of an infantile fear, but secondarily was a way of escape. The dependent factor was dominant throughout, his retreat from the life he had imposed on himself in order to combat the fear.

This case also illustrates by way of contrast an obsessional condition: for besides his hysterical anxiety he also had an obsession of "motor-cars crashing in headlong collision," which was a revival of his aggressive craving for something drastic to happen. He desired like Omar "to break this sorry scheme of things entire," and "remould it nearer to the heart's desire."

The mechanism of these cases is simple: there is the primal dread from illness in infancy; the necessity to compensate by power, success and self-sufficiency; the sense of failure when things were too much for him; and the final breakdown in which there was a return of the fears of infancy which had been kept in abeyance only by achievement and success. Yet this phobia may be not merely a resurrection of the infantile fears, but becomes chronic because it contains the desire to escape by illness from a task too great to bear, and a longing to be cared for.

The *intensity* of the emotion in these phobias is due to the intensity of the infantile experience, for the dreads of the helpless infant are far more overwhelming than any fear experienced in later life. The impossibility of dealing with the situation itself (in childhood because it was too much for him, now because he does not know what it is), turns the normal fear into anxiety, with its feeling of an awful unknown dread. It is therefore projected on to an objective phobia of a close place.

The precipitation of the symptom. The precipitating conditions in anxiety hysteria are very like those of conversion hysteria. The precipitation comes (*a*) when any situation occurs which revives the primal fear, e.g. being shut up in a lift may revive a suffocation at birth; (*b*) anything which weakens the super-ego of self-sufficiency such as failure in trying to achieve success, or illness which incapacitates him. Illness indeed is a very common precipitating cause because it (i) may revive an infantile illness, (ii) weakens the super-ego, and (iii) offers an escape from the effort of keeping up to the impossible standards of the super-ego.

The symptom in hysterical anxiety commonly takes the form of (*a*) *generalized* anxiety characteristic of the person who is always tense, worrying, anxious about his work, his health, his past, his future; in such cases we find a basic fear in early childhood to cause this. (*b*) But the fear frequently takes on a *specific* form relating to the primal fear from which the patient suffered in early childhood relating to such fears as isolation, illness, suffocation, separation, noise, loneliness, which are later precipitated as claustrophobia (from suffocation), agoraphobia (from separation), and frequently reproduce the actual illness of infancy. (*c*) Or it may take the form of the *accompaniments of anxiety* like insomnia or psychosomatic disorders. (*d*) Or it may take the form of a fear of the breakdown of his standards of success, duty or moral integrity.

Transition from hysterical to obsessional anxiety. In anxiety neurosis, whether of the hysterical or obsessional type, we find a primal source of fear in infancy. In both there is the repression of this in favour of an attitude of assertiveness, self-sufficiency and power.

But in hysterical anxiety this power is sublimated into success and achievement which usually characterizes these patients, who are often successful people. It is when this power urge fails that the breakdown takes place.

In obsessional anxiety, on the other hand, this assertiveness (which usually takes the more exaggerated form of aggressiveness, jealousy or hate) is itself repressed in favour of a more docile moral attitude, so that the aggressiveness itself is feared. This fear may then emerge as a fear of the forbidden *impulse itself* such as a fear of poisoning; or it may be of the dreaded *consequences* of the aggressiveness, say fear of insanity, or of the simple *revival of the original objective dread* in infancy now regarded as a threat to oneself as a punishment for the aggressiveness.

Thus in both hysterical and obsessional anxiety there is aggressiveness, but in hysterical anxiety the assertiveness and sense of power is the dominant attitude adopted as a barrier to keep the fears at bay, and keep them repressed; it must therefore be maintained at all costs. In the obsessions this aggressiveness is threatened, repressed and therefore feared. In both there is a fear of something in oneself, but whilst in anxiety hysteria there is a fear of fear (of failure, of illness, of disability, of inadequacy), against which the patient puts up a brave but ineffectual fight, and against which he sets a barrier of assertiveness, in the obsessions there is a fear of forbidden impulses, of sex, aggression and hate, against the threatened consequences of which the patient tries to protect himself by propitiatory acts. In both there may be a fear of a forbidden wish, but whereas in hysterial anxiety it is a fear of a wish to be ill to escape the responsibilities of life which is feared, (a dependent reaction), in the obsessions it is fear of a wish to be aggressive, to be jealous, to hate, to put to death, to hurt, which is feared. The anxiety hysteric is one who is afraid in spite of his outward show of success and self-sufficiency: the obsessional is aggressive and offensive in spite of his show of ingratiation and desire to please.

Even so, there is no reason why they should not be combined and the obsessional fear of the supposed consequences such as insanity may be used as a means of arousing pity. Many a child who has done wrong will, as we have seen, attempt to turn away the wrath of the parent by pretending a pain or illness to appeal to his sympathy; and an illness that is regarded as a threat for wrong-doing may be used to avert the consequences of that wrong. So hysterical fears, like hysteric pains, are often used (*a*) as a means of escaping responsibility and getting sympathy, (*b*) as self-punishment, (*c*) as an appeal for help because of the feared consequences of the guilt. Illness is then transformed from being a threatened punishment for guilt into a means of averting punishment for that guilt. Thus fear of illness, like an illness itself, may be an attempt at propitiation, as any other obsessional propitiation.

CHAPTER XI

OBSESSIONAL NEUROSES

OBSESSIONAL ANXIETY; OBSESSIONAL AGGRESSIONS; SEX OBSESSIONS

OBSESSIONS are *morbid mental compulsions.*

(*a*) They may be compulsive *thoughts*; such as worries about the meaning of life, the problem of evil, thoughts of death, of suicide, of revenge; doubts and questionings such as "Why am I here, and if not, when?"; obsessing thoughts of "thousands of millions and billions," of "the origin of everything out of nothing," or the false suspicions that people are against one.

(*b*) Sometimes they are compulsive *actions* in which there is a morbid impulse to act in certain ways although the act is not carried out, such as the impulse to do *harm to oneself,* to throw oneself off a height, or in front of a train; or an impulse to do serious *harm to others,* such as to push people off the pavement, to kill, to hurt, to poison, to strangle, to strike people in the face. In other cases the actions are carried out, like the compulsion to touch every lamp-post, or to step over the lines of the pavement; or the obsession may be to perform rituals or acts of propitiation like saying prayers till two o'clock in the morning, or washing the hands fifty times a day.

(*c*) Or the obsession may take the form of a *compulsive feeling or emotion,* like the feeling of inferiority, a morbid sense of shame, of self-consciousness, of shyness, of anxiety; fears of harm to oneself, such as illness, of death, of open spaces, of knives, of loneliness, and fears of doing harm to others as fear of poisoning, of raping, or strangling.

(*d*) Or the obsession may be a *compulsive inhibition,* like the inability to travel, to lift up a cup; or a general *aboulia* (lack of will), in which there is a compulsion preventing us doing the things we want to do.

(*e*) Finally, the obsession may take a *psychosomatic* form, such as compulsion to blush.[1]

---

[1] This classification of obsessions, reminiscent of Janet, is based on the differentiation of mental functions into cognitive, conative and affective processes. It is a useful one for descriptive purposes; but it is not exclusive, for most cases are mixed. A person may have a compulsive thought, say of suicide, without a corresponding impulse, but often the thought is accompanied by the

The term "obsessional" may be used in a narrower sense merely of obsessional *acts* like touching every lamp-post or counting ten before every act; but we shall use it to cover all morbid mental compulsions, whether of thoughts, acts, or feelings and emotions. A man who is the victim of a compulsive fear is just as much "obsessed" by this state of mind as the man who is given to obsessional handwashing.

Obsessions, especially in mild forms, are extremely widespread; indeed, there are probably few people who do not suffer from some mild form or other of worry or morbid fear, if it is only a tune ringing in the head, obsessionally putting the knife, fork and spoon straight on the table, getting things in line with the eye, being superstitious, having a sense of shame or humiliation about a trifling incident long since past, a feeling of self-consciousness with superiors or strangers or the opposite sex, over-conscientiousness, or a tendency to obstinacy. We worry about these matters; then we worry because we worry; until we end by thinking we are going off our heads, since the popular idea of insanity is to be under the dominance of an irrational idea or uncontrollable emotion. The mild cases are worrying enough; in severe forms they make life unbearable and drive some people to suicide. Nevertheless these are not conditions of insanity, but are due to emotional conflicts and can be cured, though with great difficulty, by psychotherapy.

The main characteristics of the obsessions are these:
  (a) They are compulsive.
  (b) They are involuntary.
  (c) They are morbid and irrational, but they are recognized to be so by the patient.

Other characteristics are that:

They are exaggerated.
They are subjective fears of ourselves.

impulse (giving rise to the theory of idea-motor action that the idea originates the impulse) and is almost certain to be associated with feelings of worry, depression and anxiety. Again, a man is compelled to perform propitiatory actions, but because of the necessity of avoiding fear. Nor is the distinction really a scientific classification of the obsessions in that it is based on symptomatology, whereas a scientific classification should be based on causative factors. Freud describes the obsessional neuroses thus: "The patient's mind is occupied with thoughts that do not really interest him, he feels impulses which seem alien to him, and he is impelled to perform actions which not only afford him no pleasure but from which he is powerless to desist" (*Introd. Lectures*, p. 219). He thus includes cognitive and conative, but not affective states.

The causes of the morbid fears are unknown.

They are therefore often objectified and personalized.

They are persistent or repetitive.

With the exception of the propitiatory acts, they are not in fact carried out.

(a) The chief characteristic of the obsession is that it is *compulsive*: we *must* perform certain actions, we are forced to think certain thoughts, we are compelled to have morbid emotions of shame, fear or depression. Indeed, when we use the word "obsessive" we usually mean that the condition is compulsive. Neither hysterical symptoms (which are mainly disabilities) nor sex perversions (unless they are sex obsessions) have this compulsive quality, the reason for which we shall see later.

Obsessions are *mental* compulsions and in this respect are distinguished from conversion hysterias which are physical disabilities, though they both originate in mental conflicts.

(b) Obsessions are *involuntary*: we are compelled to have these thoughts and do these deeds *against our will*.[1] They may appear silly and stupid, they may be loathsome like the horror of a devoted mother that she will poison her baby, or merely annoying like the compulsion to make sure continually that the gas is turned off, or see that the door is locked, or that the accounts are correct when we know perfectly well that they are.

(c) Obsessions are *morbid and irrational*. The phobia of crossing a street is unjustified, not commensurate with the danger; the compulsion to put things straight is unreasonable, serving no purpose; the feeling of inferiority has no relation to one's ability, nor the depression to the objective facts of life. We are shy and awkward when we want to appear our best, depressed when everything ought to make us happy, and are compelled to worry about the meaning of life when really we are not at all interested.

Again, obsessions are not only morbid, but are *recognized to be morbid* by the patient. When a person has a compulsion to injure the wife he deeply loves, or to fling himself over a cliff when he has no desire to die, it is not only irrational, but he knows it to be. This recognition of the irrationality of his condition adds to the distress of the patient, for he thinks he must be going mad. But this realization is not altogether undesirable, for it indicates

---

[1] What is compulsive is not necessarily involuntary, such as the compulsions of love or the pursuit of a conviction; on the other hand, what is involuntary is not necessarily compulsive, such as many undesirable thoughts which we can deal with and dismiss.

that the patient has insight into the condition, and this distinguishes the neurotic obsession from the psychotic delusion, in which there is usually no insight into the morbidity of his condition. The recognition of his abnormality is therefore not only a sign of relative sanity but also gives hope of cure.

But though the obsessional patient recognizes the irrationality of his ideas or emotions he cannot help himself. It is therefore useless to try and persuade him that there is nothing to be afraid of, no reason for his depression, or that it is silly to perform these compulsive acts. He knows all the arguments as well as we do, but what he wants to know is why they occur and particularly how he can get rid of them. In any case it is not true to say that there is "nothing to be afraid of," or to be ashamed of, because in fact there is always a real cause of fear or of remorse, although he does not know what it is since it is subjective and unconscious. The obsessions *appear* irrational, but are not so irrational when we discover the real cause; they are only irrational because they have been transferred to some trifling object or situation to which they do not properly belong.

Obsessions are always *exaggerated*: a patient will spend hectic hours putting her dressing table straight, will spend the day worrying whether she could have squashed a fly when she sat on the seat in the park yesterday, will shriek when she sees a spider: the dread she experiences in crossing the street is appalling, and the sense of shame about some trifling sin of the past may fill her with remorse and mental torture. Such dreads are out of all proportion to the object of fear or shame, and the person with claustrophobia experiences far more dread in a theatre than he does in the real danger of a bombardment: indeed real danger often comes as a welcome relief, and even temporarily cures an obsession. The appalling quality of this dread is due, as we have seen, to the fact that it is the revival of infantile experiences. In other cases it is the *consequence* of our acts which is exaggerated, like the shipping clerk who fears that if he writes a letter it will spread infection throughout South America; or the clergyman who had the obsession that if he puts his right boot on before the left a plague will break out in Australia! This patient had no experience of a plague in Australia nor any evidence that such a disaster would follow the reversal of the usual order in putting on his boots to make him fear such a disaster, yet it filled him with appalling dread.

Before proceeding further we may perhaps give a case to illustrate the psychopathology and mechanism of obsessional states.

R

A case of agoraphobia (Major X). This officer suffered from agoraphobia which made it impossible for him to cross a park, a street, or a bridge over the Thames, unless he was in contact with somebody, such as holding the hand of his little boy of nine.

The first attack he had was when he was in the Egyptian desert as Commanding Officer of the Station, crossing at nightfall between his office and the Officer's Mess. He had crossed there every evening, but on this particular occasion the darkness, the space, the solitariness, filled him with an awful dread, from which he continued to suffer for some years. Associating on this dread he traced it back to an experience at the age of six when, after being severely and unjustly reproved by his mother, he ran away from home one night and found himself in an open field. Looking up at the staring spaces above him he was filled with dread, which forced him to return home. He recognized it as the same dread he had experienced in the desert. There was the conflict between his self-will and fear of consequences: he was compelled to repress his self-will as dangerous and he became a good and obedient boy.

The recovery of these associations, together with the realization of the conflict, relieved his symptoms, but did not cure them for the conflict went back still earlier. He then revived an experience in infancy when his cruel nurse threatened him, particularly on one occasion on a deserted sea-front when he persisted in getting out of his pram and she seized him by the throat. This terror also was associated with the open space of sea and sky and isolation, without help in sight, and no contact with any human being except this horrible woman. (She was finally discovered and dismissed.) Finding himself cast on his own resources, he had to fight for himself and so became aggressive, defiant and self-willed, but being seized by the throat, he had to give in. On a later occasion when he was put in charge of an epileptic brother whom he used to wheel about, street boys jeered at his brother and the patient heroically fought them in his brother's defence. When he arrived home, his mother, seeing his clothes torn, scolded him for fighting. He felt furious at this injustice and this was the occasion and reason for his running away from home that night, which was followed by the dread; the conflict between his rebellious self-will and fear of consequences was once more precipitated. He had no option but to submit, after which he became good, amenable and ingratiating. Coming to the experience in the desert, we find a very similar subjective as well as objective situation. The objective situation was similar on all these occasions, the open shore in infancy, the open field, and the desert; and the precipitation might have been an objective one; if, for instance, he had been actually *lost* in the desert, it might have revived the infantile dread as a *conditioned anxiety*.[1] But that was not enough: he had crossed that space for months every night; why should he suddenly get this attack? Obviously mere objective circumstances were not sufficient to account

[1] P. 239.

for it. In this case the real conflict precipitating the phobia was subjective, relating to the following psychological problem.

At his Station he had under him as Adjutant a man who had previously been stationed there and had expected to get the appointment as Commanding Officer. When the patient arrived he realized the situation and wishing there to be no ill-feeling, and being a mild-mannered man (since the incident at six), he allowed the Adjutant, who was more familiar with the work, to carry on as before. But the latter took advantage of his good nature and began to dominate him. Ultimately the Adjutant submitted to him a letter to sign in which the patient was virtually made to refuse to obey orders from a higher authority, and he realized that it was time to make a stand against this domination; yet he feared to be assertive and to cause trouble with the Adjutant, as he had always feared rows, originally with his nurse and mother in childhood. He was in the throes of this conflict (Should he stand firm or should he give in?) when he was crossing from his office to the Mess and the attack came on. The subjective psychological situation as well as the objective physical one was similar to that of the age of six; and there was a moral conflict in each case. In each case he was defying authority; and in each case there was the dread of consequences, in the former case of alienating his mother on whose protection he depended, in the latter case of alienating the Adjutant who had dominated him, and of whom he stood in awe. On the other hand, he must stand up against him or risk the disgrace of court martial for breaking the regulations. It was an insoluble conflict!

Such a case presents clearly (a) the characteristics, (b) the causes, and (c) the mechanism of obsessional anxiety.

(a) It exemplifies *the characteristics of obsession*: the agoraphobia was a morbid mental compulsion; it was recognized by the patient to be morbid; it was persistent and repetitive; it was compulsive; it was involuntary, against the will of the patient; it was also irrational, there being no reason for fearing to cross the road: nevertheless there was a real but hidden moral cause of fear.

(b) *This case also illustrates the main causal factors of an obsessional anxiety.*

(i) A *primal fear* in infancy on the shore.

(ii) A strongly developed *aggressiveness* and self-will, developed as a compensation to this feeling of insecurity and in resentment at his treatment by his nurse, at his mother's injustice at the age of six, and at the bullying of the Adjutant at the precipitation of his symptoms.

(iii) The *threat of consequences* of this aggressiveness; the nurse's threats in infancy; the dark night when he ran away, and from the threat of trouble if he stood up to the Adjutant.

(iv) The adoption of an attitude of ingratiation—the super-ego —forced upon him by the fear of these consequences; his determination to be the good and amiable boy at six, which led to his later ingratiation of the Adjutant.

(v) The breakdown occurred when the moral conflict between assertiveness and fear was reactivated in his dealings with the Adjutant, which precipitated the neurosis.

This case may be kept in mind as we study the psychopathology of obsessional neuroses.

PSYCHOPATHOLOGY OF OBSESSIONS

(*A*) *The main characteristic of the obsessional as such is aggressiveness and self-will.* He may appear docile, but latently he is assertive, defiant, self-willed, full of hate and obstinate; he must always have his own way, must always dominate, and in his character is distinguished by the "obsessional drive." As the hysteric is characterized by dependence and the sex pervert by sensuousness, so the obsessional is characterized by aggressiveness.

It is this aggressiveness and self-will which gives to the obsessions their compulsive character.

The sexual element is frequently an important factor in the anxiety obsessions and propitiations and is obvious in the sex obsessions, such as the fear of raping; yet it is not sex, but obstinacy and self-will which is the characteristic feature of the obsession as such. Sex enters the picture because it is often on account of sex desires that the patient is so self-willed and must have his own way, but were it not for the aggressive element the repressed sexual desires would not emerge as a compulsion, but as a sex perversion. It is only when the sexual desire is backed by self-will that it becomes compulsive and can produce an obsession, in which case it may appear either as an obsessional anxiety, a sexual obsession, or a propitiary compulsive act. The more the sex is backed by an obstinate self-will the more compulsive it is, and the more obsessional is the symptom. Therefore, it is the self-will aggressive element which is the determining factor even in sex obsessions.

In many obsessional cases, on the other hand, the sexual element is absent or it is of no significance in the production of the obsession, the repressed feelings of hate and aggressiveness alone being the cause of the obsession.

Again, the obsessional often appears dependent, timid, panic-stricken, clinging and ingratiating, like the hysteric, but it is because he fears the consequences of his latent self-will that he must needs ingratiate and propitiate. When, therefore, a man ingratiates himself we wonder what he is up to. The hysteric, on the other hand, as we have seen, is often aggressive, self-willed and tyrannizes over the household; but he does so by means of disability, by headaches and an appeal to their pity; he too must have what he wants, but what he wants is to be loved, to be cared for, to escape responsibility, not to be aggressive and domineer like the obsessional. The final type of psychoneurosis depends on the proportions of dependence, sex and aggressiveness and the dominance of one over the others. But there are mixed cases in which it is difficult to say whether, or how much, of a condition is an obsession, or hysteria, to say where a sex perversion ends and a sex obsession begins. But it is a matter of little importance what we call them, as long as we know their nature. Man after all reacts as a whole, not in segments.

(B) *The essential conflict in obsessional conditions is the conflict between self-will and fear of consequences* (or it may be between self-will and the equivalents of fear, like shame and guilt). There is on the one hand an exaggerated self-will which refuses to give way, and on the other an exaggerated fear of consequences. One part of the personality says "I am going to have my own way!" and another part answers "If you do, disaster will follow!" It is a case of the irresistible force against the immovable post; the self-will is the irresistible force which refuses to give in because it must have its own way at all costs; and the fear is the immovable post which cannot give way because the consequences are so dreaded.

(C) *The obsessional fear is the fear of the consequences of our self-willed aggressive desires*: it is a fear of ourselves, a fear of our repressed forbidden impulses.

The conflict in the obsessions is therefore always a *subjective conflict*; it is always *endopsychic*, and unlike hysterical anxiety it is always a *moral* conflict. It is a fear of impulses within ourselves because of forbidden desires. The fear usually appears as an objective fear, the fear of close space, or of loneliness, which in fact was the original threat in childhood, but the threat persists on account of the persistence of the forbidden desires, the consequences of which are regarded as so disastrous.

The fact that the fear is a moral fear is not only proved by analysis, but is corroborated by the fact that the obsessional neurotic is not normally a cowardly or timid individual, but is often courageous and fearless in his objective relationships to life.

It was very noticeable that during the London blitz in 1943–44 neurotic people were often less nervous than the ordinary citizen.[1]

(D) Every obsessional symptom, therefore, represents a *repressed wish*. We fear these impulses because we desire them: if we had not the desire we should not have cause to fear. A man coming to London for treatment happened to meet in Piccadilly acquaintances from his home town: he reddened and burst into a sweat of shame, he did not know why. It was lest they might think he had been with women, which in fact he had not. But would he have blushed, had there not been the desire to do so? If these wishes and impulses are no longer consciously desired, they were nevertheless at one time definitely and deliberately desired, and that they are still subconsciously desired is evidenced by their appearance in the symptoms, as well as in dreams. A woman patient, for instance, who has a *horror* of passing water in public, dreams that she is doing so to her heart's content. We frequently find that what the patient consciously fears he enjoys in his dreams, revealing his latent wish.

(E) Since it is far easier to deal with a known than an unknown fear, an objective situation like a close space than an unconscious forbidden desire, these morbid fears of ourselves are often *projected on to objects of the outside world* connected in any way with our fears. So we fear open space either because such was the primal fear in infancy at the moment of conflict, or because space means isolation and desertion which is the consequence of our persisting in forbidden desires.

Not only so, but these repressed impulses are so active that it is not surprising that being repressed and unrecognized they are often *objectified and personalized*, so that the patient feels as though he is assailed by outside forces and not from his own impulses, that he is possessed by devils, the victim of malignant powers compelling him to do what is alien to his will while he remains a slave to their demands. (The psychotic patient believes that he *is* so possessed.) So morbid complexes appear to be dissociated personalities forcing their will upon us; or as the devil

[1] Four times in ten days were the windows of the author's house (temporarily repaired) blown in by the explosion of bombs and rockets, but on no occasion did a patient being treated show any sign of anxiety, nor cease to carry on with free association on account of the raid overhead: and only two patients, both of whom lived over fifty miles from London, ceased to come for treatment on account of the bombing. Their fears were subjective, not objective. On the other hand, many of the patients in the 41st Neuropathic Army Hospital who had personally had *traumatic* experiences at Dunkirk, Norway and elsewhere, showed marked terror even of the gramophone record of a blitz. But in this case the original fear was objective.

who is the projection, objectification and personalization of our repressed complexes. These we shall consider later as paranoid obsessions (p. 332 f.).

(F) Although the self-willedness is repressed, it is still active with the result that *every time the repressed self-will asserts itself*, so constantly is the patient thrown into a state of anxiety and dread. The wretched and harassed patient is now in a pitiable state; he must assert himself and be successful to keep down his fear; but if he asserts himself he is threatened with punishment: thus he is deprived of the very means by which alone he can fight against these fears. He is assailed on every side, yet his very fears rob him of the strength to meet the difficulties of life. No wonder he is driven to make overtures with fate by means of over-conscientiousness, and develops propitiatory obsessions to avert the consequences of his forbidden desires.

This conflict between self-will and fear of consequences is of course extremely common in early childhood, and yet all children do not become obsessional. This is true, though in point of fact there are few people who altogether do escape from some form or another of obsessions or morbid anxiety however mild (if it is only a tendency to worry, to be obstinate or to be over-conscientious), which may be due to the prevalence of this moral problem in early childhood. Such a problem is unavoidable since the child is compelled in ordinary life to conform to social demands, and the clash between the individual will and the will of society is inevitable.

Normally this conflict between self-will and fear of consequences is solved by the child in one or another of several different ways.

(i) One child threatened with disastrous consequences is *frankly defiant* and rebellious, determined to do what he likes and be damned to the consequences. This happens when the child is constitutionally of an aggressive temperament, when there is no previous predisposition to fear, where the threatened fear is not too severe, or when the parents do not carry out their threats. When the defiant child discovers that nothing happens, he is confirmed in his self-will and continues to be defiant. If circumstances are propitious he follows his own line and makes a success of life: if circumstances are bad his defiance may turn him into a delinquent; only if this defiance is later repressed by further threats does he become neurotic and an obsessional.

(ii) In another child the fear is so strong that, dreading the consequences, *he abandons his forbidden desires*, suppresses his temper, sex or hatred, and becomes well-behaved, good, obedient and amenable, as indeed the parents intended. He finds some outlet for his assertiveness in doing things that are approved, and all is well. This happens when the child is of a more docile temperament, his aggressiveness less developed, or when the threat is too severe for him to defy. So he gives in and becomes good, but sapless.

(iii) But suppose both his fear and his self-will are so exaggerated that neither will give way: the self-will refuses to give in because it must have its own way; but the fear also refuses to give in because the consequences are so disastrous. Then we have the situation already described, of the irresistible force of self-will against the immovable post of fear. The child's personality is torn between the rebellious demands on the one side, the threat of disaster on the other. Neither side will give in and the child is left with an unsolved and insoluble problem. The perpetual conflict reduces his whole personality to a state of impotence; he can do nothing, he can decide nothing, because whatever he decides to do with one side of his personality is immediately resisted by the other side of his divided personality.

In the obsessions there is always an unsolved moral problem.

The results of this moral conflict are: (*a*) First, that the child lives in a constant state of dread, and yet, because he represses his forbidden desires, he is unaware of what these fears are. This is the situation in the *obsessional anxieties*. (*b*) In other cases the forbidden desires may be so strong that they thrust themselves into consciousness, and the child has constantly to be fighting them down, so that he suffers from a perpetual fear of his tempers, his hate, his jealousy, his impulses to hurt, his sex impulses. This corresponds to what we shall call the *obsessional aggressions* and *sex obsessions*. (*c*) But the child cannot continue to live in this state of distress everlastingly; that is beyond human endurance; for human nature is able to stand anything except doubt. But since neither side will give in, a compromise has to be made between these two conflicting tendencies.

The result is that a *pact* is made by the child with itself, with its parents or with God: it allows itself to indulge the forbidden desire, but with the promise to be extra good in everything else. He becomes over-conscientious and will sometimes develop a "confession mania," which makes him confess every trifling fault except the real one. He allows himself to continue masturbation, but is punctilious in doing everything his mother tells him. At first this may be consciously and deliberately done; in the obsessional patient the problem has become unconscious so that he is possessed by an irrational compulsion to confess, but he no longer knows why he has to confess, nor what he has to confess. So he develops *obsessional character traits* like punctiliousness and over-conscientiousness; and *obsessional propitiations* like hand-washing to compensate for the stains upon his soul.

There are many modifications of these main reactions. For instance, an individual will blithely continue with his sin, but refuses to admit any guilt with regard to it. Feeling guilt nevertheless, he projects his guilt on to some trifling error, which he knows is undeserving of the sense of guilt, such as having swindled the railway company out of sixpence ten years before. So a man who has abandoned his wife and child, and "married" another woman, feels no guilt whatever about this, but has the morbid fear that if he does any trifling wrong, like leaving a knife on the table, some disaster will come to his "wife" or their child, which is the punishment for the guilt he refuses to admit.

The three main elements in the construction of an obsessional neurosis are (A) Fear—together with shame, inferiority, etc., (B) Self-will and aggression, (C) An exaggerated super-ego. We must consider these in turn.

(A) The sources of morbid fears in the obsessions

Morbid fears appear at three stages in an obsession: the primal fears in infancy; the threatened fear of consequences of one's forbidden desires; and finally the fear as it is precipitated in the symptom. These three are commonly combined in the production of obsessional anxiety.

(i) *The primal fear in infancy.* In most cases of obsessional anxiety and phobias we find a primal source of fear in infancy, usually in the first year of life, which we do not find in the same consistency in other forms of psychoneurosis, nor even in the obsessional aggressions, but which we do find in the hysterical anxieties and phobias which we have already discussed. *It is often on account of these primal fears that later threats cannot be defied.*

The basic conflict in the obsessions, as we have seen, is between self-will and the fear of consequences. But in many cases such threats would have no effect were it not for this deeper primal fear in infancy. One child, threatened with illness or desertion, defies the parents and chances the consequences. Another child dare not take the risk and be defiant, for it already has experienced the dread of being alone, ill, feeling deserted, or being suffocated. That is why of the many people shut up in a building on fire, only one may suffer thereafter from claustrophobia. The primal objective fear in infancy is therefore a potent factor in the production of the phobia. It is on account of these dreads, as we have seen, that the child is compelled to be aggressive in order to defend itself; and, on the contrary, it is on account of these fears that the child has later to repress its aggressiveness, for fear of consequences.

These primal fears are, therefore, both the cause of the aggressiveness and the reason for its repression. Because of the need for security the child must stand up for itself and be self-sufficient, but because of the need for security it must repress this assertiveness since it must have the goodwill of others. The primal fear must therefore be regarded as an actual *causative factor* in the production of the neuroses, and not merely a symptom from the past borrowed to express our subjective fears, as some would have us believe.

There are *numerous causes of primal dread in infancy*, such as illness, difficult birth, anxiety derived by suggestibility from the anxiety of a mother (a very common cause), the punishments or threats of a mother, the fear of objective dangers such as a fall, loud noises, suffocation and not least of all nightmares. Some fears are innate, others are acquired.

Watson[2] and others have demonstrated two forms of primitive stimuli of fear in the new-born infant, noise and falling (or withdrawing of support), which are regarded by them as the only primal sources of fear. These are amply confirmed in analysis as causes of infantile fear, the fear of falling accounting for the very

---

[1] *Atavism.* It has been suggested, and was for a long time held, that these dreads were *atavistic tendencies*: that the fear of falling are reverberations of our past going back to our ancestral life when we lived in trees; that our fear of thunderstorms and winds comes from the same source: that claustrophobia comes from the time when we lived in caves, and the associated danger of agoraphobia and isolation from becoming lost in forest or plain. But this theory does not explain why one person suffers from anxiety attacks and another is free, since all possess the same ancestry in that respect; nor why one suffers from loneliness, whereas another has agoraphobia and another claustrophobia. Moreover, if they are innate could we cure them, as we do, by psychotherapy? Yet the atavistic theory may be true to this extent, that there is probably within us a native predisposition to respond by fear to certain situations such as falling, suffocation or isolation, but it requires traumatic experiences to precipitate them into complexes and to produce neuroses, and the release of these complexes are found to cure the neuroses. Ancestral they may be, but only in the sense that we have an ancestral predisposition to such fear, not an inheritance of the morbid fears as such. Incidentally it is curious that some who are most sceptical about the possibility of the recovery of infantile memories find no difficulty in accepting the theory of ancestral memories going back tens of thousands of years!   [2] *The Psychology of a Behaviourist.*

prevalent *fear of heights*. The morbid *phobia of noise* is less frequent perhaps because we have become more acclimatized to it.

But there are other causes of dread which in the nature of the case cannot be experimentally produced in the laboratory and which are found in analysis to be at the root of many anxiety states, such as *fear of suffocation*—indeed it would be strange if the child deprived of air did not get into a state of dread. But we cannot very well suffocate a child in the laboratory to observe whether it is terrified, but we can observe it in babies taking anaesthetics, and in analysis we often find suffocation to be one of the most terrifying experiences in infantile life directly contributing to the development of later anxiety states, especially claustrophobia. Indeed a number of children dislike having their clothes put on over their heads because of the suggestion of suffocation.

Fear of separation, isolation and loneliness, appears to be an innate fear, for there is in the child a strong stereotropic tendency to keep in close contact with the mother; in fact the tendency to cling is the predominant reaction of the infant to a situation of danger. Separation from the mother therefore produces a state of tense anxiety, which has received the specific name of "separation anxiety." It was found in the last World War that the two situations which caused fear in the evacuated child were separation from the mother, and the anxiety of the mother. Bombs and explosions alone (unless the child's house was actually bombed) did not affect them: in fact they enjoyed the thrill provided the mother was calm. On the other hand, so strong was this stereotropic attachment that they often preferred to be with a bad mother (in one case who used to burn the child's hand as a punishment) than with a good foster-mother.

Many other fears like *fear of the dark*, which are said to be atavistic and innate, are found not to be so, but acquired. Children are not naturally afraid of the dark as such, though they can easily be made to be so, so that in such cases the fear must come from actual experiences: they are conditioned fears. A child suddenly awakened by a loud crash in the middle of the night, or who has a bad nightmare, will develop a conditioned fear of the dark associated with it.

Many of these fears, therefore, which later appear as symptoms thus arise from objective and *impersonal experiences* such as suffocation, separation, isolation and illness, and conditioned fears of the dark.

But many fears arise from *abnormal relationships to people*. A common cause of morbid anxiety, already mentioned, is derived from the mother's anxiety which is often transferred to the child, who is most susceptible to the mother's moods. The mother who in an air raid keeps asking the child: "Are you afraid?" "Are you all right?" gives the child who was otherwise quite confident the feeling that there is something dreadful to be afraid of; and as the mother is obviously herself afraid, he cannot get protection from her. A child ill with pneumonia had no anxiety until the mother began to look anxious and worried: then the child hated the mother because she made him anxious. Suggestibility is a common source of all kinds of fear.

Cases of actual ill-treatment from jealous mothers, drunken fathers or cruel nurses, and quarrels of parents are almost too obvious causes of fear to require illustration: but they are none the less important. These fears are the worse because they are fears of those on whom the child depends for protection and security. But neglect may be just as harmful as threats, especially when the child feels unwanted; when one child is born too soon after the other; when the father is seriously ill and the financial outlook poor; when a girl is born when a boy is wanted; when the mother is a "career woman" so that the child is felt to be a nuisance; and when the child is illegitimate. These children have a poor start; they may or may not have all that is physically necessary done for them, but not the love which is most necessary for their health and happiness. The mother who wants a girl and has a boy tries to make no difference, but the boy easily senses her attitude, feels disappointment, tries to be a girl and if for any reason this coincides with a physiological immaturity, it is likely to become a homosexuality. Like Institutional children they lack personal and individual love, and tend to grow up capable of fulfilling their functions in life, but with a sense of something missing and an inability to enjoy life to the full.

Morbid fears and other affective states like depression often arise out of *false interpretation of ordinary experiences.*

A boy of fifteen suffers from bad depression dating back to the time when after giving birth to another child, his mother died, of which event he was not told for several years. He could only interpret this as that the mother had no more use for him, as she now had another baby whom he preferred. A curious case was a man with an obsessional horror of baldness which would make him unattractive to women. This was traced back to an experience when he was suckling at the age of two [sic] at his mother's breast whilst she brushed his hair, a good deal of which came out: then she stopped suckling him. He did what so many children do, put two and two together and made a neurosis, for a child unacquainted with logic continually commits the fallacy of *post hoc ergo propter hoc*. So in this case when his hair came out and his mother stopped suckling him, he assumed it was *because* his hair came out that his mother stopped suckling him. The growth of hair was therefore a symbol of his mother's love and therefore essential to secure the love of other women. He therefore dreaded any sign of baldness as a mark of inferiority for which women would scorn him. Many a child carried off by strange people for an operation, and then suffocated by a weird man in a white robe feels that his mother has basely deserted him, and when he returns from hospital is cold and indifferent towards her. At all operations the mother if possible should be present to reassure the child until the anaesthetic is given and again when the child awakens. One child hearing a roaring lion in the night first looked under the bed and then went timidly in the direction of the sound into the next room: he found it was his father, snoring in fact, but the boy did not understand that. He realized that his apparently kindly father had in him this roaring animal and thereafter the slightest irritation on the father's part was interpreted as a signal warning of this raging animal ready to spring out at him. His fear of his father was transferred to all men, schoolmasters and others, against whom he was always on the defensive. Being on the defensive made him aggressive which made him unpopular, and twice he ran away from school.

It is not fully realized how much of a child's fear can be derived from circumstances which appear normal to others, but which he misinterprets; and that accounts for the fact that in some cases a person gets a neurosis in apparently the best of circumstances and with the kindliest of parents, who because of an outburst of temporary anger may appear to be ogres. This is the problem depicted in the story of Little Red Riding Hood, in which what looks like the kindly grandmother really turns out to be the wolf. In several of our cases the fear of the "evil eye" originated in the glaring eye of the angry mother or nurse. The child tries by fairy stories of this kind to work out its problem. In other cases the angry punishing mother is transformed in dreams into the revenging witch; but the fairy godmother, representing the mother in her kindly aspect, is reassuring to the child that all will be well in the end, because she is stronger than the witch. For a child, therefore, such fairy stories have a therapeutic significance, but they should end well, for by such means the child is reassured. It is possible that the office of godparent, psychologically speaking, was designed for this very purpose, since the child cannot trust the parent whose moods are variable, and needs a godparent or fairy godmother, who free from responsibilities for the child and under no necessity to discipline him, can afford to be more uniformly kind. Similarly the dragon and ogre often represents the father in his angry moods, but there is the St. George to slay the dragon and the Prince Charming waiting to rescue the helpless maid. Thus myths and fairy stories represent not only the childhood of the race, but common psychological experiences in the childhood of the individual, which account for their popularity and prevalence.

But why do children repeat or like to have read to them tales ending in disaster and tragedy, and love blood-curdling stories? This reiteration of dreaded experiences has the therapeutic effect of acclimatizing the child to the terrifying experiences, and the child's playing at bombing after he has been bombed out is designed to accustom him to this situation, in case he be subjected to it again. It also reassures him by giving him the sense of command over such experiences which he produces himself in play, instead of being their victim.

In many cases the dread from which the patient suffers is traced back in free association to *birth itself*, incredible as this may seem.[1]

Erasmus Darwen, Freud and Rank have pointed out that many cases of birth trauma are associated with the feeling of anxiety (*angst* = a narrow space), of appalling catastrophe, of impending doom, and these are symptoms commonly reproduced in nightmares and in anxiety states, as well as in the specific feeling of suffocation or air hunger so characteristic of claustrophobia. The phobia of passing through a long tunnel and never coming to the end, or that it ends in disaster, is very common in dreams, and has often been ascribed to the psyiological sensations of the movement of the bowels. No doubt physiological disturbance can play an important part in the phobias as we shall see when we analyse nightmares. But these cases usually trace themselves back in analysis to a prolonged birth, the horrors of which the patient re-experiences during analysis. Those who relive these infantile experiences in analysis are convinced that they can have no other explanation. Nor is there any theoretic reason why the experiences should not be retained or recollected: indeed that the experiences of a difficult birth should leave its traces upon the child is to be expected considering that the brain of the infant is so plastic and impressionable.[2] If it is said that it is impossible for the infant to

---

[1] "The Reliability of Infantile Memories" by the author, *Lancet*, June 16, 1928, p. 1259.

[2] An objection sometimes raised is that an infant's nerves are not myelinated and therefore it cannot possibly remember. That begs the question in assuming that non-myelinated nerves do not function, whereas in fact the nerves of the sympathetic nervous system are never myelinated and yet function.

retain such impressions we have only to point to the fact that an infant of a few days old can form conditioned reflexes with regard, say, to sucking at the breast, which reflexes involve the functions of retention, reproduction, recognition and of differentiation.

It is not that these infantile experiences are "remembered" as we remember the experiences of yesterday, but they are relived in analysis and reproduced with the original intensity. There is, as it were, a "physical memory" in which the original physical sensations are reproduced with their accompanying horror; the interpretation is of course added later. Another fact of considerable interest is that these patients who know nothing of the facts of birth yet revive the experience with its medical details correct. Some have felt themselves being born feet foremost without knowing that this is possible, and the memory has proved correct. In several other cases the patient has revived the *shock* of being slapped (to produce respiration at birth), but have stated that curiously they experienced no pain with this slapping, although they were quite unaware that a new-born infant has no cutaneous sensation, and their recollection was therefore medically correct: for the infant experiences protopathic sensibility and shock but not epicritic sensibility. Therefore those obstetricians are well advised, who choose methods of resuscitation other than those which produce such shock.

Further evidence of the reality of these memories is that when these fears are revived in analysis the patient often experiences the most appalling dread of precisely the same nature as the phobia from which he suffers at the present day, which leaves no doubt in his own mind of the genuineness of these infantile experiences, and of their connection with his present symptoms. The causal connection is finally confirmed by the fact that when these early experiences have been revived and the patient realizes of what he was originally afraid, he is cured of his phobia. Imagination would not do that.

Another indication of the infantile origin of these experiences is the fact that these dreads, such as claustrophobia, are far more overwhelming to the patient than any objective fear he may experience in adult life. In adult life we have emotions of anger, sex and fear which are strong and even overpowering, but short of conditions of insanity, these emotions and feelings are automatically controlled by the organized personality as a whole. The infant, on the other hand, has not this power of control and, therefore, in states of intense excitement, the emotions completely overwhelm him and possess his whole personality so that he becomes himself, as it were, a mass of fear or of rage. He can neither escape from his fear, nor react adequately to his rage, so that all his emotion is dammed back into his organism and fills him with that dread which is so characteristic of neurotic anxiety, and in the face of which he is helpless in the grip of an overwhelming passion. It is no ordinary fear: it is a terror which seizes his whole personality, possesses him and overwhelms him like some great monster from which he cannot escape. Indeed it often appears as such in dreams. It is this feeling of paralysis which he experiences in anxiety attacks and in nightmares in which he is rooted to the spot and frozen with horror, which are reproductions of infantile dread.

In many cases the patient is able to confirm the fact that he had some marked cause of fear in infancy, and deeper investigation by analysis may prove the connection between such experiences and these present morbid fears. In other cases we are not able to get a history of this infantile cause of fear from the patient, nor even from the mother who may not recollect anything of the kind to cause it, and may even deny it.[1]

But whether we can confirm it or not, when we come to analyse out these original causes of obsessional anxiety, we invariably find such experiences of dread in infancy. These primitive experiences are of the greatest importance in the production of anxiety states for they are the prototype of all later attacks of anxiety.

It is possible that this accounts also for the prevalence of neurotic anxiety amongst savage tribes. It is said that the savage is without psychoneuroses and the popular picture of the "happy savage" gives support to this view. This picture, so contrary to the fact, may be due to the envy of civilized man of the "freedom" of the savage; but it would be truer to say that the savage is in a perpetual anxiety state, as evidenced by his fears of taboos under which he constantly lives, with dread of unknown but sinister forces, which he has perpetually to propitiate.

The fear of the savage is often said to be due to the terror of the "mysterious forces of nature," which he personalizes. But after all man in the course of time becomes accustomed to clouds and

---

[1] But the memories of mothers are notoriously unreliable, especially when the experience makes any reflection upon their functions as mothers. A striking illustration was that of a young man who visualized that he had had the trauma of two circumcisions in infancy. This was stoutly denied by the mother, who was Jewish and for whom circumcision was an important event, which she was bound to remember. Quite accidentally she later discovered a diary she kept of her children's childhood, and there found that the son's reproduction in analysis was quite correct and that her recollection was incorrect: he had been twice circumcised because something had gone wrong with the first.

storms and in time thinks little of them: in fact most of them have a poor opinion of their gods, who are but exaggerated human beings if they exist at all, and are not beyond being bribed. The prevalence of neurotic fear amongst savages is more probably due to the occasions of dread in infancy, for the primitive child is undoubtedly submitted to more terrifying environment and rough handling than the civilized child, as well as to the sudden alarms and the violent passions of those around, which develop a sense of insecurity towards life. For such a child, whether savage or civilized, life is a dangerous thing, insecure, uncertain: he feels the world to be a dreadful place inhabited by foes, evil influences and malign forces which fill him with superstitious dread, as in the case of the anxiety hysteric.

At the same time he is impelled by passions within himself which he cannot adequately curb but which are threatened with terrifying consequences. The fears of primitive man are therefore not merely the objective fears of life, of ill-health, of starvation, of shocks: he will without hesitation leap into the sea to attack a shark, as the author has often personally seen in his childhood.[1] His fears are of the "unknown," of unseen evils, of mysterious powers, of malignant spirits, of superstitions and dreads which arise out of his own *moral* conflicts. His taboos and ceremonials are designed to avert the disastrous consequences just as are the obsessions of civilized man. If primitive man appears to escape the psycho-neuroses, it is because he avoids the precipitation of the psycho-neuroses by substituting for them these ceremonials and taboos to which he transfers his anxiety: but that *is* his neurosis. Like the propitiating acts of the obsessional, these taboos must be observed perpetually if he is to escape some unknown disaster. In savage and civilized child alike, therefore, the conflict between aggressive-ness and fear of consequences is the cause of obsessional fears, taboos and propitiations.

Nor can it be merely a lack of knowledge which makes the man fear these things: for even the philosopher has such dreads. Indeed the philosopher often seems particularly prone to such irrational dreads since in his determination to rationalize every-thing he fails to do justice to the irrational in life, especially the emotional within him. Since the irrational is not permitted a place in his life and yet demands expression, it becomes a hostile force,

---

[1] A diary kept by a runaway Englishman named Diaper, living amongst and as a cannibal, who was known to the present writer in boyhood, was published under the title of *Cannibal Jack* (now out of print). It records the life of the native savages amongst whom he lived as a savage over a hundred years ago.

which he fears. Indeed, it is sometimes (to judge from philosophers we have analysed) the necessity to solve his inner problems which has led him to be a philosopher in the first place, and the failure to solve it makes him the neurotic.

But these primal fears in infancy, though predisposing to later fears, do not necessarily of themselves produce neurotic fears in later life. It is true that without these primal fears a child would probably not develop a hysterical or obsessional anxiety, but all children who have these fears do not become neurotic: otherwise obsessional or hysterical anxiety would be far more prevalent than it is. The child comes to realize that life is not as bad as he thought, provided later conditions of life are favourable. But sometimes circumstances perpetuate the fears, for the child may be so crushed by perpetual fear that he never develops the self-confidence necessary to face life, and grows up timid, dependent, puny-minded, shrinking, cowardly, anxious and ingratiating. Feeble protests, petulant irritability and grievances are as far as he ever gets in the way of assertiveness. Again these early fears are sometimes forgotten but reactivated, and a child who has had fears of suffocation at birth or from an anaesthetic may have these revived when as a soldier he is buried in a trench or as a civilian under debris: it becomes a *conditioned anxiety*. In other cases these fears are repressed by an attitude of aggressiveness and self-sufficiency as a barrier against the fear, but when this breaks down the old fears are revived, as in *hysterical anxiety*. Or again this aggressiveness may be so exaggerated that it has to be repressed and comes to be feared, as in *obsessional anxiety*.

(ii) *The secondary fear* is the threat of the consequences of the forbidden desires. To revert to our basic conflict: "I must have my own way" is met with the threat "If you do, disaster will happen." The secondary fear is the fear *on account of which the forbidden impulses are repressed*.

The primary and the secondary fear are related, for, whilst these threats may be so severe as to repress the aggressiveness, as a rule, if it were not for the early fears already experienced, the later threats would not have such a disastrous effect, but would be defied, as we have seen. It is on account of the infantile dreads that the later threats are so effective in repressing the forbidden impulses. On the other hand, the infantile fears, so common in childhood, usually pass away were it not for the later reinforcement and threats. Fortunately, it takes a good deal to make a neurosis.

The secondary fear and consequent threats have various sources.

Sometimes these repressing fears are the *actual consequences* of our self-willed acts: the child disobeys the mother and falls downstairs or burns itself; so he learns that disobedience is fatal and represses his self-will. But commonly the repressing fear comes from the *threats of punishment* from the mother, or a beating from the nurse, or being left alone in the dark, or being locked in a cupboard for naughtiness. These personal fears coming from those whom the child looks to for protection, are particularly dreadful. But fear may arise from the *direct effects of the child's own rage* both mental and physical. A child in a state of rage may be so possessed by its fury as to become terrified of its overwhelming passion, a frequent origin for the phobia of going mad. Fear comes from the sense of obliteration, and the child feels its personality obliterated by the strength of its own emotion, since its personality is as yet so poorly organized. The *physiological effects* are no less terrifying. In rage there is the feeling that his head will burst, the weakness in the legs, the pounding of his heart; in fear, the feeling of faintness and giving way of the limbs; in sex, feelings of sickness and nausea. These ill-effects being the consequences of rage or other emotions tend to repress them. The feelings of physical nausea associated in the child with sex feelings of an overwhelming nature, may account for the feeling of "disgust" so often connected with sex, and this "disgust" then tends to repress the very feelings arousing it, which are now regarded as morally disgusting. The self-repression tends to create a prudish attitude towards sex, and people who find sex "disgusting" are often those in whom these feelings have been aroused in earlier sex experiences and followed by feelings of nausea, as we discover in analysis. It is a common cause of frigidity and impotence leading to disaster in married life.

Such experiences whether of rage or of sex may also produce *nightmares*, which are the reproduction of subjective dreads in dramatic and hideous form, and these also are a common cause of repression. Dreams tend to accentuate the experiences of the day: the threatening mother turns into a revengeful witch, the child's rage into a monstrous form overwhelming him, so that when forbidden impulses are not repressed by the threats of the day, they are repressed by the horrors of the night. The self-willed child may defy the former, but dare not defy the latter.[1]

[1] A boy threatened by his mother hated her and wished to hurt her, but dared not. At night he dreamed that he rolled down huge boulders which killed her, and that lightning struck her house. He was so terrified of the results of his omnipotent rage that he repressed his aggressiveness and was for ever after docile.

Such a natural form of repression, that is to say the repression of a primitive impulse by the consequences of its own excess, are quite apart from any cultural or moral influences. This is an interesting fact, for it may account for the almost universal taboos regarding sex, even in the most primitive tribes.

Incidentally these two causes of repression (the overwhelming nature of the emotion, and the subsequent nightmares) are a very good reason why the child should be discouraged from the free indulgence of sex, or indeed of any emotional excess. One of the most anxiety-ridden children we have ever met was the child of parents who considered that a child should be allowed to masturbate as much as it liked. Such practices are not as "harmless" as they are sometimes regarded.[1]

(B) Source of the aggressive element in the obsessions

The obsessional, as we have said, is characterized by self-will, hate, jealousy, and aggressiveness.

It is this aggressive element which gives to the obsessions their compulsive character, and so distinguishes them from the hysterias and sex perversions. It is because we *must* have our own way, that the fear of consequences is also compulsive, because we must take our revenge that the fear of hurting is compulsive, and because

[1] *Castration complex.* Freud maintained that the repression is due to the fear of castration on account of incestuous sexual wishes towards the opposite parent. "Castration" in the sense of loss of one's sex organs is a common cause of anxiety where it is associated with a threat by a nurse or mother for masturbation. But far more commonly in our experience it follows circumcision which is regarded by the child as a punishment for masturbation which itself often arises from the need for a circumcision. This "punishment" will lead to the repression of sex, and commonly results in impotency. But we cannot agree that it is the only source of repression.

The "castration complex" in the girl comes about in this way. The little girl who finds that her baby brother gets more love than she does (mothers so often prefer boys), wonders why. The only difference between them is their sex organs: it must therefore be that his mother prefers him for this. Then she wonders why she has not the same, and concludes that it must be that she has been castrated. In neither the boy nor girl is the castration fear necessarily due to an Oedipus situation. In the girl it is the basic need for love, not of sex, which originates the castration complex. Similarly in Adlerian psychopathology, we do not find that the child gets the inferiority complex because of an "organ inferiority"; but because it feels unloved it wonders why and then says, "It must be because I am lame or weak or red-haired." The organ inferiority is not the primary cause of the complex but the reason the child gives itself to explain the lack of affection.

Some psychoanalysts have later interpreted "castration" in a broader sense to represent all "deprivation." With this conception of "deprivation" we do not quarrel since it agrees so far with our insistence on the deprivation of love as the most important factor in the neuroses. But to continue to use the term "castration" in this symbolic sense is simply to invite misunderstanding and confusion.

our sex desires are so compulsive that we must propitiate to avoid their threatened disasters. To quote one patient: "It is not merely *if* I do this that the disaster will happen, but I *must* do it, so that the disaster *must* happen. I had to do it: but if I did as I had to, the horror must come." This inevitability of fate is characteristic of Greek tragedy. If there were merely the fear of doing it we should give up the idea, as indeed frequently occurs. If there were merely the aggressiveness and no fear we should be defiant. But if there persists an unconscious refusal to give up what will bring upon us disastrous consequences, the fear persists, even if the desire as such never appears in consciousness and remains entirely unrecognized, and produces an obsession.

Assertiveness is a normal constituent of life: it is the personality in its conative aspect. It is not an isolated "instinct," but is the utilization of energy in any effort of the personality to attain its ends. The milder forms we may call assertiveness; the exaggerated forms, aggressiveness or self-will.

This assertiveness may express itself in specific forms which we call an impulse—to fight, to love, to run away. It is the raw material of the *Will* which is the functioning of the personality as a whole directed towards the pursuit of its ends. Assertiveness may be sublimated and directed towards the higher social and cultural achievements of mankind. It can be exaggerated and it can be crushed.

If we lack assertiveness, whether temperamentally or because it is suppressed, we suffer from weakness of will and lack of confidence. If it is frustrated it may be perverted into sullenness, resentment, spite, revenge, or a sense of grievance. If repressed it may be transformed into psychoneurotic character traits like outbursts of temper, or into obsessional neuroses like the fear of hurting people.

The origin of exaggerated aggressiveness. (i) Assertiveness is innately present in all normal people, but it appears to be natively stronger in some people than others who are of a milder, gentler temperament. Some people are *temperamentally aggressive*. We might therefore expect the man of bull-dog breed to be more obsessional. This does not appear to be the case, perhaps because such a man defies the fears which would otherwise repress the aggressiveness. The temperamentally aggressive child usually makes the strong-willed and successful business man.

(ii) On the psychological side aggressiveness is usually derived from three sources, over-encouragement, frustration and reaction to deprivation.

Obsessionals are often found to be those who in childhood have their self-will exaggerated and over-developed by being spoilt and pampered, a case of *exaggeration by encouragement*. Such a child will brook no interference and hates everyone who frustrates it. "How *dare* my mother," says one such patient, "stop me from doing *anything* I want!" Such aggressiveness conflicts with the demands of its parents and invites repression, to appear later as an obsession. This is the simplest cause of obsessional aggression, the fear of doing harm to others.

The sense of omnipotence is characteristic of the child and may be observed in children's play, as in a boy of three, who when thwarted in his desire to go to the shops to buy a certain toy, said, "I'm going to smash up the whole world," and then looked a little startled at his outburst and its possible consequences on the world! Such phantasies of omnipotence in children must not of course be taken too seriously, for it is only when the assertiveness is repressed that it may emerge as an obsession. Otherwise it tends to pass or develops into practical achievement. But to the child himself it may be real enough for he believes in the omnipotence of his wish. Therefore if he wishes a person dead and that person dies he may suffer from a violent sense of guilt and fear of the consequences of what his wish has brought about and may later suffer from a fear of injuring people, or shudder at the thought of cruelty to animals. This belief in the omnipotence of the wish originates in infantile experiences, for if the infant, whenever he wishes anything (his food, his napkin changed, to be carried, or to be put down), immediately gets the gratification of the wish, he is bound to develop the idea that he has only to wish for anything and it occurs without any effort on his part. This appears in fairy stories like the "Magic Carpet," and in novels like Balzac's *Peau de Chagrin*. In the child who continues to be pampered, the *wish* therefore becomes a substitute for the *will* and in many persons remains so in adult life, so that they expect everything and do nothing: they cannot tolerate frustration, and spend their time grumbling at the way life has treated them. They are unhappy people.

Another cause of aggressiveness is *frustration*. Indeed there are some psychologists who say that aggressiveness is experienced only when we are frustrated; for when we are denied a thing we want it the more (p. 75). The exaggeration is doubly strong when there is both encouragement and frustration, when the child is at one time allowed his own way and at another threatened; pampered by a mother, and scolded by a nurse; treated leniently by a father and frustrated by a jealous mother. Both the encouragement on the one side and the thwarting on the other exaggerates his aggressiveness. This dual treatment is often found to be the cause of delinquency; for the one makes him feel he can do what he likes, and the other by denying him what he wants, makes him want it the more. In Greek mythology Paris was first unwanted by his parents and exposed to die, and later was pampered by them; and he made all the trouble about Helen and caused the Trojan wars.

Exaggerated assertiveness may be a *reaction to earlier fears*, which compel a child to stand up for itself and be prematurely self-sufficient, in the way already described under anxiety hysteria.

But in our experience by far the commonest cause of the abnormal aggressiveness is found to be a reaction to a *feeling of deprivation of love*. Since the child's most fundamental need is for protective love, the denial of this love fills him with jealousy, resentment, rage, hate and fury, as we may observe any day in the nursery, for both love and rage are means of self-preservation. It is the typical reaction of the two-year-old child who is in the self-willed phase. Jealousy is natural in a child, as it is based upon the need for safety; indeed such behaviour is observed in animals like a favourite dog, who barks and protests when his master pets his own child. Every child wants to be first in order to be assured of protection and security. But such jealousy is of course greatly exaggerated if the child has previously been pampered and then feels thrust out.

There are many *occasions of the feeling of deprivation of love* leading to jealousy and hate found in the analysis of obsessional patients. The most common is perhaps the jealousy of a child who has hitherto received all the affection, but is pushed aside in favour of the baby who steals the picture; or it may be the jealousy of a younger child for an older child who is getting all the privileges; or the jealousy of a girl for the boy who is the mother's favourite; or of a boy for the sister who is the father's favourite, which makes him feel inferior; or it may be the jealousy of a healthy child for an invalid child who is getting all the attention; or of a parent towards his or her own child for stealing the love of the other parent. Inasmuch as the parent usually has a greater affection for the child of the opposite sex, the attachment of the child is usually returned towards the parent of the opposite sex, therefore each parent is jealous of the child of the *same* sex who robs him or her of love, and may treat the child with a polite indifference if not dislike.

Nothing therefore is more calculated to arouse rage and aggressiveness than the feeling of being left out or unloved.[1]

The evidence of this aggression in the obsessions appears at every turn.

(a) In going into *the early history* of these cases we usually find that about the age of two (the self-willed period of childhood) these patients were obstinate, "had a will of their own," and were very naughty, sulky, jealous, obstinate and bad-tempered; later they become difficult, tomboyish, rebellious or defiant and exhibited other manifestations of aggression. The parents may assure us that "he was always a good child"; but that is because they are recalling the time after the self-will had been repressed and the child adopted its good super-ego.

(b) The assertiveness also appears in the *character* of the obsessional. It is this which gives to the obsessional his "obsessional drive": he is often a person who has an exaggerated power psychology, is successful, ambitious, earnest, conscientious, efficient and capable. This character is derived from that part of his aggression which has escaped repression and has been sublimated as the ego ideal into forms approved by others.

In other cases the obsessional patient, more of whose aggressiveness has been repressed, outwardly appears to be timid, clinging, submissive and helpless, but we do not need to go far below the surface to discover his self-will. His intimate friends will confirm that he has a will of his own, his wife tells you he can be thoroughly obstinate if he likes, and usually manages to get what he wants. The patient does not recognize his assertiveness as much as others who know him better than he does himself. This state of tension in the obsessional is well illustrated in the capable business man, who full of self-pity was describing the hardness of his life, and reported that last evening he returned home tired after a troublesome day's work "and to crown everything I found that the maid had put my slippers out of reach under the bed and I said to myself 'My God! What next!'"

(c) Another indication of the aggressiveness of the obsessional is the fact that he *cannot be hypnotized*. The milder and more dependent forms of obsessional anxiety are open to *suggestion*, and indeed this is a valuable form of treatment to alleviate the anxiety, restore the self-confidence, and give the sense of security. But it

---

[1] Anal-erotism is said to be a cause of aggressiveness and obstinacy. We have not found it to be so, although it may be a mode of expressing obstinacy. The holding in of faeces is one of the few ways in which the child can defy the parent, and so far is a way of expressing aggressiveness, but does not originate it.

is the general opinion of those who have wide experience of hypnosis that whilst most conversion hysterics are easily hypnotized, those suffering from obsessional states cannot be brought into deeper hypnotic states. Hypnotism, like hysteria, is characteristically a condition of dependence, a return to a state of passivity, and its main feature is suggestibility, or psychic dependence, which means that the subject accepts without question whatever is suggested to him. The obsessional is aggressive and above all things dislikes being dominated and therefore even though he may ask to be hypnotized, and indeed may want to be in order to satisfy the deeper sense of dependence which lies beneath the assertiveness, he cannot be, because of the stubborn resistance to being dominated by anybody.

(d) The aggressiveness also appears *in the symptom itself*, especially those we have called obsessional aggressions, such as the fear of strangling, the impulse to plunge a knife into someone, the thought that we have poisoned someone we love, or spread disease.

(e) If any further doubt about the matter remains, it is completely dispelled by the manifestation of *aggression in the course of analysis*. As we unearth the cause of the fear, it is dispelled (since it is realized what is the real cause of the fear, and that it is no longer applicable), and the fear having now been abolished, there is nothing to hold back the aggressive tendencies which it had repressed, so that these surge forth in their crude and primitive form; as the fear goes, the rage, the anger, the hate, the bitterness, the jealousy all surge up. This is a common phase in the treatment of obsessionals, at which point the patient feels more confidence in himself whilst his friends complain that treatment has made him worse—"he used to be so nice and considerate."

(f) Sometimes this hate and aggressiveness is directed towards the physician in which case we have the *negative transference*, which is particularly liable to occur in obsessional cases in which aggressiveness and hate are the dominant features, whereas a positive transference is more likely to occur in the conversion hysterics where the craving for love is dominant.

This basic aggressiveness explains the characteristics of the obsessions. (a) In the first place it explains the *compulsiveness* of the obsession, as we have explained. It is because we *must* have our way that the consequences must happen. (b) But it also accounts for the *persistence* of the obsessions: for these repressed self-will impulses being repressed, are never satisfied and are therefore subject to perseveration; as long as the self-will persists, so long will the fear of the consequences remain. We are compelled to wash our hands and in half an hour must do so again, although we know it is silly. This is because the moral problem is not solved by its projection on to a physical plane and therefore persists. That is why obsessions tend to be chronic. (c) It also accounts for the *repetitive* nature of the obsessions, for so often as the aggression is revived, so often is the fear or need for propitiation reactivated. (d) The self-willed aggressiveness also accounts for the *exaggerated* nature of the symptom, for the greater the self-will to do the forbidden act, the greater the fear which is out of all proportion to the supposed objective cause; and the greater the guilt the greater the urgency to carry out the propitiations. (e) Because the self-will compulsion is repressed these obsessional fears are *involuntary*, being opposed to the dominant will, contrary to the accepted character of the personality. (f) Because of their projection on to irrelevant external objects and situations, obsessions also appear *irrational*.

Certain popular theories regarding the aetiology of obsessions may be mentioned. It used to be thought that the obsession came about in this way—that the *idea* of something, say a knife or a cliff, came into our mind, and this then produced the *impulse* to throw ourselves over, or to stab someone. There is an element of truth in this, the theory of "idio-motor action," for although the idea did not create the impulse, it nevertheless aroused the impulse and was the stimulus to this particular attack. But such a stimulus could not produce such a response were it not that the disposition was already present, ready to be aroused to such a response. The nature of the response depends not primarily on the stimulus, but on the latent disposition. (p. 41.)

Another popular idea may be exploded, or rather explained (for like most popular fallacies there is much truth in it); namely, the idea that we feel impelled to do something horrible just because it is horrible, the suggestion being that in some way the very fact that it is the one thing we do not wish to do which impels us to do it. It is in fact the very things the obsession most dislikes which he has the impulse to do. But it was not because it was horrible that a man has the morbid impulse to murder his mother; the impulse and desire were already there; it was because it was horrible that he repressed it, and being repressed it emerges as this horrible impulse. It is merely another way of saying that the super-ego is the opposite of the impulses it represses.

Minor instances of this are the compulsion to be rude or tactless; like the lady who having invited an interesting gentleman and his boring wife to dinner, let him in at the front door and unwittingly shut out the wife! *Tactlessness* is not always as innocent as it appears; and the person who is always "saying the wrong thing" is probably saying what she really intends to say: innocent naïveté is often a cloak for intentional spite.

A lady is buying some scent and being in doubt as to which was the best of two scents said to the beautiful young man serving her, "I don't suppose you would know." He replied, "Madam, I do happen to know." She said, "You would!" and then could have sunk with shame. The latent aggressiveness is obvious in these cases.

Closely akin to this is the common experience which most children feel and many adults have, namely, the desire to do things just because they are forbidden or "naughty." Why is there so much zest in doing things that are forbidden with the result that to forbid things is often an invitation to do them? This may have a simple explanation, namely, that so many desirable things are forbidden us in early childhood that we naturally conclude that all nice things are forbidden, and therefore that all forbidden things are desirable. There is an acquired association between naughtiness and desirability. But that is also why so many forbidden things which look desirable turn out to be disappointing, for we do not in fact want them except that they are forbidden.

There is, however, an added reason, for we are so hedged about with social taboos that there is a general desire to rebel and do as we like; and therefore whatever is forbidden is a good occasion for revolt, to throw off restraint, to demonstrate one's defiance, irrespective of what the occasion or the object may be.

All these illustrations demonstrate the basic self-will in man, and the causes of its exaggeration.

Repression of aggression. If the child succeeds in sublimating most of his assertiveness all may be well. But if the jealousy, hate and aggressiveness are disapproved, or if the child meets with one of the consequences or threats to his aggressiveness already mentioned, he must repress them. It is because of the deprivation of love that he becomes aggressive, and it is because of the need of love and security that he must repress it. He therefore has to adopt a super-ego of conformity to the will of others. Thereafter he fears the consequences of his aggressiveness as in the obsessional anxieties, although the aggressiveness and hate themselves do not appear in consciousness, but only the fear. Or he may suffer from obsessional aggressions in which there is a fear of the impulse itself, like fear of poisoning, although he is quite unaware of any desire to do so; or the symptom may assume the form of taking measures to propitiate for it as in the propitiatory obsessions, although he does not know why he feels guilty nor for what he is propitiating.

(C) The super-ego in the obsessions

In the obsession the aggressiveness or sex is repressed by the fear of consequences, with the result that a moral attitude is adopted, the purpose of which is to keep the fears at bay, to keep the forbidden desires repressed, and to compensate for the forbidden desires by a life of rectitude.

The nature of the super-ego depends on the nature of the conflict. If it is stark *fear* that is repressed then an attitude of self-sufficiency, power and success must be adopted to prove to oneself that one is strong and not afraid. If the forbidden impulse is *aggressiveness*, hate or jealousy, then it is obvious the super-ego must be one of ingratiation, being amenable and co-operative. If the *sexual* element is dominant the super-ego commonly takes an ascetic or prudish form; if the forbidden impulses are condemned as "dirty" the super-ego may take an aesthetic form; if the tendency is to be dishonest or lie, the consequences of which we fear, then we have a super-ego of scrupulous honesty and truthfulness. By these ultra-moral characteristics people therefore reveal the undesirable qualities they are trying to hide.

It is on account of the super-ego that although the obsessional patient feels the compulsion to commit these dastardly or dishonest acts, such as the impulse to strangle, *he does not in fact do the acts he fears*; he does not give way to his fears of poisoning or impulse to rape, because the super-ego which represses these impulses also sees to it that they are kept in check. In the propitiating acts, on the other hand, which are themselves activities of the super-ego, the acts are carried out to combat these impulses, as we shall see later.

The function of the super-ego in the obsessions is therefore to keep the forbidden impulses repressed, and sometimes it succeeds in doing so, as in the case of men and women of the highest moral rectitude who never sin and never make a mistake. But their very desire to be perfect becomes an obsession, and so great is the strain that in some cases such perfect characters end by a complete moral collapse (like the missionary in Somerset Maugham's *Rain*) or suicide (like the perfect Captain in Conrad's *Lord Jim*).

The subjective and objective problem. The establishment of the super-ego repressing forbidden desires raises moral issues, and transforms the objective to a subjective problem. This transition is very clear in our case of Major X. It was on account of the objective threats in childhood that he first experienced dread and which made him react by self-assertiveness. But when the self-willed rebellion was repressed by the fear of consequences this made him repress and fear his assertiveness, and assume an attitude of ingratiation and conciliatoriness. Thereafter, the impulses themselves which incur such consequences are regarded as morally wrong.

Thus it comes about that what was an *objective* danger becomes a *subjective* danger: what was at first a matter of social relationships between the child and the reproving mother, between the individual and society, becomes a *moral* problem concerned with individual attitude towards himself and the standards he has now adopted. He condemns himself concerning things for which other people no longer condemn him, and becomes his own severest critic. Not only so, but because he represses all the forbidden desires, he now has a sense of guilt but is unaware of why he feels it or of what he is guilty, so that the problem becomes a *psychopathological* one. This is an insoluble problem from which he can only escape by a neurosis. He is so absorbed with this endopsychic problem that he is unable to face his objective difficulties in life and having repressed his assertiveness which he regards as wrong, he is deprived of the courage which would enable him to cope with his problems and the means whereby he can stand up to them. The essence of the obsessional anxiety was therefore a present-day subjective moral conflict; but the moral conflict would not have arisen had it not been for the objective fears of his early childhood, which compelled him to submission.

The relations between the objective and subjective fears between the physical and moral danger is often observed in the child. One who spent his childhood in Africa has the fear of noise of wild animals at night. This might be considered natural under the circumstances: but his fear was that he would be abandoned by his parents and left to their mercy. But why should he fear this? It was not, as it might have been, that his parents were indifferent. It was because he persisted in being disobedient and therefore *forfeited their protection*. This is a typical obsessional anxiety in its simplest form. To tell such a child that there is nothing to be afraid of, or to tell him "not to be silly," is to fail to realize the moral significance of the fear. A child who is always asking "Am I a good boy?" is not necessarily pious, nor reflecting the severity of the mother, but the extent of his own feeling of guilt. Probably most of the morbid fears and nightmares from which so many children suffer are of this subjective type, fear of their own conscience, and that is why night terrors commonly start about the age of three when conscience and self-consciousness are developing.

When a man developed a claustrophobia (in the tube train which stopped in the tunnel), it was not merely a revival of the time when he was shut into a cupboard as a child, as it would be in hysterical anxiety. That punishment was for his self-willed disobedience and brought him to heel. But now the assertiveness was reactivated as a latent revolt against his father, the head of the firm of solicitors, who kept him down, but whom he dared not defy because of his earlier fears. He felt his personality suffocated by his father. He "must get out" of this intolerable situation: he could not bear to be "shut in" and the underground incident symbolically represented this fear of being obliterated. When he recovered an experience in childhood when his father unjustly punished him, his rage was released and he said, "My God! he will never do that again!" He thereafter stood up to his father, started a firm of his own, and was later honoured for his service to his country. It was as necessary to recover the original punishment which made him repress his assertiveness as it was to resolve the present-day moral conflict with his father which precipitated the claustrophobia. Once rid of the infantile fear of his father he could assert himself normally.

Psychopathologists seem divided between those who find the cause of the psychoneuroses in objective experiences and fears, such as claustrophobia due to being shut up in a cupboard, or even a fall on the head (a first favourite of the older neurologists); and those who find the essential causes in subjective conflicts present or past. These views are not incompatible, except in so far as they claim to be exclusive: indeed in all deep-rooted psycho-neuroses we find a combination of both objective and subjective factors, both of which have to be discovered for a complete cure. It is true, as we have seen, that the essential cause of the neurotic breakdown is a present-day moral problem. But we maintain that there would not have been the present subjective moral problem were it not for the objective experiences in early childhood. It is true that were it not for the present-day moral problem he would not fear; but were it not for the original problem he would not have had *cause* to fear. Those psychopathologists who deal only with the present-day moral conflict ignore the material facts which originated the moral conflict: those who consider only the environmental factors of childhood ignore the factors which make that conflict persist, and perpetuate the neurosis. Both play a necessary part in the production of the neurosis, and both require to be resolved to produce a *radical* cure.

Precipitating causes. From the foregoing discussion it will be obvious what will be the main causes of the precipitation of the breakdown. (*a*) The breakdown, as in hysteria, may be precipitated by anything which is capable of *arousing the repressed complexes and emotions* into activity, whether aggression, fear or sex; so that once released they refuse to be repressed any longer and give rise to the breakdown. (*b*) Secondly, anything that *weakens the super-ego* so that it is no longer capable of keeping the repressed and forbidden emotions at bay. Either of these upsets the balance that has been more or less successfully maintained for many years, and the result is "the nervous breakdown" by which we mean the "breakdown" of the established balance of the personality as maintained by the super-ego.

(*a*) According to the nature of the super-ego will be the precipitating cause. If the super-ego is one of *power*, then failure in business, failure in love, illness, or loss of an appointment or failing in an examination may be the precipitating cause: if it is one of *goodness*, it may be the arousal of whatever meets with the disapproval of others, such as jealousy, selfishness, or other moral failure: if it is *asceticism*, it may be any arousal of a sensual or sexual desire. All these are a threat to our super-ego.

(*b*) Sometimes the breakdown comes about by the *general weakening* of the super-ego with the lapse of time and experience, since the old motives no longer operate: at other times when the strain of living up to this super-ego becomes too burdensome. Sometimes the super-ego meets with a direct rebuff from others, as in the case of the woman whose ideal was to be self-sacrificing for everybody, but was told by her employer that she was merely a busybody, as in fact she was, her super-ego being based on self-importance. This blow to her pride precipitated an attack of depression and bad-temper, the former being due to the original arousal of the need for affection, and the latter derived from repressed hatred in childhood for which she was punished, as a result of which she developed her false super-ego. The very exaggeration of the super-ego which always occurs in obsessional states, invites failure. Perched on the pinnacle of his exaggerated ambitions or moral ideals, the obsessional patient is a fair target for criticism and at the same time is in constant danger of falling; he is therefore in a constant state of anxiety.

One such patient got an attack of agoraphobia in Regent Street one lunch hour for no apparent reason: but the reason was that his "conscience" smote him because he was taking off an extra quarter of an hour from the Government Office for purposes of his own. His attacks were always when he was doing something wrong, associated with a voice saying "Take care!" This was the voice of his nurse in childhood who taught him that the devil was round the corner ready to pounce on naughty boys. Indeed, he was once vouchsafed a glimpse of the devil in the person of the cook, who for the purpose of frightening him out of his naughtiness impersonated the devil, requiring only a small quantity of burnt cork to transform her into his perfect image. Ever after he lived a life of strict rectitude and as long as he did so he was free from overt symptoms: but unfortunately he was temperamentally strong-willed, and when in the course of time he began to outgrow not only his childhood fears but his childhood moral standards, his self-will surged forth in revolt, with the consequent dread of disaster. The essential feature in this case was obviously an exaggerated and morbid conscience.

Curiously enough in some cases an obsession may be precipitated when a person *abandons* what he considers to be wrong. This is because these forbidden desires put up a last fight and precipitate a more acute conflict. It is not uncommon for a girl to develop propitiatory obsessional acts when she ceases auto-erotic practices about the age of sixteen in favour of more natural heterosexual desires. Because she suppresses them the frustrated desires become more active, precipitating anxiety and demanding propitiation.

In other cases the breakdown occurs with the *repression of guilt*, that is to say with the repression of the super-ego. In one case a man and his wife agreed on "free love," but when at his suggestion his wife went to spend a weekend with a man friend, he precipitated an anxiety state, which greatly embarrassed and humiliated him! These problems cannot be solved by repressing a sense of guilt any more than by repressing forbidden impulses. That is why we cannot cure these obsessional conditions merely by telling the patient to give vent to his forbidden repressed desires. A repressed sense of guilt can be just as harassing as a repressed impulse of sex or aggression, and anything which arouses the sense of guilt or reminds us of some misbehaviour of our past is enough to precipitate an obsession.

Once the breakdown is precipitated almost anything, subjective feeling or objective conditions, even remotely connected with the conflict or suggesting it in any way, is sufficient to precipitate an attack: a warm room is enough to suggest suffocation or perspiration, a knife suggests murder, a harmless miss of a heart-beat suggests death, reading of a train disaster in the morning paper suggests impending doom. It is not surprising that the patient complains that the symptom comes on "for no reason at all."

(c) It will be obvious that there are certain conditions in life which tend to precipitate breakdowns more than others, since they are prone to rouse the latent conflict; especially illness, the resulting anxiety of which may be far more terrifying than the occasion warrants. *Illness is a very common precipitating cause of phobias* because in the first place there is a real and objective cause of worry, since the illness affects our life and work. It also may arouse fears of earlier experiences of illnesses, the primal fears in infancy; but most of all if it is associated with punishment for forbidden desires. So the boy who fainted in church after diphtheria, felt this to be on account of his masturbation, about which he has been threatened in his earlier childhood, and now everyone would know of his guilt. An illness comes to such as a nemesis.

Again, illness strikes a blow to the power psychology, to the self-confidence and self-sufficiency which we have set up as a barrier against primal fears, a threat to the integrity of the personality. But illness also provides us with an excuse for escaping from the strain of living up to these exaggerated standards as well as our excuse to get sympathy, but this unconscious desire for illness acts as a still further threat which we fear and must resist at all costs.

To these psychological factors we must add the fact that illness is a common precipitating cause because of its toxic effects, which lowers resistance of the patient, encourages psychosomatic disorders which give him real grounds for believing he is ill, and renders him incapable of coping with his responsibilities and problems.

The Symptom as in all the psychoneuroses represents the emergence of the repressed tendencies. But it is a *compromise* of these conflicting forces and the super-ego. The form of the final symptom depends on the predominance of one or another of these factors. The most obvious illustration of this compromise is in the fear of hurting or poisoning, in which is expressed the impulse to hurt, the fear of its consequences, and the super-ego's horror at the very idea. This compromise is derived from elements from all three strata, the aggression, the fear, and the super-ego. The man who had the phobia that if he put his right boot on before the left a plague would break out in Australia, was demonstrating the fear of consequences but also gratifying his sense of omnipotence: he was a veritable god whose slightest act had far-reaching and

T

disastrous consequences. Yet his super-ego was shocked at the idea.

A girl had an obsessional hate of her mother to whom she is devotedly attached, but feels guilty for having such feelings and deserving of punishment. So she develops a phobia, namely, that she will be punished for her guilt by her mother being killed in an accident: a beautiful compromise satisfying both her desire that her mother should be killed and her moral sense. As, unfortunately for her, no accident occurred, she later developed the fear that her mother would commit suicide, which would also free her and exonerate her from blame. Her self-will, her fear of consequences, and her moral ego ideal are all gratified! She was a most devoted daughter, but a very sick woman!

So with obsessions in which the moral super-ego is dominant, like the shame or remorse at some sin or imagined sin of the past, which gives one the gratification of thinking about that sin: the persistence of the remorse is due to the fact that the desire persists. It enables the patient to think continuously of the lost joys of sin, the loss of which contributes to his sadness! A public confession of sin is often a form of self-display and the persisting thought of the past sin gives expression to the longing for the good old times, as well as to true repentance. The obsessional fear of inferiority is often to excuse oneself from making an effort, but is coupled with the omnipotent feeling "If only I had not this inferiority complex what great things I could do." Thus the inferiority complex gratifies the feeling of superiority without the necessary effort of achievement, and self-depreciation is often an excuse for laziness. The inferiority complex is the only one of which people boast of possessing; that is because it is a back-handed compliment to themselves since it implies that they think much less of themselves than they really are! The obsessional psychosomatic symptom of blushing represents the shame in not conforming to social demands, but it also represents the anger against having to conform to these social demands, and an excuse to avoid the society which makes us feel inferior by not treating us with the consideration and respect we were led to expect in childhood.

The symptom in obsessional conditions is, therefore, as in all psychoneuroses, *an attempt to cure the patient* by giving expression to tendencies of the personality, especially assertiveness, which should never have been repressed, and without which the personality cannot be strong and free. The fact that they emerge in pathological form is not the fault of the impulses but of the super-ego which has repressed them, or rather of the circumstances which resulted in the formation of the super-ego. The obsessional symptom is a revolt of the natural self against the exaggerated moral demands of the moral self. But in many cases it is the expression of a sense of guilt to which we ought to be paying consideration.

The Specific Symptom. There is no purpose in discussing the various phobias in detail because the conscious object of fear, whether of cancer, crowds, loneliness, of flies or of hearing an organ, are comparatively unimportant and often accidental. Indeed we frequently find the symptom shifting from one object to another, so that in treatment we may find ourselves chasing these symptoms around instead of getting at the fundamental causes of fear. The specific phobias are significant only as being an index and a guide to the more deep-seated cause of the trouble, and we therefore take them merely as the starting point of our analysis to discover the deeper causes.

Some are derived from the *primal fear* in infancy, the fear of loneliness, of isolation, of separation, of suffocation, are all infantile fears, without any reference or consciousness of forbidden desires. In other cases the symptom comes from the *threatened fear*, fear of harm to oneself as a result of the forbidden impulses, such as fear of madness, fear of Hell and death, fear of castration. In other cases the *fear is of the repressed impulse* itself, as in the fear of hurting, or the fear of sexually assaulting. In still other cases the *moral element* is dominant and we have abnormal character traits like over-conscientiousness and obsessional propitiatory acts, associated with anxiety if these are not carried out. The symptom in all these cases can be traced to a specific phase in the development of the neurosis.

Again, because the cause of the fear is unknown and repressed we tend to *project the anxiety* upon specific objects or situations in some way connected with the fear: so we fear illness, open spaces, closed spaces, life, suicide, but still without in the least knowing why we fear these things, the real object of fear being not these things, but the impulses within ourselves; so the anxiety states turn into specific phobias. Or again we *personalize these dangerous impulses* and project them into fear of animals, of ogres, of robbers, of burglars. So the fear borrows its shape from any fear we have experienced (p. 262).

Finally, because the real cause of fear, shame or guilt is unknown, the fear may become *transferred to the symptom*, so that, for instance, the psychosomatic accompaniments of fear or shame such as blushing, irregularity of the heart and perspiration may themselves become the objects of fear, whereas in fact they are the results. The transference of these fears to specific objects or situations serve a useful purpose to the patient, for it is easier to deal with a material than a moral danger, since we may devise means of avoiding it. It is easier to avoid a close space than to avoid the consequences of our self-will which we refuse to abandon; to cling to someone in our fear of loneliness than to face up to the consequences of a sin which is deserving of these consequences; to perform some ritual, than to become moral, to wash our hands than to clean our soul, to say our prayers than to repent.

But because these fears are transferred from the real moral problem to these objects or acts, the latter become invested with far more emotion than they warrant. Thus the fear of blushing is so fraught with shame that people have been known to take their lives because of it: and if they fail to carry out the slightest ritual they are obsessed with the most terrifying fears.

Mechanism and types of obsession

We see in the obsessions the *threefold mechanism* characteristic of all the psychoneuroses, two primitive tendencies conflicting with one another, both of which are repressed in favour of a moral attitude. In the case of the obsessions there is a strongly developed self-willedness; this is repressed by fear of consequences; and therefore the individual develops a super-ego of being good, to avert the fear.[1]

The specific type of obsession is determined according to which of these three phases of the conflict is dominant: the aggressiveness, the fear of consequences, or the super-ego.

(a) *If the fear element predominates,* it alone may appear in consciousness, and these are the *obsessional anxieties* and phobias, characterized by the *fear of harm to oneself,* like the fear of insanity, or the fear of loneliness, which are, however, threats on account of our forbidden desires. In such cases the aggressiveness or hate is so repressed that it does not appear at all, but only as anxiety.

In many cases, however, it is not fear, but shame, disgust, humiliation, disappointment or depression which repress the forbidden desires, in which case the symptom takes the form of an obsessional shame, depression or sense of inferiority instead of

---

[1] In addition to these phases we often find in obsessional anxieties a primal fear in infancy, on account of which the later threatened fear of consequences is regarded as so disastrous. But this is not essential to the obsessional conflict as such, nor does it usually occur in the obsessional aggressions.

fear or anxiety. These we may group as *obsessional affective states.* In such cases the more self-will there lies behind the persisting desire, the stronger and more persistent will be the depression, shame or inferiority, which is the result or consequence of the desire.

(b) *If the aggressive impulses predominate* they themselves appear in consciousness as part of the symptom, so that we have a compulsion to hurt, or a fear of poisoning or strangling. These are what, for want of a better name, we call the *obsessional or compulsive aggressions,* in which the idea of doing *harm to others* is the chief motive. In these conditions we are aware of the impulse to hurt, but we are not aware that it is wished. The man who has the impulse to strike every nurse in the face has no conscious desire to do so, nor has the mother who has the obsessional fear of poisoning her child: but an analysis always reveals the unconscious desire and why it is desired.

In other cases it is sex which is the repressed forbidden desire, in which case the obsession may appear as a *sex obsession,* such as the fear of raping or of taking off one's clothing.

(c) *If the moral super-ego is dominant* in the causation and symptom, we have the *obsessional propitiations,* such as the compulsion to be tidy, to say prayers, or *obsessional character traits,* such as being over-conscientious, over-scrupulous and punctilious—the purpose of which acts is to avert the dreaded consequences of our forbidden desires. Henceforth all anxiety becomes transferred from the forbidden impulses, of which we may now be quite unaware, to the carrying out of these moral and religious demands, which themselves become compulsive and which *must* be performed with the greatest exactitude, punctiliousness and sense of duty. Everything which prevents us carrying out these acts, or any failure in living up to these moral standards will fill us with distress and alarm because of the threat of disaster: hence the anxiety which is associated with the carrying out of all obsessional acts, ceremonials and rituals.

(d) But the conflict may be so severe that the patient suffers from indecision and other *obsessional inhibitions* which prevent him doing anything lest he shall do anything wrong. He will spend hours deciding on which tie to put on. It is perpetually the case of "to be or not to be"; that is the question and remains a question which is never satisfactorily answered. Whatever one side of his personality decides the other side refuses to comply: so he lives in a permanent state of never being able to make up his mind and suffers from aboulia, lack of will. Usually these inhibitions are on the part of the super-ego to prevent him carrying out the forbidden desires; but they may be on the part of the ego refusing to carry out the demands of the super-ego.

To illustrate these various reactions and their relation to different types of obsession we may take a hypothetical case. A girl has a *fear of killing* her mother. This came from a momentary impulse, immediately repressed, to be rid of her mother, as the girl resented her interference in a love affair. But such a latent desire might have taken various forms. (i) It might have taken the form of an *impulse* to kill her mother to whom she was, however, consciously devoted. (ii) It may have appeared simply as a dread of something happening to herself, in which the idea of hurting her mother is entirely repressed, and only the fear of consequences to herself appears in consciousness. This is an *obsessional anxiety or phobia*. (iii) On the other hand, it might have appeared as the *thought that the mother may be killed* in an accident (when there was no reason whatsoever for thinking she would be) which is a mixture of fear of losing a mother on whom she depends, and a desire that she should be killed so as to get free of her; but the phobia also relieves the girl of the responsibility of having killed or wished to kill her mother, and the wish remains undetected. These are *obsessional aggressions or compulsions*. (iv) The fear that *she might go mad and then kill her mother* is another thinly disguised form of the same desire, but it also exonerates her from blame, for if one is mad one is not responsible for one's actions. The obsessional fear of insanity, however repellent, often represents such a desire, but in the form of an obsessional anxiety. (v) To counteract the forbidden desire, she may develop an *over-anxiety* about the mother's health, though the mother is in perfect health, or an exaggerated feeling of responsibility for her, when the mother can quite well take care of herself. These attitudes she consciously accepts: they are obsessional *character traits*. (vi) But the guilt may be more conscious, though the reason may be unknown, and she may feel it necessary to confess everything to her mother (everything except that she hates her) and develops a confessional mania; or she may have to count ten before performing any act (to keep a check on her impulses) which are forms of *propitiatory obsession*. (vii) Or she many develop an *obsessional inhibition* that she cannot touch her mother, which is a precaution of the super-ego to prevent her "laying hands" on her mother.

We shall consider these clinical types in greater detail in the following chapter.

CHAPTER XII

CLINICAL OBSESSIONAL TYPES

(A) Obsessional anxieties and phobias

Obsessional anxieties are fears of the consequences of our forbidden impulses, in which the *fear of harm to oneself* is the dominant feature and this fear alone appears as the symptom. The phobia is compulsive for the self-will insists on the forbidden desire, and every time the forbidden wish is aroused, so often is the fear precipitated, as we have already demonstrated.

The obsessional anxieties are akin to hysterical anxieties, and indeed they may all be clinically grouped as "anxiety hysteria," since they are both characterized by a fear of harm to oneself. They may both originate in infantile fears and may assume the same form, so that the symptoms are often identical.

Thus phobias such as fear of illness, fear of loneliness, fear of open spaces, fear of close space, fear of death, of some impending catastrophe, of heights, of the dark, of the future and of the past may be the mere emergence of infantile fears threatening the integrity of our personality, as in hysterical anxiety, but they are very commonly fear of the consequences of forbidden unconscious desires, as in obsessional anxiety. Some further notes on common obsessional anxieties may be added.

Agoraphobia is said to be a fear of open space. But as we have pointed out, on closer investigation it is found to be not so much a fear of open space as a *fear of isolation,* fear of loneliness, fear of separation, of lack of contact. The space as such is important in that it accentuates the sense of isolation. Animals separated from the herd suffer this dread; man suffers it when lost in the desert or forest; infants suffer from it most of all. We frequently find that the agoraphobia relates back to the separation at birth itself, or at least in infancy. In hysterical anxiety this infantile fear is repressed but emerges when the barrier of self-sufficiency breaks down. In obsessional anxiety this fear assumes a moral nature, for by his anti-social aggressiveness the obsessional cuts *himself* off from his fellows, deserves to be isolated.

Claustrophobia is the so-called fear of close spaces. But it is associated with a large number of other symptoms such as a dislike of being shut in, of being thwarted, of having a dress or shirt put over the head in dressing, in being kissed on the mouth, the dread of an anaesthetic, of being buried alive, or travelling in underground trains, of being in a stuffy atmosphere as in a church, theatre or cabin of a ship.[1]

Another instance is that of a patient who feeling stuffy in a small bedroom, got up in the night, broke the window and slept peacefully; only to find in the morning that he had broken the glass of the bookcase! An American patient got claustrophobia whenever he came to England, because it was so small a place to live in! There was not enough room for his global personality.

Claustrophobia basically represents a fear of suffocation. We can live without food for weeks, without drinks for days, but we cannot exist without air for more than a few minutes. It is often traceable back to birth or the giving of an anaesthetic for an operation like the removal of tonsils, and the discovery and release of this fear often cures the phobia.

But there are other origins of claustrophobia. A patient had a horror of anything being over her face, which originated when she was put in her cot as an infant and being in a rage twisted about till her face was buried in the pillow from which position she could not extricate herself: this was a result, and was therefore regarded as the punishment, for her rage. In a similar case the claustrophobia originated in her head being pushed under the water in the bath; in two other cases from being overlain by cats (who seem to like the warm spot of an infant's face and have been known to suffocate children to death). In another case the fear came from being overlain by the mother, and the patient during the analysis went through the struggle of agony in the attempt to push away the great wall of flesh. In another case the child's cries were suffocated by the mother pressing the child's face to her bosom to keep him from waking his irritable father, which besides producing a claustrophobia, gave rise to a compulsive tic of the mouth when talking, that is, expressing himself.

All these experiences were the prototypes of the later claustrophobia. They may themselves be momentary and leave no observable results except the temporary protestations of the child, but it may fill the child with continuing dread if it is related to any disobedience or forbidden desire, which gives it a moral significance.

---

[1] One individual suffering from claustrophobia, but compelled to cross the ocean, wrote asking the chief steward for a comfortable "birth." She received the reply that he would do his best but could not guarantee that she would not suffer from "mal de *mère*!"

Equally important, though less recognized, are the cases in which the suffocation comes from an *overwhelming passion*, whether of sex feeling or of anger, even in infancy, the child "choking with anger," or being overwhelmed with a terrifying orgasm. For in these cases also the terrifying experiences come about as the result of one's own behaviour.

The importance of all these objective sources of fear for the prevention of anxiety neurosis must not be overlooked. At the same time it must be stressed again that these fears alone do not make a neurosis, and granted that the child is given subsequent reassurance the fear passes.

But these fears often lead to a power urge to counteract them and thereafter the fear is of losing this sense of power. The patient cannot bear to be shut in, thwarted, obstructed, hindered; he must be free, he must have ample space for his personality to move in with nobody crowding in upon him. He has a sense of omnipotence and cannot bear that his power should in any way be limited: he is intolerant of all restriction even that of a tight collar and cannot brook any restraint even to sitting in an inside seat in a theatre, and when in a stuffy room he feels he must get out. Anything in fact which savours of frustration fills him with panic. "The trouble about a claustrophobic," said a patient suffering from it, "is that no space is big enough for him!" He appears to be timid; he is really arrogant, but he fears the consequences of his arrogance because of threats in childhood.

It is his insoluble problem that he cannot live without asserting himself, but that if he asserts himself he is threatened with disaster. Therefore when his assertiveness is aroused he gets into a panic: but equally when his assertiveness is threatened he gets in a panic. It is not surprising that he is in an almost constant state of dread. The fear of a close space is therefore symbolic of the frustration, suffocation of the personality.

The fear of falling is probably, as Watson would have us believe, an innate fear. It is a very common symptom, and of some complexity. There is, for instance, reason to think that astigmatism with the production of giddiness may be a factor; others think that it is due to lack of co-ordination, for whilst your eyes tell you that you are 100 feet from the ground, your feet tell you 5 feet from the ground; but when you are sitting in an airplane, you do not suffer from fear of falling because sitting gives you the sense of firmness and security. Psychologically, it may be an objectively conditioned symptom originating in a terrifying experience of an actual fall in infancy. But such experiences usually pass unless reinforced, or reactivated by a fall or accident in adult life, or reactivated by a moral problem which is precipitated. The fear of falling symbolically represents a *fear of falling from our pedestal*, whether of our ambitions, as in the Adlerian psychopathology, or of a *moral lapse*, a "fall" of a sexual nature. On the other hand, the fear of falling in some cases is found to be a *desire* to fall, to come down from the pedestal instead of perpetual striving to live in the giddy heights of idealism, effort or ambition, or it may be an unconscious urge towards a sexual lapse.

Even the fear of the impulse to throw ourselves in front of a train which is obviously not consciously wished but fills us with horror, is sometimes due to a subconscious wish to let everything go. It often occurs in people who are overstrained and have an unconscious urge to "put an end to it all." In others we have found it to be a masochistic sexual desire to be "less than the dust beneath thy chariot wheels."

Since the problem is basically a moral one, it cannot be solved by avoiding such objective situations. Therefore a man cannot escape a fear of heights by becoming a tea planter in Assam, where he lives in a bungalow, for he is perpetually harassed with the thought that on his next leave five years hence in Calcutta he may be put on the second floor in the hotel.

(B) *Obsessional or compulsive aggressions*

This is the name we give to those obsessions the characteristic feature of which is a compulsion or *fear of harm to others* as distinct from the obsessional anxieties and phobias which are fear of harm to oneself.

Self-will is, as we have seen, the most characteristic feature of the obsessions. In both the obsessional anxieties and the obsessional aggressions there is a fear of one's self-willed impulses, but in the former the fear is of consequences of harm to oneself, in the latter, fear that one's aggressiveness will do harm to others. In the former the primal fear so dominates the picture that the self-will and aggressiveness does not appear in the symptom except to give it compulsiveness. In the obsessional and compulsive aggressions, the aggressiveness is primal, and is repressed by threats of consequences, with the result that the aggressiveness itself appears in the symptom together with the fear, as in a fear of hurting or of strangling. The simplest illustration is that of an *obsessional impulse*, such as the man who had the impulse to strike every nurse in the face. But as a rule there is a fear without the feelings of compulsion to do it.

The most common instances of the obsessional aggressive phobias are of hurting, of killing, or poisoning. In every such case we find an early impulse to hurt or kill, very frequently as a result of jealousy, but this becomes repressed either by threats of punishment, fear of the further loss of protective love, or by nightmares which often objectify the rage as monstrous furies threatening the child, and so emerges as the fear of the impulse.

It is sometimes said that the over-anxiety of the mother about her child is always an unconscious *wish* that the child should be ill. This is frequently the case: but not necessarily. It may be an ordinary justifiable anxiety concerning, say, an actual illness of the child, or it may simply be that the mother herself was the subject of the same kind of anxiety in her childhood. Again, her present over-anxiety may be concerned with her personal moral conflicts which have nothing to do with the child, but only projected on to it. In other words, the mother's anxiety may be objective, conditioned, hysteric or obsessional. So too, a child's fear of losing his mother may be because he wants to be rid of her; but it may also be that he cannot do without her, a conscious or repressed dependence on her.

Mrs. B. (p. 192) who prided herself on being a perfect mother (the exaggerated super-ego) had the phobia that she would leave on the gas in the little girl's bedroom and so suffocate her, and this fear was regarded as the natural anxiety of the good mother for the safety of her child. On analysis it was found that beneath her devotion there was a bitter resentment against this child because she stood in the way of her ambition, which significantly enough was maternity and child welfare work! The wish to be rid of her child so that she should fulfil this ambition was interestingly shown in the fact that on two occasions when she went in to make sure the gas was turned off she actually turned it on! So strongly may unconscious motives work. Her anxiety for her child was natural in view of her own unconscious impulse to get rid of her.

A woman has an obsession that she will poison her child, and that she will leave wires in the kettle which will give cancer to her husband. She also was the "perfect mother" and the devoted wife. She had been the spoilt child of her mother and developed strong narcissistic and omnipotent ideas: she used to kiss her own body. Going too far she got a thrashing from her father which humiliated and infuriated her. She would like to have murdered him. But she was helpless and her anger had to be repressed, so that she became a sweet docile girl. The phobias were precipitated when she had a baby, and her husband naturally paid some regard to the child: her furious jealousy and hate were aroused, but she could not give vent to it, for was she not the perfect mother, the sweet wife. So the revenge took the form of a fear of injuring both the child and the husband (taking the place of her father). The child later died, but her hate pursued the wretched creature even to the after-world, for she feared that something she might do would harm the child in heaven! The repressed aggressiveness and hate, the fear of consequences and the unconscious wish are all obvious in this case, and combine to form the symptom.

The fear that harm might happen to others has the same motive. The woman who feared an accident might happen to her husband was repressing an unconscious wish arising from the fact that the man she had always been in love with was now free to marry her, but she could not marry unless "something happened" to her husband.

In another case, a patient, during the release of her aggressiveness in analysis, was learning to drive and suddenly got a panic of driving, lest she smash into things. This was not mere timidity, but represented a feeling of power, rage and fury which she has repressed. Now that she has all this power at her disposal, she is afraid it will get out of control, and force her to smash into people.

The man who had the fear of stabbing a knife into his wife, discovered that this was related to an impulse to do so to his mother, whose favourite he was, when she was ill-treating his older brother. He could not give expression to his anger because his mother would have turned on him, so he repressed it; later he transferred this repressed hate against his domineering wife when she was scolding one of their children, but against whom he was afraid to stand up, as he had been of his mother.

A girl of thirteen suffered from the fear that she would, in writing letters to her mother from school, transmit germs which might contaminate or injure her mother. In her mother's presence she was asked if she was self-willed as a child, but immediately her mother replied, "Oh, no! She was the sweetest child." But the girl replied, "Oh! Mother, but you didn't know!" As a small child she had a furious jealousy against a baby sister, and hated her mother. Later she developed tuberculosis and found it paid to be "patient and sweet" because people brought her more presents. But when her mother came to sit with her in the open-air balcony she used to say, "Mother dear, don't stay here, it is so cold for you! *I* am used to it." Such consideration on the part of the sick child was most touching: but her real reason was that she wished to be rid of her mother and preferred to read her books undisturbed. Her present-day phobia was a revolt against having to write letters to her mother, combined with a subconscious wish to get rid of her mother in this microbic manner! But the meaning of her symptom that every letter she wrote would be contaminated and spread disease which would kill her mother and her sister went further than that, for she was not only giving vent to her hate against her mother, but to her contamination complex (the unconscious desire to be "filthy"), and also giving vent to her phantasy of power (that so slight an act of hers can produce such disastrous and far-reaching results). Yet the fear of killing was not *merely* the desire to kill, but the fear of losing her mother and her protection if she were to get rid of her. The symptom (as Freud says) was over-determined, with several motives. This patient was quite cured of her obsessions by the revelation of these causes. Obsessions are difficult to cure and some we have in fact not been able to cure: but to say, as some do, that they are incurable is contradicted by facts; indeed the adolescent type often cures itself.

Obsessional tics are of this order. Tics may be reflex spasms due to irritation, say of a slight injury to a vertebra through a fall producing a tic of the neck, or an irritable tooth which may produce a tic of the mouth. But a tic is often an obsessional compulsion. *A psychological tic is an aborted action;* we have an impulse to act but the act is checked.

A woman has a spasmodic shrug of the right shoulder. It was a "habit spasm" revived from an experience at the age of three when from being the favoured child she was discarded for a new baby. She became furious, attacked the baby, and was locked up in her bedroom. Screaming in rage and desperation she tried to lift the window with her shoulder to get out, but failed. She had to give in and ever after became the "good girl." The tic of the shoulder represented the aggressive self-willed determination which was repressed, and was revived every time she felt angry or annoyed or resentful or jealous. It was an aborted impulse.

Another woman has a blinking or rather squeezing of the eyelids: which related to an incident about the age of two when she was persistently naughty in the bath, till her mother in exasperation pushed the sponge full of soap into her face and hurt her eyes badly. This injury and her mother's anger made her repress her assertiveness, and she ultimately became a nurse. The spasm of the eyes represented the suppression of her self-will, and appeared whenever her self-will was aroused.

Such obsessional acts are obviously different in origin from propitiatory acts, the one being a manifestation of the repressed ego, the other the super-ego.

Stammering and stuttering are most unpleasant symptoms frequently associated with a marked sense of shame and humiliation. The difference between them has been described thus: stammering is a stoppage that you cannot move; and stuttering is a movement that you cannot stop! In some cases it is a hesitation due to indecision, the demand to say something, to blurt out what one really feels, accompanied by the fear of doing so because of rebuff or humiliation, a case of obsessional inhibition to which we shall later refer. In other cases the unconscious motive is to elicit sympathy as in a conversion hysteria; or a means of avoiding unpleasant tasks. There is almost invariably an unconscious motive and that is why mere vocal exercises and breathing so often have only partial results.

A boy of six, whose phantasy of himself can be judged from the fact that his father nicknamed him "Pure Gold," made a contemptuous remark about a street boy who thereupon fought him and gave him a bloody nose. A crowd collected, asked what was the matter, but the patient stammered, unable to give a correct explanation because his humiliation was the result of his own arrogance. He continued to stammer whenever his temptation to arrogance was met by the fear of humiliation. Stammering like other psychoneuroses has its purpose.

In another case a small boy new to a class was asked a question in spelling which he should have learnt and stumbled in his reply, where-upon the teacher thinking he was a stammerer passed on to the next. So he discovered in this an easy way out of unpleasant tasks. Another found his stammer useful on occasions when people were inclined to be angry with him, and his stammering would turn their annoyance into pity. These motives were of course unconscious.

But stammering we have often found to have as its motive a desire to attract attention, which it certainly does. That is one reason why stammerers do not stammer in public speaking, or singing, because they are then already in the limelight.

A boy much repressed at home made friends with another boy who stammered. Seeing the notice the other boy got for his stammer (people turned round in the street), he decided to do the same. Another value of stammering is that unpleasant as it is in consciousness, it is obvious that as long as a patient stammers he holds the field, and everyone has to wait and keep silence till he is finished.

These motives for stammering are not surmises, but have all been found in actual cases.

Clinically, though stammering is so obviously a functional condition (other contributing conditions like left-handedness not-withstanding) it is not easy to cure, and our results have been poor if the condition started in the earliest years before the patient ever learned to speak correctly. Those originating later are more hopeful, and those which are recent, as in traumatic experiences of war, are comparatively easy. In the war cases one nearly always found that the patient was actually speaking at the time of the accident or bomb explosion, a case of association. The difficulty in the treatment of stammering may be that speech being so refined an instrument of the emotions, it requires that there must be a more effective adjustment and more complete resolution of the causes before the patient's speech is cured. In many cases a combination of analysis and speech re-education is required when neither is itself sufficient.

Nail biting is a common compulsive expression of repressed aggressiveness. Biting is a primitive mode of attack, still used by children and adults in extreme cases. The child who cannot let off its aggressiveness against others, lets off its aggression by biting its own nails, which has the added advantage that it can feel the effect of its biting (even taking pleasure in injuring itself) and also that its hand cannot, like its toys, be taken away from it.

Suicide is often due to an impulse of the same nature, as we learn from cases in which the attempt has not succeeded. It is sometimes heroic, as with Arctic explorers, sometimes due to sheer despair, but in other cases it comes of rage and frustration, which failing to find outlet against others is turned into destructiveness against oneself. We may see this self-destructiveness in the child who bangs its head against the wall: it must hurt something! That is particularly so in cases where the suicide takes a violent form like shooting or cutting the throat, as against more passive forms like drowning and poisoning. This destructiveness against oneself is accentuated when there is a marked duality between the ego and the super-ego such as we find in the obsessions: for on the one hand the moral super-ego may so rage against the immoral ego that it turns in destruction against itself. Men of the highest moral integrity have been known to commit suicide sometimes because of the too great strain of living up to their high ideals, or perhaps from some sense of guilt. On the other hand, the ego may be so enraged at the super-ego for keeping it perpetually frustrated that it cannot tolerate the restraint and commits suicide.

(C) *Sex anxieties and obsessions*

These are the conditions in which the fear or compulsion relates to a sexual impulse or desire. As in the obsessional aggressiveness the fear of hurting is due to a desire to hurt, so in the sex obsessions there is the fear of committing a sexual act, because there is a strong unconscious urge towards it. The sexual factor, like the aggressive, may not appear in consciousness but only as the fear: so that whenever sex is in any way aroused there results an attack of pure anxiety or dread. These we may call *Sex anxieties*. It is therefore sometimes impossible on the face of it to tell whether an anxiety neurosis has a sexual, an hysteric or an aggressive basis since the basic factors may be completely repressed and appear only as anxiety or a phobia. In other cases the feared sex impulses like the impulses to hurt appear in the symptom. These we shall call *sex obsessions*.

Cases of sex anxieties

A married woman who had had a "good time" with men friends before marriage developed her first attack of violent agoraphobia when motoring to a picnic in the country with a man friend. At birth she suffered suffocation and was unloved by her parents who favoured the sister, so that she found a necessary solace in sex and in later flirtations to satisfy her sense of security. In the car the desire arose to have "a good time" with this man; but if she did she might lose the love and security of her husband, which in view of her early anxiety she must at all costs keep. But she revolted against having to spend her life with a dull though devoted husband. The attack of agoraphobia saved the situation; by compelling her to return, it came down on the side of her security, and so solved the moral problem. At the same time it called for the attention of her husband. But the guilty desire persisted so that the fear which made her cling to her husband also persisted.

Another woman had a phobia of the deep tones of an organ, because, as she discovered, they represented the deep angry voice of her father who had beaten her for being wilful and disobedient: but in beating her he had aroused her sex feelings, so that the symptom was an unconscious masochistic yearning, and her violent shakings partly a fear and partly a reproduction of the pleasurable experience of being beaten. We have had not a few patients in whom the feeling of being overwhelmed by fear itself gave them masochistic sex pleasure. For a similar reason some women have the obsession that people are blaming or abusing them, because the thought of being abused arouses these same masochistic feelings. One such who feared the hostility of her servant maid, visualized her in free association as "springing on me, overmastering me, abusing me and beating me, and that increases my sexual desire; and I imagine her masturbating me as she abuses me." In other cases the compulsions which appear to be purely aggressive such as the impulse to strangle or to stab with a knife may be sexual in origin, and closely allied to sadism.

The fear of cancer is commonly the fear of the moral cancer within us, and it is at the same time a punishment for it. Such symptoms are often precipitated in adolescence when the inevitable arousal of sex brings with it the fear of syphilis, insanity and other supposed disastrous consequences of sex.

Sex obsessions. In other cases the sexual element appears in the symptom itself in precisely the same way as the aggressive element in the obsessional aggressions; such as the fear of a father that he will rape his daughter, the fear of a woman that she will tear off her clothes in public (exhibitionist compulsion); the compulsion to mutilate oneself or others sexually, to shout out obscene words, or being obsessed with sex thoughts. These may be further associated with compulsive feelings of shame about sex, although the patient may not be aware of being in any way guilty about sex. The "contamination complex" is most commonly of a sexual nature, such as in the case of the young man who had the obsession that if he touched a door handle, book or other object this might convey semen and cause some young woman to have a baby. This safeguarded his morals and avoided the consequences of sex, but also satisfied his power fantasy of having any woman he wanted and being the father of millions.

In such cases the patient cannot but admit the sexual nature of his obsession, but would be the last to admit that there is any *desire* to do the thing he fears or is ashamed of: but if there were no desire there would be no shame. In obsessional shame or disgust it is usually sex which is repressed, for the simple reason that such terms are usually applied to sex and not to manifestations of aggression. There are, however, other non-sexual activities of which we are made to feel shame and disgust, such as interest in our motions as children, which later may produce obsessions such as that the body smells.

If these sex activities are not exaggerated but threatened and repressed in childhood, it may lead to sex impotence in adult life: if they are strongly developed and then repressed, it may lead to arrest of development of sex so that they later emerge as the sex perversions: but if the sex is backed by self-will and repressed by fear of consequences there will result a sex anxiety or a typical sex obsession. This is the difference in psychopathology between sex perversions and sex obsession: *what is desired in the perversions is fcared and abhorred in the obsessions.*

A professional man has the impulse to strangle any girl to whom he is making love, and on two occasions has had to rush off and have himself certified in a mental hospital, on his own initiative. This related back to infantile life when he was furious with his mother's breast, to which he was sensuously attracted but which did not give him the milk he wanted; so he "strangled" it in his efforts to get what he wanted. This is sadistic, but it was no conscious pleasure but the horror of the compulsion which dominated his mind.

(D) *Other obsessional affective states*

As we have seen[1] there are other affective states besides that of fear, namely disgust, shame, humiliation, inferiority, guilt,

[1] P. 244.

U

depression and disappointment, which are as obsessional as fear, and which, like fear, may be the *result* of a child's forbidden impulses, *repress* these impulses, and appear as *symptoms*. If a self-willed child's desire to mess itself is met with disgust, or to show off is met with shame and humiliation, the disgust and humiliation tend to repress the desire; but any later arousal of the forbidden desire even unconsciously will be accompanied by the precipitation of shame and humiliation as an obsession.

In all such cases, we find the same conflict as in obsessional anxiety but instead of a conflict between self-will and fear, the essential conflict is between self-will and shame, inferiority or disgust, "I am going to have my own way: if you do, you will be humiliated, or disgusting, or shameful." The self-will is repressed because of these consequences, but the latent determination to gratify these desires, which refuses to be silenced, perpetuates the conflict so that there persists either the obsessional *compulsions* to do these things (to be dirty, etc.) or the fear of doing them or being them, like the phobia that one smells, or it may be simply the obsessional feeling of shame or disgust which are occasioned by them, but the cause of which is unknown. The forms these obsessional affective states take are therefore similar to those of obsessional fears. There is the same inevitability about them because we cannot escape from them, and there is the same compulsiveness about them which marks them out as obsessional. These obsessions of inferiority, shame and depression are often called "anxiety states," but this is a misnomer since they often exist with an entire absence of fear or anxiety. They are "anxiety" equivalents only in the sense that they correspond to obsessional anxiety in their origin and formation. So we call the whole group *obsessional affective states*, and individually obsessional depression (in contrast to both constitutional and reactive depression) and obsessional shame (as distinct from normal shame). In all these conditions there is the idea of degradation of the personality, just as in the phobias there is the fear of harm to oneself. It is therefore unnecessary to discuss them in detail, for when we are confronted with such cases we can simply apply the same psychopathology, substituting the shame or depression for the fear.

A patient suffers from shame and blushing, originating in an experience when he was snubbed for showing off as a child, since when any impulse to show off is accompanied by blushing. But the unconscious desire to show off persists, and its frustration makes him more determined and aggressive. But every time the desire to show off is aroused it is immediately and automatically checked, and gives rise to an attack of blushing. Another patient is obsessed with the humiliating feeling of inferiority that he is a "little boy" even amongst his contemporaries: it represented the wish to be young, for then whatever he does is wonderful for one so young, and he could do what he liked, and be excused, for he is such a pet! The obsessional feeling that one is stupid is not one which on the face of it suggests any wish: but one may make oneself deliberately stupid in order to avoid facing facts, and in some people this persists as an obsession. The fear that we shall make fools of ourselves may relate to an unconscious urge to make fools of ourselves, to break loose, to defy convention, to "go native," to "go berserk," to be silly for once, to say something shocking. But we are deterred by the opinion of others who would be shocked and that is alien to our super-ego: therefore we are afraid or ashamed of this our wish.

Depression may be endogenous and constitutional as in cyclo-thymia or involutional melancholia; it may be "simple" when there are adverse circumstances and life seems hopeless; it may be a reaction when a child has been spoilt, expected too much and so been disappointed and depressed, even though circumstances are not adverse. Finally, a depression occurring in infancy, which is often associated with digestive troubles, may be repressed and later emerge as a psychoneurotic depression, although the patient will tell you that he has nothing to be depressed about. The treat-ment of each type is obviously different. Depression in infancy is most commonly associated with the deprivation of love. It is later precipitated by not getting the love he wants, perhaps from his wife, and this revives the old depression, a condition similar to an hysteric anxiety. But the depression may be due to the frustration of forbidden desires which leads to despair. Every time the desire is aroused even unconsciously, the depression follows. The difference between depression and anxiety is that anxiety persists as long as there is effort and hope of fulfilment, depression when all hope is abandoned.

(E) Propitiatory obsessions—obsessional character traits, obsessional acts and obsessional inhibitions

IN the obsessions there is a threefold mechanism, the aggressive-ness, repressed by fear of consequences, which gives way to a super-ego: and we have discussed those conditions in which the fear is dominant (the obsessional anxieties) and those in which the forbidden impulses emerge into consciousness (the obses-sional aggressions and sex obsessions). Now we must consider those in which the super-ego is dominant, taking the form of obsessional character traits and propitiations as a set-off to the forbidden desires.

Propitiatory obsessions are the activity of a morbid conscience. They are not primarily, like other psychoneuroses, the emergence of repressed impulses, but the efforts of the super-ego to keep them repressed, and it is the super-ego which in these disorders determines the nature and form of the symptom.

All the psychoneuroses, as we have seen, may be regarded as due to the essential conflict between the ego or natural self and the super-ego or moral self. But whereas hysteria, sex perversions and tics are the rebellion of the ego against the dictates of the super-ego, the propitiatory obsessions are the effort of the moral super-ego to compensate and propitiate for the sins of the ego. The other psychoneuroses are "immoral"; the propitiating obsessions are "moral." The super-ego is of course active in the other psychoneuroses, not only in repressing the forbidden impulses, but play some part in the symptom; in the propitiatory obsessions, the abnormal super-ego is the dominant factor in the symptom. That is why, in the obsessional aggressions, although we may have the impulse to poison or to strangle, we do not in fact carry it out, since the act is prevented by the super-ego; whereas when it is the moral super-ego which is called upon to act, as in the propitiatory acts, the action is permitted, so that we carry out the rituals or ceremonial acts, like saying prayers and hand-washing. Obsessional actions, therefore, almost always belong to the propitiatory group of obsessions, and indeed the term "obsessions" is by some psychopathologists confined to such acts. But as we have observed, thoughts and feelings can be just as compulsive as acts, and we prefer to use the term in this broader sense, using the term "propitiatory obsessions" for these where there is a compulsion to act under the dictates of the super-ego.

Psychopathology. The relation of the propitiatory acts to other forms of obsession may be stated in this way. There is first the self-willed impulse of the personality to do what it wants: "I must have my own way!" This is followed by fear of consequences: "If you do disaster will happen!" But as the impulses of the organized ego are irresistible, and the threatened consequences are inevitable, something must be done to stave off the disaster. *The propitiatory obsessions are designed to avert the threatened consequences of our forbidden self-willed desires.*

The obvious solution of the problem would be to give up the forbidden desire; but that is precisely what the self-willed obsessional refuses to do. Not only so, but he no longer knows what are these desires of which he feels guilty and for which he must propitiate, since they are now repressed and unconscious. The obsessions therefore are a method of solving an unconscious moral problem by symbolically side-stepping it. If the patient feels "unclean," yet persists in his "uncleanness," he must wash his hands fifty times a day to get rid of his guilt: if he feels "sinful" he must be very pious and continually say his prayers: if he is sensitive about his guilt, he develops a mania to confess: if he feels crooked in his moral character, he must get everything straight in line with his eye, or put his knife, fork and spoon straight before he begins a meal: if he is disobedient, he must develop a mania of punctilious obedience in the minutest thing; and he must "touch wood" to give him security. All these are compensations to propitiate for a forbidden desire and to avoid its consequences. All these things he *must* do or else suffer the dreaded consequences. The compulsion of the propitiation is made necessary by the compulsiveness of the forbidden desire and the inevitability of the consequences.

This self-willed persistence of the forbidden desire is the explanation of the common obsession that one has "sinned against the Holy Ghost" which never hath forgiveness. It is not merely that we sin against the light, for at times we all do that, and yet claim forgiveness. The sin against the Holy Ghost is never forgiven because one part of our personality refuses to give up the sin, and therefore since repentance is impossible forgiveness is impossible. The problem is not made easier by the fact that we are not aware of what the sin is, nor why we feel guilt, and therefore cannot repent even if we would. Our problem is therefore insoluble and the doom inevitable, until by analysis both the nature of the sin and the morbidity of the guilt are revealed.

The severity of the super-ego. We have already discussed the formation of the super-ego and its motive forces (p. 284). The conflict between the ego and the super-ego produces a state of tension in the personality which results in various types of psychoneurosis according to the nature of the conflict. In the propitiatory obsessions we have to do with an *exaggeratedly severe* super-ego, so that the patient may be completely obsessed by his compulsion to carry out these propitiatory acts.

The exaggerated severity and compulsion of the super-ego in the obsessions is derived from various sources:

(a) First, from *the severity of the parents* with whom identification is made; the more severely the parent scolds the child as very wicked for some fault, the more the child (by identifying itself with the parent and incorporating these demands by introjection into its own personality), calls itself wicked and filthy.

(b) But curiously enough the super-ego in the obsessions may be even more severe than the parents themselves and the child far more severe with itself with regard to cleanliness, religiosity and scrupulousness than ever the parent insisted upon. The most care-free parents sometimes have the most guilt-ridden and obsessional children, pursued by threats from a vengeful god pursuing the wretched child with his terrors. This is because a function of the super-ego is to keep repressed the forbidden impulses, and there-fore *the more self-willed we are, the more ruthless must be the super-ego* which keeps them in check and the more necessary the pro-pitiation by which we must atone for them. Not only so but the function of the super-ego is to keep the *fears* at bay, so that the more terrifying the fear the stronger must be the super-ego to repress them or propitiate for them. The child who is made to feel that it will go to Hell unless it is good, naturally exaggerates its efforts at goodness.

(c) But the most important reason for the strength and com-pulsions of the super-ego is that the self-will and aggressiveness of the ego, when repressed, are *transferred to the super-ego, and turned against the ego.* The obsessional is always self-willed and aggressive, and when the individual turns from being "bad" to being "good" he does not cease to be aggressive, but becomes as aggressive in his moral demands on himself as he was previously in demanding satisfaction for his self-will. So the super-ego becomes so tyrannical, bigoted, severe, domineering, and even cruel in its demands upon the luckless victim, that his life becomes unbearable. We all know people of this ruthless moral and religious type, violent in their condemnation of the sins of others. In the obsessions this moral violence is turned against the patient himself. What Freud refers to as the "raging super-ego" is no poetic figure but a terrible reality to its victim, who is hag-ridden by his conscience and persecuted by its intolerance: his life is made unbearable; he is pestered to perform rituals day and night; he is forced to be excessively punctilious and over-scrupulous; he is prevented from doing what he decides to do by this cruel power within. Every cautious step he takes in life is fraught with dread and his personality is the unwilling battlefield of outrageous forces within him which are stronger than himself. It is not surprising that some of these obsessionals are urged to suicide. Whilst there-fore the super-ego takes its *form* and character from others by identification, it takes its·*material* from the primitive impulses of the ego, but in doing so it takes over the ruthlessness and other of the qualities of the ego which it has repressed.[1]

In the propitiatory obsessions the super-ego is itself repressed with the result that we may feel guilty about things for which we do not rationally feel guilty as well as having to propitiate for sins of which we are entirely unconscious. Both sin and condemnation are repressed and unconscious, and both may appear in the morbid symptom. A sense of guilt and wrong may therefore arise either from a conscious sense of guilt that we have done what is contrary to our conscious ego ideal, or from a buried super-ego of the past, long since outlived, which is for some reason reactivated and revived, so that the person has a sense of guilt, but is quite unaware of having done anything shameful or being at all guilty. The former is normal and a valuable corrective for life and conduct; the latter is what is most commonly met with in the obsessions, which arise from a repressed sense of guilt. The propitiatory obsessions therefore are motivated by a super-ego of the past which is quite inconsistent with the standards of the present day. It is repressed for the same reason that any impulse is repressed, because it is objectionable: we do not like to be made to feel conscience-stricken and perpetually guilty, and therefore bury the super-ego which makes us feel so. But though the old super-ego may have been long since forgotten, long since superseded by more rational standards, it may still be active, so that like any other complex it may emerge in the form of a symptom, as a compulsive sense of guilt. It is therefore true to say, as the

---

[1] *Guilt.* In the full sense of the term we feel guilty when we have fallen short of the standard we have ourselves adopted and therefore it presupposes the recognition of such a standard. But we may accept a standard unconsciously without recognizing what it is. Patients recovering experiences in infantile life, often revive what they describe as a feeling of guilt, when, for instance, at the breast-feeding period they bite the nipple and are pushed away or smacked. Obviously this cannot depend on consciousness of a standard of behaviour, but what they describe as a sense of guilt appears to arise from the experience of *disastrous consequences following one's own act*. This is more than just fear. If a child is hurt purely as the result of another's action it experiences fear, without a sense of guilt; but when the painful event follows an action of one's own, it is quite a different experience: the pain is associated with and *referred to one's own act* and is described by patients reviving the experience as a feeling of guilt. Thus a feeling of guilt of an embryonic type can apparently be experienced in infancy, long before the infant can have appreciated any moral standard. The origin of guilt and the sense of "wrong" are therefore extremely primitive and that is why guilt and the rudiments of the super-ego so often reside deep in unconsciousness. Indeed because of the accidental association of pain following one's own act, a child may feel guilty and inhibit behaviour and feelings which were in no sense wrong nor were regarded as such by the mother.

psychoanalysts have said, that *there is not only a conscious conscience but an unconscious conscience*, and it is from the latter that obsessional guilt arises, giving rise to a *morbid* sense of shame, guilt, humiliation, disgust with oneself, and the need to perform propitiatory acts against them, all of which now appear so irrational.

The contrast between the conscious conscience and the unconscious conscience may be illustrated. An individual is quite normal in his conscious attitude towards sex, and yet is sexually impotent, the reason being that any sexual expression or wish on his part may be accompanied by the unconscious sense of guilt or anxiety from some threat of the past, which may be so strong as to frustrate his natural desire. He is forbidden sex not by his conscious conscience but by his unconscious conscience. Another instance is that already mentioned of the man who agreed with his wife that each could live in "free love" with anyone else at will. But when the husband encouraged the wife to spend the week-end with another man, and she did so, he had a nervous breakdown as the result—much to his annoyance. He suffered from a repressed sense of guilt for his "free love" defiance of a repressed super-ego.

The same contrast between conscious and unconscious guilt is exemplified in dreams. Usually we regard dreams as a means of expressing repressed wishes: but they may also be an expression of guilt. For instance, a young widow dreams of making love and being made love to, but with anxiety and moral resistance; which is in contrast to her day time, for she has no hesitation in going much further in love-making than she permits herself to do in her dreams, thus proving that subconsciously she feels more guilt than is present in her conscious mind. She has repressed not her forbidden desires, but her sense of guilt.

Jung has laid more emphasis on this aspect of the neuroses than Freud. He long ago maintained that there is *a moral conflict in the unconscious*, which therefore cannot consist only of sexual wishes. Guilt may, like primitive impulses, be repressed and emerge to produce symptoms.

The moral sense, giving rise to guilt is often regarded as innate; but in our view morality as such is not hereditary nor ancestral, nor is there an innate moral sense. What is ancestral and innate is the child's sense of dependence on others and therefore its identification with them, which compels the child to adopt their standards. We do not inherit a moral sense, but every child has a need for others which makes the development of a conscience inevitable, irrespective of any teaching. Out of this dependence both social life and a moral sense is developed.

There are *various types of propitiatory obsessions*. These are (A) Obsessional character traits, (B) Obsessional propitiatory acts, and (C) Obsessional inhibitions. They are all designed to keep at bay forbidden desires in ourselves.

(A) Obsessional character traits

Obsessional character traits like over-conscientiousness, over-scrupulousness, over-punctiliousness (often associated with intolerance, hardness of character and bigotry), are common instances. In these the super-ego is consciously accepted, although its original source and motives are forgotten. The super-ego, as we have said, is always abnormal because it exists at the cost of repression. But in obsessional character traits it is the *accepted* part of the personality and therefore may not be regarded as abnormal by the patient. Indeed his exaggerated attitude of over-conscientiousness is his safeguard against the forbidden and threatening fears. One man belonging to a strict religious sect came because his particular church forbade him not only to play games on a Sunday but to play his favourite game of tennis on public courts; and he came because his conscience worried him that he often broke this rule. "Mind you," he said, "I am always careful only to play with Christians!" We replied that he must sometimes find it hard to get a good game!—to which he replied that the real difficulty was that a partner might *say* he was a Christian and then turn out not to be. In such a case it is not the function of the analyst to tell such a man that his standard is absurd, but to find out why he thus "sinned." It was a basic rebellion against a super-ego which he found too rigid for his personality, but to which he held. Not only so, but it was found that the real guilt concerned a sexual sin he would not previously acknowledge even to himself, and which he transferred to his tennis.

The trouble about obsessional character traits is that as the patients may not be aware that they are in any way abnormal, they are not so accessible to treatment; they have no insight, though they are not psychotic. The house-proud woman does not realize that in perpetually putting things in order to the distraction of her husband, she is really symbolizing the need to put things in order in her own soul; she rationalizes and says it is so that she knows where things are. Nor does the pacifist realize that in his craving for world peace he may be compensating for a sense of dispeace in his own inner life and expressing a yearning for peace which he finds unattainable. Like so many other people, he is striving to work out in the objective world problems which he finds insoluble in his own soul. Many people take up social work as a flight from their own moral and psychological problems. Others become politicians to put their country right because they cannot solve their own domestic unhappiness.[1] The same mechanism has been observed in the projection of a moral fear on to an external object like a fear of tunnels.

Other instances of obsessional character traits are over-conscientiousness, over-scrupulousness, over-punctiliousness about details, pettifogging over trifles, splitting hairs, over-tidiness, fussiness about punctuality, about correct behaviour, exaggerated accuracy, intolerance of oneself and others, over-devotion to religious exercises and moral scrupulosity. These are all propitiatory character traits, the compulsion of which reveals the strength of the forbidden impulse, and the necessity to perform which proclaims the extent of the inner sense of guilt. The Scots have a word for it; the "unco-guid" are always suspect. The idea that the greatest saints are most conscious of sin may not be without justification: in fact many of the greatest saints have previously been the greatest sinners and it would be surprising if they did not look back on their past with regret in more senses than one. In so far as the desire still persists even unconsciously, the necessity to propitiate and compensate is still active. Not only so, but their remorse concerning sins and trifling faults of the past proclaims their ultra-righteousness to the world.

Obsessional character traits may be observed to originate in early childhood. As we have seen, when the child is confronted with the conflict between self-will and fear, and neither will give way, it resorts to various compromises: the child may make a private pact with itself, with its parents or with God, to be very good in everything else, provided it is allowed to continue the one forbidden sin, commonly that of masturbation. It becomes over-conscientious, over-scrupulous, very obedient, anxious to please and to be good. These are obsessional character traits by means of which the child hopes to propitiate for its sin and to keep the goodwill of the mother on whom its security depends. When a child continually says "Am I a good boy?" "Have I been an obedient girl to-day?" it is usually a sign that he or she are none too good. The confession mania in which a child feels com-

[1] It would be interesting to get a census of the domestic life of Members of Parliament and of Congress.

pelled to tell the mother everything reveals the fact that the child is not telling all.

In other cases the conflict in the personality between the ego and the super-ego gives rise to *morbid self-consciousness* which is simply the one part of the personality being conscious of the other, the super-ego being conscious of the ego, and having a poor opinion of it. We may regard as obsessional character traits tendencies like self-deprecation, being apologetic, being ingratiating, and habits of self-condemnation, which may all be super-ego judgments upon the behaviour of the ego or natural self. These take on a more morbid form and may become symptoms of which the patient complains, in which case the type of judgment commonly reveals the nature of the impulses for which they propitiate, such as the obsession that one smells (usually a condemnation of anal erotic tendencies), that one is ugly (repressing vanity), that one has hair on the face (repressed masculinity), that one is awkward, a fool or stupid. They represent a demand of the ego to be erotic, vain, and the right to make a fool of oneself if one wants to; so that they become a perpetual menace to our moral and social self, which is correspondingly ashamed of them.

The purpose of the self-condemnation or self-depreciation is to keep the forbidden desires repressed by going to an extreme of condemnation. Yet even here the forbidden impulse cannot obliterate itself completely and the Publican may easily fall into self-righteousness and congratulate himself that he is not a hypocrite like the Pharisee. The conceited man who "modestly" begins every speech by the remark that "of course he knows nothing about the subject" is not only proclaiming himself superior to others who are not so modest, but at the same time guarding his conceit against possible criticism. In Adler's case a man in a crowd at a religious festival fell on the ground and shouted out, "I am the chief of sinners." He had to be chief of something!

(B) Propitiatory obsessional acts

But the problem may become more acute, and the forbidden impulses of the natural self may be so strong and persistent that they cannot be allayed by such an obvious compromise as the adoption of compensating character traits. In such a case we have to guard against them by taking positive precautions against them, such as the performance of rituals, ceremonials and other propitiatory acts which we are compelled to perform, though against our will. The purpose of these propitiatory acts is to avert the consequences of our forbidden desires.

But both the nature of the forbidden desires and the super-ego may be repressed. Therefore most obsessional propitiations the patient recognizes to be abnormal. The obsessional feels the necessity to pick up every bit of paper on the floor, which becomes the bane of his life and yet he is compelled to perform it. He must put his hand deep in every envelope he opens but does not know why: he regards these acts as silly and irrational.

Other instances of propitiatory acts are having to make sure the door is locked, that one's accounts are perfectly right, that one has turned off the light, saying prayers until two o'clock in the morning, touching between every pair of banister legs on the stair, washing one's hands numbers of times a day, making sure everything is sterilized, counting ten to avoid making any rash decision, putting things exactly in line with the eye, stepping on or over the cracks in the pavement, touching every lamp-post and innumerable other compulsions.

The classic instance is of *hand-washing*; the soul is guilty of something impure: but the individual refuses to repent or give up the desire, and represses her sense of guilt. Therefore it transfers itself to her hands and she must wash them. But this does not solve the problem for it does not get rid of the stain on her soul; so the wretched victim has persistently and repeatedly to wash her hands. This propitiatory act of hand-washing is often necessitated by a sense of moral uncleanness of which the patient is quite unconscious: and the same applies to the contamination complex, the super-ego being dominant, the fear of dirtying oneself, or the fear of contaminating others, referring to an unconscious wish.

In one case a boy wrestling with another boy had sex feelings. This filled him with dread owing to certain childhood sex experiences. Thereafter he could not bear to sit near a boy in class lest he felt sexual; and when he came for consultations he would creep round the walls to be as far away from the physician to avoid being contaminated. His condition was cured by analysis.

A young man of high moral reputation, already referred to, who had a "contamination complex" that if he touches his sex organs, then he might deposit semen on a door handle, so that if a girl touches the handle it might give her a baby, found its origin in an occasion when by physical contact with a girl he feared that he had given her a baby. This obsession persisted long after the possibility of such a result; but it aroused the whole sexual conflict between his desires and his moral fear. If it had occurred, and because of his strong sex instincts he could not guarantee that it would not occur again, his whole reputation as a high-minded, pure young man would fall. The symptom therefore was to defend this self-righteous super-ego against the possibility of such a downfall; it warned him, "keep clear of all sex." On the other hand, the obsession perpetually gratifies the unconscious desire to impregnate every girl he meets.

But *simple everyday illustrations of such obsessional propitiations* are not difficult to find, one of the most common of which is "touching wood." When a man is boasting of his good fortune, e.g. "that he has not had a day's illness in five years," he ends with "Touch wood!" Why must he observe this obsessional formality? Because he is vain, he is boastful, he is arrogant, he is defying Providence, and such defiance of fate (as in the case of Ulysses with Polyphemus) courts disaster. He must therefore "touch wood" as a means of averting disaster. Moreover, touching, since early infancy, is a symbol of contact, of security, of something to hold on to.

Superstitions such as that of *sitting down* 13 *to a meal* (Christ and the 12 disciples) threatens impending disaster to those who have the Judas in them. The superstitious fear of *going under a ladder* (derived from the ladder of the Cross beneath which, as in the old paintings, the devil is lurking ready to steal one's soul) is based on a fear that the devil will get one for one's sins. But one does not fear the devil getting hold of one, unless one feels that the devil has reason to do so. By precautions and avoidances of this kind we hope to assure ourselves that all is well. It is only those who feel guilty who are superstitious.

Another instance is the *carrying of mascots* as in the case of airmen and others on a hazardous voyage; the idea being that in being adventurous they are defying fate and inviting disaster. The same conflict between defiance and fear of possible disaster which the airman (who insists on tempting Providence) can do nothing more about, makes him resort to a means of averting the disaster, and so gives himself this sense of security. The carrying of the mascot serves its purpose if it succeeds in giving him more confidence, for the increased confidence may in fact save him from disaster. It is a case where the belief itself (in this case that the mascot confers some immunity) is a dynamic force producing objective results: faith can override mountains.

Sometimes the propitiatory obsessions are *symbolic precautions against the emergence of the forbidden impulses*. The necessity of the clerk in a business house to return continually to see that the accounts are correct symbolically represents a sense of guilt that there is something wrong with his moral account which he feels he must put right; but because he refuses to do so, he must perform the ritual symbolically and perpetually. The necessity to return time after time to see that the gas fire is turned off is due to the fear that there will be an explosion, but for different reasons. In one case of a woman it was symbolic of the explosion of her sexual passions, the fear that the "flames of passion" would get out of control. On the other hand, the mother previously mentioned who had continually to see that the gas light in her child's room was turned off had, it transpired, an unconscious wish to get rid of her child so that she could pursue her career; her sense of guilt therefore compelled her to take these anxious precautions against that impulse. But on one occasion, as we recall, she found the gas turned off and left it turned on, thus giving expression to her unconscious wish. Obsessional *anxiety* occurs where there is a fear of these forbidden impulses; the obsessional *acts* occur when they are so strong that specific precautions must be taken against them. Therefore if these people are prevented from carrying out their propitiatory acts they are thrown into a state of great anxiety, distress, shame or guilt which the propitiations were designed to avert. A woman's precautions to see that the door is bolted may be a normal fear of burglars; but if she has to go time after time and then finding it bolted begins to worry that she may then have unbolted it, it makes one suspect not only that the condition is pathological, but that the idea of leaving it unbolted represents an unconscious invitation! She has to keep the door firmly barred against these threatening sexual imaginations. The compulsion to step *on* the cracks in the pavement or to step *over* them, may be an atavistic trait going back to the times when we were liable to meet with snakes in the grass; but there are other types of snake in the grass, and its emergence in certain people as an obsession is due to the fact that it is utilized symbolically, and may represent the need at one time to *stamp* on the serpent of sin, at another to *avoid* it by stepping over it.

A case illustrating the causes of the propitiatory obsession is that of the middle of the three brothers already mentioned.[1] A business man, not at all religious in his ordinary life, has to take off his hat as he passes every church and bow four times: he also has the compulsion to put his hand into every envelope he opens and rummage about till he is quite sure nothing is left, and then must suddenly withdraw his

---

[1] One "good," one "bad," and one neurotic.

hand. He also takes ages in putting his arms into the armholes of his coat, and his legs through the legs of his trousers—not to speak of many other such obsessions. Analysis revealed that he was a premature child, delicate and weakly, his one comfort being at the breast: when his mother, a rigid woman, deprived him of this, he felt it must be wrong to want sensuous pleasure and he must taboo it if he is to keep the protective love of the mother which he so sorely needed. He also felt in a rage with his mother, and as he got stronger and less dependent on her his resentment against her increased, and he became self-willed and disobedient. He was then told that bad boys went to Hell, which affected him little till he saw a picture of Hell and the souls in torment, and then he became preoccupied with death. At six he got pneumonia owing to disobedience in going out without a coat. He pathetically wanted to make peace with his mother before he died (to make it up with God was impossible, as his fate was sealed). But before he could do so he lost consciousness and was in fact at death's door for several days (the doctor said he could not live through the night). During his delirium he had vivid hallucinations of Hell. When he recovered he felt God had let him off this time, but it would be his last chance. He must be good and obedient, and his whole life was lived under threat of death and Hell if he did anything naughty. But when adolescence came with assertiveness and sex he could not be so submissive and the conflict was precipitated. When he got married he felt (like his older brother) that to enjoy sex was sinful and applied this to his marriage; but (like his younger brother) he said, "To hell with it, I am going to have sex if I want to," and therefore would prowl about looking sensuously at women. The sense of guilt for these forbidden desires compelled him to propitiate to God by baring his head and bowing whilst passing the church. Putting his arms and legs in his clothes represented sexual intercourse, which was forbidden; hence the hesitation. The obsessions of fiddling inside the envelopes arose when once his attractive secretary was in his room and he had the impulse to put his hand between her legs from behind. He had to do this with the envelope as a propitiation for the now unconscious wish; but the action also symbolically gratified the desire, until he had then to withdraw suddenly. The cure took the form of his having to defy the fictitiously angry God, and to face up to his moral issues.

The characteristics of the obsessional propitiations are illustrated in such a case, and may be recalled.

(a) As in all obsessional conditions there are repressed forbidden *self-willed impulses* the consequences of which are feared.

(b) The obsessional propitiations are *compulsive* because there is the compulsion of the ego to do the forbidden thing, there is also the compulsion to propitiate for them. Therefore the patient *must* wash his hands, say prayers till two in the morning and make sure the door is locked, and if he fails to do them he is filled with anxiety because of the penalties threatened.

(c) The propitiating obsessional always represents an *unsolved* moral problem because neither side will give in. The aggressiveness refuses to give up its self-will, but the fear is too great to be ignored; therefore since the consequence of our self-will is inevitable something must be done to avert the consequence. The individual who refuses to give up his guilt compromises by symbolically avoiding them by doing propitiatory acts.

(d) Moreover the problem is *unsolvable* because the forbidden impulses for which it is necessary to propitiate are themselves repressed and *unconscious*: we feel a profound sense of guilt for what we know not: we feel self-conscious without being aware of any cause for shame: we are compelled to perform certain rituals to avert the consequences of sins which we are not aware of having committed. It is not that one consciously feels one ought to repent of certain sins: but there is the involuntary compulsion to do these acts to propitiate for sins of which we are unaware. This too is illustrated in the case above.

(e) But this super-ego which condemns and propitiates *is also repressed*. It is a super-ego of the past, long since discarded and forgotten, which condemns sins which he would now view with common sense devoid of any guilt whatever. The propitiations are not, therefore, the expression of a normally accepted moral standard, but always of a *perverted super-ego*. It is the operation of an unconscious conscience, which harasses us. If it were the conscious conscience which passed judgment on the wrongdoing we should either give it up or adopt new standards as we are perpetually doing. But even though we see the stupidity of the act and want to be rational about it, the buried super-ego representing the voice of the father, which is often taken for the voice of God, threatens us with disaster if we do.

(f) That is why the compulsions seem so *irrational*, and are so regarded by the patient himself, and also why those obsessional propitiations are themselves involuntary though compulsive. Although the obsessional feels compelled to carry out these propitiating acts, he recognizes only too well the stupidity of his actions, and is driven nearly crazy in being unwillingly compelled to perform acts which he knows to be irrational and unnecessary, and by kind friends who tell him it is so silly to do them, as if he were not sufficiently aware of the fact!

(g) Although in the propitiatory obsessions the sin and guilt originate in the past, *there is always a guilt for an unrecognized sin of the present day*, which the patient refuses to admit or to relinquish. Were there not a present desire to keep alive the threat, the need for propitiation would pass. If a man feels remorse over a sin of the past it always means that he still has the desire; otherwise having repented and given it up there would be no more guilt or remorse. He cannot forgive himself for the past sin, because he still desires it. The "sin" may turn out to be something trifling which the patient with his present standards would not consider sinful and therefore when discovered the feeling of guilt and the need to propitiate are abolished.

(*h*) Because the desire persists, the guilt and threatened consequences persist; the propitiations do not solve the moral problem and therefore must be constantly repeated. Hardly has the obsessional ceased to perform his propitiatory act than he must do it again. This explains the *repetitive* nature of the obsessions and why the relief of doing the hand-washing is short-lived, for the obvious reason that the forbidden desire is still active, and washing the hands or doing religious rites does not wash away the sins of the soul, and any amount of bowing to churches does not abolish the sense of guilt. The personality cannot bluff itself all the time and the feeling of guilt therefore makes the repetition of the act compulsory.

(*i*) Because the moral problem is repressed and unconscious, the propitiation is transferred and projected on to a material object or action: they are the symbolic representation of an inward moral conflict: *propitiatory obsessions are the outward and visible sign of an inward lack of grace.* The washing of the hands is to wash the soul of the guilt: picking off every spot of fluff from one's clothes is to be morally spotless: getting things straight in a line or on the table is the need to get things straight in our moral life. The reason for this projection and symbolization is not simply because the real problem is hidden, but also because it simplifies the problem for the time being. It is far easier to bare one's head than to bare one's soul, to make the sign of the Cross than to bear the Cross, to wash the hands than to cleanse one's soul; to pick off bits of fluff than to remove the spots on one's moral character; to say prayers than to repent. In any case our self-willed ego refuses to allow us to reform and repent. But as this leaves the moral problem unsolved there is the constant necessity to repeat the propitiatory act, so that the hand-washing is recurrent and persistent and the religious ritual and ceremonials must be regularly performed to keep on the right side of God.

(*j*) But another very curious feature of many propitiatory

X

obsessions is that it is a compromise and *gratifies the forbidden wish for which it propitiates*. To propitiate for the sin of masturbation a woman must press her hand up between the legs of the banisters as she goes upstairs, which is obviously only a symbolic masturbation: and if she misses one she must start again from the bottom, so prolonging the subconscious pleasure. To punish herself for sexual desires a woman must press her sex organs to produce pain: but this, she admits, sometimes produces an orgasm, and she must repeat it until it ceases to do so—after her sex is thoroughly satisfied. The compulsion to touch every lamp-post is often a phallic masturbation symbolically gratifying the desire. A mother insists that a self-willed child must clean her teeth: so the child has a compulsion to go on cleaning her teeth until they are *perfectly* clean (the need for moral cleanliness from masturbation); but by this persistence she becomes a perfect nuisance to her mother, thus paying her out for forbidding her the pleasure. A woman with repressed hatred had the compulsion, whenever she sat down on a seat in the park, to go the next day and hunt for hours to make sure that she had not squashed a fly and left it suffering (not dead). All that time she was unconsciously enjoying the thought of its suffering, the original object of hate being her younger sister of whom she was jealous and wished to make suffer. The man's rummaging in the envelope and his lingering over putting his arms and legs into his clothes were symbolic acts of sexual intercourse. From these illustrations it will also be inferred that the majority though not all obsessional propitiations are of a sexual nature, and that we find, in fact, to be the case.

We conclude, therefore, that the *propitiatory obsession is not only a propitiation for sin, but is a gratification for the sin for which it propitiates*. The propitiation therefore corresponds to all the psychoneuroses in that it is a compromise in which not only the moral super-ego, but the repressed ego is gratified.

(C) *Obsessional inhibitions*

Just as in conversion hysteria there is a physical disability or paralysis, so in the obsessions there may be mental inhibition which prevents us using our mind and exercising our will as we wish. This occurs when the conflict between self-will and fear of consequences is so evenly divided that neither will give way and each side operates *by preventing the other from carrying out its will*. Thus obsessional inhibitions are either the inhibitions of the forbidden impulses of the natural self by the condemning super-ego, or the refusal of the ego to allow the super-ego to carry out its demands.

In some cases the obsessional inhibitions take the form of a positive symptom, and are the means resorted to by the moral super-ego to defend itself against the dangers incurred by the forbidden impulses. The super-ego guards itself against the forbidden impulses by avoiding the situations which produce them. Take such a case as a woman's *fear of leaving home*: this fear may be a simple reproduction of an infantile fear of separation (hysterical anxiety); or it may be fear of the consequences of forbidden desires (obsessional anxiety): but in fact it was a means adopted by the super-ego to prevent her leaving home (obsessional inhibition), because she had the secret desire to leave home for sexual adventures, but her moral sense inhibited her by producing an inability to leave home, and so preventing her from carrying out the forbidden desire. Adler mentions a case in which a bank clerk had the fear of crossing the ocean which he intended to do after embezzling. The super-ego utilized the fear to prevent him from carrying out his intentions when ordinary moral prohibitions failed.

Another illustration is that of a highly-sexed but moral girl who developed the obsession that there is something wrong with her sex organs; the object of this phobia is that she can tell herself it is impossible for her to have sex relations and thus defends herself against her temptations. So the super-ego gains a false victory over the impulses of the ego and averts a moral catastrophe at the expense of producing a neurotic symptom.

Sometimes the super-ego resorts to physical symptoms like *aphonia*; which may be an hysterical symptom designed like any other illness to get sympathy: or it may have an obsessional motive and be designed to keep undesirable thoughts under control. A case of the latter type occurred almost before our eyes. A girl patient was taken by the author to a consultant in endocrinology, misunderstood his verdict, and thought that they were fooling her. She was furious and wanted to tell them what she thought of them and that they were a couple of humbugs, but dared not as she was afraid that further treatment would be refused. So afraid was she of the urge to blurt out her resentful feelings that she suppressed *all* speech and developed aphonia. This was cured some days later in analysis by writing, when the reason was discovered and the misunderstanding rectified.

In stammering the motive is similar. As we have seen there is sometimes a strong urge to say what you want, to let out your aggressiveness, but the fear of doing so checks it, and produces the hesitation. A stammer is due to a compulsion to say, and an equally strong compulsion not to say: the stammering speech therefore represents a stammering personality. We may regard stammering as an obsessional tic if we look at the compulsive part (the ego), or an obsessional inhibition if we consider the repressing part (the super-ego).

Obsessional indecision is a form of obsessional inhibition. So strong is the rebellion of the ego against the dictates of the super-ego and the will that it only requires the individual to say "I will do so and so" for the repressed ego to say "No you don't!" It is the revolt of self-will against the will. One result of such a conflict is that it is impossible for these people to decide anything, for whatever one side of the personality desires is opposed by the other side; and whatever is willed by the one side is resisted by the other, so that the patient may take an hour deciding what tie he should put on, whether to take his waterproof or not; and no sooner has he decided, than he feels he has made a profound mistake and must go back to change. This is also a common cause of *aboulia*, or lack of will; the patient can decide but is quite incapable of carrying out his decision. An individual resolves to do a morning's hard work, but cannot settle down, for the ego refuses to allow him to. He then sides with the ego and decides to slack, but no sooner has he turned on the radio than his super-ego makes him restless and feel he ought to be working. Mild obsessions of this kind are common, as seen in the man who has habits which he considers reprehensible, such as meanness, tempers, greed, malice against others, sensuality, jealousy, conceit—but his will is quite incapable of surmounting them, not so much because they are themselves strong impulses, but because there is some self-willed obstinacy within him which refuses to give them up and says "Why should I?"

Thus the obsessional inhibition is not always an inhibition of an impulse by the moral self. It may be the other way round, the ego checking the super-ego. As the moral self refuses to permit the natural self to do what it wants, the latter takes revenge by frustrating the former in every moral decision it tries to make.

There was the case of the youth whose father, himself frustrated by financial considerations from taking Medicine, foolishly determined that the son should fulfil the father's ambitions. In spite of hard work and effort the boy failed each time in a different subject, which was his way of saying that he did not want to become a doctor. Allowed to be an engineer he passed his exams. Another patient has a compulsive inhibition regarding paying his debts, which he recognized as irrational, especially as it only applies to people to whom he otherwise owes an obligation, including the analyst! This related to a complex of childhood, for when he was delicate and ill his mother made him feel that he was a nuisance and greatly indebted to her, which he resented. He then transferred his feelings to anyone to whom he owed an obligation, and showed his unconscious resentment by a compulsion not to pay his debts.

Weakness of will may therefore be due to inherent and constitutional weakness; or it may be due to a poor character from bad discipline; or it may be due to a dissociation in which one part of our personality refuses to allow the other part its way, and prevents it from carrying out its will.

Treatment. What hope is there for the patient caught in this vice of self-will and fear? What do we aim at in treatment? When enquiry is made into the causes of the guilt and fear it is found that in fact the "sins" which are made to appear so appalling are usually trifling peccadillos of childhood, which have nevertheless been made to appear dreadful crimes and condemned with appalling but fictitious disasters by ill-educated parents and guardians whose only method of producing good behaviour is by threats. In analysis the patient *revives* both the primal fears and the threatened fears, and discovers the causes of these fears; when he sees this he feels anger and resentment against those who thus unfairly made him afraid and this anger abolishes his fear; finally he readjusts his attitude to the whole experience, getting rid of his unjustifiable guilt and fears. Thus the repressed self-will is released and is transformed into confidence and strength of will; and the repressed sex desires are released to fulfill their normal function in adult love. This is not theory but fact.

If, on the other hand, there is a real sin of the present day, of which he is consciously ashamed but refused to recognize (like the tennis player mentioned, whose sin was really sexual), he is made to face up to the moral issue.

The mental hygiene and prevention of the propitiatory obsessions lies especially in the avoidance of exaggerated moral standards far beyond the child's capacity to live up to; for these give the child an abnormal sense of guilt. Unfortunately children, owing to their dependence upon us, are only too ready to believe that comparatively innocent acts are as wicked as we say they are, and believe the threats which we ourselves do not believe. The well-intentioned lies of the parent become the obsession of the child.

CHAPTER XIII

DISORDERS OF PERSONALITY

FUGUES and dual personalities are better known in popular than in medical literature; the former being frequently reported in the Press as "loss of memory," and the latter in R. L. Stevenson's *Dr. Jekyll and Mr. Hyde.*

An instance of a fugue was that of a rubber planter who hated his work, which was unsuited to his temperament, but which he was bound to stick to. One day he slipped away into a jungle, lost all memory of his work and where he was, and enjoyed himself wandering about and watching the birds. A search-party found him twenty-one days later, in an exhausted condition with complete amnesia. The analysis revealed that in childhood he had had to give place to a more attractive young brother and felt socially inferior: that was why he was ill-adapted to manage the people on the plantation. When visitors came he therefore slipped away to a wood at the foot of the garden and spent his time listening to the birds (as he did in the jungle). The essence of his disorder was an escape; the natural self revolted against the social demands laid upon him and he played truant.

Fugues as we see from this case have much the same motive as occupational neuroses (p. 222); but whilst the latter are localized disorders of function relating to the particular work, the fugues are revolts of a more repressed part of the personality against conditions of life.

These conditions of fugue and dual personality thus differ in certain respects from the other psychoneuroses, which justifies us in classifying them separately.

In all the psychoneuroses there is a conflict between specific impulses of the natural self, like self-pity, aggressiveness and sex, and the moral self or super-ego which represses them, the form of the psychoneuroses depending upon the nature of the repressed impulse. In dual personality and fugues the ego is more highly organized before repression so that the conflict is between two well-organized "personalities"; there is therefore a much deeper segmentation or splitting of the personality in these conditions as compared with the psychoneuroses. That is why we have taken the liberty of calling them specifically "disorders of personality," although in fact all psychoneuroses and behaviour disorders are such. The more organized is the ego before repression and the more strongly motivated the super-ego which represses it, the greater the split and duality in the personality.

Each of these well-defined and well-organized "personalities" is then capable of acting as a separate entity with its own way, its own aims, its own demands, its own will. When one of the personalities becomes repressed by the other, the individual may live for many years according to the dictates of the dominant personality without the presence of the other being suspected, until the repressed personality suddenly emerges. So we behave at one time as the Dr. Jekyll and another time as the Mr. Hyde. To such an extent does each "personality" act as a complete unit, that when we meet with an individual in a fugue state there is nothing to suggest that we are not conversing with an ordinary person, nor do we detect that there is anything abnormal about him or his behaviour. We have had patients wander for days in a fugue state without the abnormality of their behaviour being suspected. "The police," says Charcot, "don't stop them." Indeed, in the alternation of personalities it is not easy to say which is the "real" personality and which the "secondary," which is the normal and which the abnormal.

Duality of personality in greater or less degree exists in most people, so that the sweet person has outbursts of temper, the arrogant person of self-pity, the saint of meanness and the hypocrite has bouts of sincerity. Indeed, the appeal of Stevenson's novel is probably because it corresponds to what most people find within their personalities, heroism side by side with cowardice, sentiment with brutality, generosity with greed. But such duality in the personality is not the same thing as "dual personality" which is usually reserved for those conditions in which the dissociation is such that *at least one of the personalities is unaware of the other.*

In the majority of cases it is the moral super-ego which has been dominant before the crisis, and the natural self repressed. But not invariably, for in cases of religious conversion it is the "good" self which has been repressed and the natural self dominant, and the conversion takes the form of the "good" self rising up and taking possession of the personality and ousting the "bad" self. Sometimes the "fall from grace" in the reverse direction takes place as suddenly. Usually, however, it is the natural self which has been repressed by the moral self, until it rebels against the demands of the super-ego, and takes possession of the personality as in the fugue or dual personality. We have already discussed the causes of such dissociation.[1] They are sometimes due to physical stress or fatigue, which Janet has emphasized, and sometimes, as Freud has pointed out, to repression. In either case there is the subsequent splitting of one part of the personality from the other, and the automatic functioning of the dissociated part. The cases we shall have under consideration are those in which there is no physical shock or strain, and the conditions were discovered under investigation to be due to purely psychological causes.

This rebellion of the repressed personality against the dominant one takes different forms in fugues and in dual personalities. The rough difference between the two appears to be that whilst in dual personalities the ego revolts and takes possession of the personality which therefore assumes a *different character*, in fugue states the ego refusing any longer to be under the dominance of the super-ego escapes from the intolerable circumstances imposed upon it by the super-ego and *takes to flight*, as the name "fugue" implies. It is in this case not so much a change in character as a change in environment and sphere of operation; it is an escape from an intolerable situation.

Dual personality. In dual personality the two "personalities" or characters are both so well organized and of such equal strength that neither will give way, so that when the inevitable conflict is precipitated they take turns, as it were, in dominating the actions of the personality, which at one time functions as the Dr. Jekyll and at another time as the Mr. Hyde. This involves a complete change in character.

Cases of dual personality are illustrated in Morton Prince's Sally Beauchamp and in other cases mentioned by Janet. Genuine cases of dual personality are in our experience rare: indeed we cannot recall ever having met a "typical" case. The fact that Janet regarded America as the home of dual personalities, whereas America regarded France as the natural nursery of these disorders, lends support to one's impression that these cases are more popular than populous.

The nearest case to a dual personality we have investigated is that of a woman (Mrs. M. M.) who would go into a trance, and in that state impersonate certain characters, now a little girl, now a priest of the Middle Ages, now an Irishman. These were her so-called "controls,"

[1] P. 228.

in whose personality for the time being she would live and act. In the "person" of the priest, Father Power, she took services on Sunday evenings in a London theatre, and preached sermons considerably above the level of her ordinary intelligence. We personally investigated her case for the purpose of a law suit, since she was charged by a London newspaper with being a fraud. (The charge was proved to be false.) The opinion we formed was that these impersonations were in fact identifications with people she had known in childhood. So completely does a child identify itself with others and impersonate them in thought, speech and manner that for the time being she *is* that person. The sermons may have been memory traces from sermons she had heard in childhood which had made an indelible impression on her mind whilst in a state of semi-trance. In the services she deliberately put herself in a state of trance.

One might ask, were the "multiple personalities" of Sally Beauchamp, and others of that nature, due to a *multiplicity of unconscious impersonations and identifications* with people in childhood?

Fugue states are much more common, in which the patient disappears and suffers from "loss of memory." These fugue states usually occur in people who find themselves in *uncongenial circumstances*, but from which they cannot escape; in work which they loathe but which they must dutifully carry out; in a profession they find irksome, or faced with domestic situations which are repugnant to them.[1]

A fugue is a flight, as the name implies: and the name is given because the individual disappears from his ordinary surroundings and is later found suffering from loss of memory. But on analysis it is found to be also a psychological flight, a flight not only from one's circumstances but from oneself.

As in obsessions, the fugue represents an escape from a moral problem, in this case by obliteration and flight from the situation which arouses it. The stories of Cain, of Oedipus and of the Wandering Jew, all of whom wandered over the face of the earth, symbolize man's eternal attempt to escape from himself and from moral problems which he has failed to solve, but from which he can never escape by physical wandering.

Man devises all kinds of methods of solving the moral problem

[1] Cases of psychopathological fugue must be distinguished from epileptic automatic states, in which an individual may assume another personality and even commit a murder in his epileptic state with subsequent loss of memory: also from states of pure confusion due to shock or exhaustion: and from simple loss of memory from a psychological obliteration of some unpleasant experience, but without active flight to another type of life. The term "loss of memory" is therefore an inadequate description.

of having to adjust himself as an individual to the material and social demands made upon him. The most rational way is deliberately to throw up his uncongenial work and take other work, but that takes courage, because of the uncertainty of a new career, or because family, friends and one's own sense of duty oppose it. Many men and women remain failures because they have not the courage to change their jobs, and many remain among the unemployed because they have not the initiative to take work outside what they are accustomed to. Others refuse to give up uncongenial work because their pride will not admit failure. Others, unwilling to face disapproval, find excuses for leaving work, like politicians who cover their failure by retiring from office "on medical grounds." Another develops an hysterical pain to escape from the situation, whilst yet another goes into a fugue state in which he obliterates the whole of the past from memory.

Several types of fugue may be mentioned. (a) In the first type it is a flight from a simple *insoluble problem*, resulting in "loss of memory" which is an obliteration of the whole problem from the mind, a refusal even to think of the problem. Such cases are those of "wandering with loss of memory" rather than definite flight.

The most recent case we have had was of a soldier who was found wandering with loss of memory in Portsmouth, without any idea how he got there. He remarked that he thought he had a letter in his pocket which had something to do with it, but he would not look at it. This was a letter from his wife to say that she had left him. Bewildered, he had wandered about, obliterated his memory for the whole thing, and was returning to his mother in the Isle of Wight, when he suffered this fugue state. His memory was recovered, the dissociation reduced, and facing up to his problem he decided to divorce his wife, and became normal and happy.

(b) In another type it is a flight from *uncongenial circumstances* in which a person finds himself, a flight from an intolerable situation accompanied by forgetfulness, of which the rubber planter was a case in point.

(c) In the third type, it is a flight from a type of life which an individual has *voluntarily imposed upon himself* and which he therefore cannot voluntarily relinquish, but against which his natural self unconsciously revolts. In this case the conflict is more subjective.

The minister was a case in point. On his way back from church he disappeared and three days later found himself in Edinburgh where he had never been before, but which he recognized from photographs.

He was well fed, shaved and neatly dressed and aroused no suspicion. His father had been in the ministry and his widowed mother had induced him to do the same. This was with his consent, but against his nàtural inclinations. The fugue state was the assertion of his natural self and its revolt against continuing work in a sphere which, however successful, was uncongenial to him.

In such cases the super-ego forces its demands on the personality; but instead of the ego and super-ego taking turns, as in dual personality, the ego refuses any longer to be subject to these demands, abandons its task, says "I'm off!" and takes to flight. Such a fugue may therefore be described as *a flight of the ego from the demands of the super-ego.*

(*d*) Sometimes the fugue is an attempt to solve a problem of the past, not to escape from it.

That was so in the case of the officer who after the war developed fugue states, sometimes for days, sometimes for only minutes at a time, in which he imagined himself back in France, where he felt he had failed in his duty, and with the desire to return to the scene to retrieve the past. In one of these fugue states, thinking he was in France, he committed a crime. He was charged at the Police Court but had a complete loss of memory of the incident. Between that and the Assizes to which he was committed, he not only recovered his memory of what he had done under hypnosis, but saw the reasons and motives for his action. This was pleaded so convincingly that in spite of his admission of the act, and the initial scepticism of the jury, he was acquitted.

Somnambulism (sleep-walking) is a minor form of fugue, for if we analyse out the motive in sleep-walking, which we can do best under hypnosis, we find it to be an attempt to re-enact a situation, to do something that has been left undone, or to solve some problem as yet unsolved.[1] Ordinarily an attempt is made to solve our problems in dreams—indeed, that, in our opinion, is the function of dreams—but sometimes the dream takes the form of actually re-enacting the situation, in which case it is somnambulic. The case of Lady Macbeth is classical and typical. A patient, a married woman, would leave her bedroom, go to another room, move about it, and then return to bed. This re-enacted the scene when she nursed her father, and often at night used to go to his room. But it also touched on the unsolved problem in the prefer-

---

[1] We do not agree with Janet in classifying somnambulism with hysteria simply because there is dissociation in both; for as we have said there is dissociation in all neuroses. The difference between hysteria on the one hand and somnambulism and fugues is in the massiveness of the dissociated part.

ence she had for her father to her husband. In her sleep-walking, she was returning to care for her father. A child, lacking affection from her parents, would sleep-walk to try and find the affection she craved. Sleep-walking should always be regarded as a neurosis and if possible its causes discovered, as it indicates a deep-seated problem in the child's personality.

De-personalization. This condition is closely allied to the other disorders of personality. In fugues the patient may completely forget himself and what he is. In de-personalization the patient has the feeling that he is unreal, or it may be that the world around him is unreal. The classic instance is that of J. M. Barrie's *Mary Rose*, who in childhood lived in a world of phantasy ("The Island that likes to be visited") and later became a "ghost," unreal, who did not recognize her own son.

The condition is of course common in physical illness and states of weakness like fevers: "Who am I, and where am I?" are common questions. We are concerned only with those which are psychologically caused.

The basic cause of this feeling of unreality is that the patient has superimposed on himself a fictitious personality, a *persona* or mask, a super-ego which is alien to his natural self which he repressed. Thereafter he is literally "not himself" and therefore has the "feeling of being unreal." In truth, *he feels unreal for the simple reason that he is unreal,* he is not being his real self but a fictitious superimposed self. In most cases we find that in his early days there was a strongly formed personality which has been repressed in favour of the *persona,* which for so many years has dominated the patient that he believes it to be his true self; but in time it wears thin and the real self begins to assert itself. The patient then begins to feel that the life he has been living is unreal, not his true self, and that *he* is unreal, which in fact is the case.

In other cases he feels that *the objective world is unreal.* This is because it is undesirable or too hard for him to face, and he therefore makes it unreal because he wants it to be unreal. In the fugue states he escapes from the objectionable world by flight, but when he cannot escape from it, he may ignore it and protest that it does not exist, and makes it unreal, just as many people hearing a bad piece of news say, "It can't be! I won't believe it!" So when these people say the world around is not real, it is just another method of man's escape from his eternal problem of his adjustment to life.

Paranoid states may also be considered amongst the "disorders of personality," for in them one of the "personalities," the repressed one, is projected and made to appear in the form of another personality which is persecuting one, or of voices accusing one. These are the voices of our other personality.

True paranoia as such is probably a constitutional disorder, although neither its causes nor its cure is yet discovered. It is a psychosis and conforms to any definition of psychosis we choose to give. It is marked by suspicion, ideas of reference (that people are talking about one), hearing accusing voices, and delusions of persecution. But apart from its probable constitutional basis, the psychology of the paranoic is worth considering, since there are paranoid conditions of an obsessional type.

The paranoid individual is characterized by a *power psychology* and is *deficient in love*: or what love there is, is egocentric and narcissistic, which accounts for the tendency of the paranoic to be homosexual. It is because of his claim to override others that he feels that others are hostile to him; it is because he has designs against others that he is full of suspicion that they are plotting against him. Like the Priest of the Grove of Nemi[1] who became Priest-King only by murdering the last occupant, the paranoic goes in constant fear of his life from those who wish to murder him and succeed him: he fears murder because he himself is a murderer; for him danger lurks behind every tree.

Sometimes it is the super-ego or moral self which is repressed and projected on to the outside world; sometimes it is the repressed ego or natural self which is so projected.

In *paranoid obsessions the super-ego or unconscious conscience is projected* on to the outside world, and therefore condemns one.

To take an instance, that of a woman university lecturer in aesthetics. As a child she was innocently indulging in sex, was discovered, called a "filthy thing," and had her hand slapped. She was furious, but then by identification adopted the mother's attitude, turned against herself and called herself a filthy thing; but this being unpleasant she repressed it. She then transferred the complex to her dolls and made them do the same thing (satisfying her desires), and then punished them for being filthy (satisfying her super-ego). She then developed a super-ego with a "clean" attitude of mind and became lecturer in aesthetics. But she later suffered from various obsessions, due to the emergence of her repressed impulses; (*a*) that people would think she was a prostitute (the revival of her early sex desires), (*b*) an over-scrupulousness about bathing and cleanliness (propitiatory obsession), (*c*) an obsession that the girls in her class thought that she had a dirty body, which was the original judgment passed on her by her unconscious conscience. This

[1] Frazer's *Golden Bough*.

paranoid obsession came about originally from the objective condemnation of her mother; then being accepted, it became a condemnation of herself; then she projected the self-condemnation on to others, who, she said, regarded her as filthy. She complains that others are accusing her of sins which she is not aware of having committed, whereas in fact she is condemned by no one but her own conscience: it is really self-accusation.

Mild paranoid projections of this kind are common in ordinary behaviour.

A professional woman complains that people do not respect her, which is not the fact. The explanation is that she has undesirable characteristics of which she is unconscious but which she despises in herself. She therefore thinks that other people will think the same; so she says they *do* think the same and do not respect her. She then goes a step further, for since she is unconscious of her sins, she resents their supposed criticism and so perpetually justifies herself before others: but the more she justifies herself the more she exposes herself to criticism. By thus projecting her own criticism on to others she spares herself the humiliation of admitting her own failings, but it is at the cost of the imaginary adverse judgment of others.

In other cases it is *the repressed ego which is projected*. So the patient, obsessed by his guilty self-condemnation, but refusing to acknowledge his guilt, conveniently projects it on to the devil, the source of all evil, as the cause of her being made to do evil things. The devil is the projection, objectification, and personalization of our own complexes—a very real and active being, born of a cleft personality, if not with the cloven hoof.

The projection and personalization of the *rejected ego* and its impulses is illustrated in the case of the boy patient who rages against an imaginary foe, strikes and punches his own body, especially in the sexual region, shakes his fist at an imaginary foe and shouts, "Don't come near me," "Don't you dare to touch me," etc., and a moment after is talking as a normal individual. He is actually downing his sexual feelings which he has rejected, but which are projected and personalized as an outside tempting agency against which he shakes his fist. He has no conscious objection to sex, but experiences in childhood had made him afraid of his sex feelings and repress them as foul and horrible, but when they were reawakened in adolescence he had to fight them and did so, not as internal forces or impulses, because he refused to admit them, but as external foes. His super-ego condemned them and literally shouted insults against them. He made a difficult but excellent recovery when these complexes were revealed and released, in spite of the apparently "psychotic" nature of his symptoms.

Alternatively, the patient projecting the forbidden impulses on to others, becomes ruthless in his condemnation of sins to which he is unconsciously addicted, but of which the person in question may be quite innocent. They are the people of hard, rigid, bigoted personality, fanatics in a cause in which they are really fighting against themselves. They criticize other people and therefore become excessively sensitive to the criticisms of others, for obvious reasons. They do not for a moment realize that they are really condemning themselves, and that in passing judgment on others they are revealing their own faults; that in judging, they are being judged. Mild cases are of those who like teasing others, but themselves hate to be teased.

Sometimes the personalized projections are so vivid that they appear in the form of "voices" from outside. These may come either from the projected ego or the projected super-ego. So common and so realistic is this experience that the term the "voice of the devil" and the "voice of conscience" are variously used of the one and the other. Both ego and super-ego, we must remember, may be repressed and unconscious.

The projected voice of the moral super-ego is heard condemning us for sins of which we are unaware—"You are a thief!" "Everyone knows what you have done!" "You are a bitch! a snob, a liar, a humbug!" These voices are the condemnation of the natural self by the repressed and projected moral self, even though the individual is unconscious of any sin or guilt: it is the activity of the unconscious conscience.

In other cases it is *the projected voice of the repressed ego* which makes itself heard, and being personalized appears as a voice saying, "Murder him!" "Strangle her!" Or if the individual is going to do something good and moral says, "No you don't!"

In true psychotic paranoia these are taken for actual external real voices; in obsessional paranoia they are recognized as imaginary or at most as subjective; it is "as though" a voice is heard. The psychology is the same; the difference may be that where there is an unstable constitution, the patient may be unable, on account of the strength of the conflict, to cope with the compelling ideas and so develops true paranoia in which he does not differentiate between the real and the imaginary. In obsessional paranoics there is the same violent unconscious conflict going on but the man of more stable constitution retains his balance.

We have said, and rightly, that these apparently external voices are merely the *voice of the super-ego* projected on to the outside world: it is ourselves condemning us. But we must remember that these voices were originally voices from outside persons; they were derived from the original condemnation of parents or others whose personalities have been introjected by identification into ourselves to form our super-ego or conscience, giving us the sense of guilt and shame. It is natural, therefore, that these voices should again be heard as from without, because they originally were from without: in being projected, therefore, they are simply reverting to type. By ascribing the accusations to the original source we may often get rid of them.

If the voices accuse us of certain sins it is probable that we are in fact guilty of those sins though unconsciously, for these voices would not condemn us were it not that we had these forbidden desires. That is why it is wasting our time to attempt to prove to the patient that he has *not* done these things; he knows better and feels guilty. A reference to the lecturer in aesthetics will illustrate these facts. It is more to the point to bring to light in these patients what are the forbidden desires of which they feel guilty. It is still more necessary to bring to light the morbid conscience which originally condemned them and which in all probability was greatly exaggerated, than the morbid sins which were probably trifling. Where the patient is psychotic and believes in the truth of these voices analytic treatment is of course impossible, since apart from other things we cannot get his co-operation.

CHAPTER XIV

SEX PERVERSIONS AND ABERRATIONS

I⊤ is strange that an instinct so strong and deep-rooted as the sexual, and so necessary to the continuance of the race, should be so commonly perverted from its normal and natural ends, and subject to so many aberrations. One would have thought that in a matter so urgent as the reproduction of the species, nature would have secured that nothing should stand in the way of these impulses fulfilling their natural functions and reaching their natural goals. That indeed is more or less the case with the lower animals amongst whom perversions, though they exist (as in the case of homosexuality amongst rams when they are segregated too long), are rare. Yet in man, far from that being the case, the sexual instinct is subject to all kinds of abnormalities and perversions.

There are thousands of our fellow men and women, otherwise apparently normal, whose sexual feelings have no relation whatever with the opposite sex, and whose sexual impulses are so perverted that they are quite incapable of reproducing their species. Some have no desire at all towards the opposite sex: others have the desire but find themselves impotent to perform the sex act: whilst others have their desires directed to all kinds of other objects.

There are those, for instance, whose sex feelings are aroused only towards inanimate objects, like shoes or corsets, as in *fetichism*, or even dead bodies; or towards themselves alone, as in *narcissism*; or to those of the same sex, as in *homosexuality*. In others it is the sexual impulse or activity that is perverted, such as in those who have sexual pleasure in inflicting pain on others, strangling, cutting off hair, beating, thrashing, or inflicting mental cruelty on others, all of which are instances of *sadism*. Others find their only sex pleasure in having pain inflicted on themselves, in being beaten, in submitting to others, having others angry with them, blaming them or ordering them about, or having their hands tied up, all of which are instances of *masochism*, the essential feature of which is the sexual pleasure in being overmastered at the hands of the loved person, even to the extent of suffering pain. The *exhibitionist* desires only to expose himself, whilst the *observationist* desires only to gratify his desires by seeing others exposed.

Y

Sometimes the sexual perversions are of a more bizarre type, like the young man whose sexuality could only be aroused by shaking hands with an old man: or the one who could only be sexually aroused by the thought of a vomiting horse, or again by seeing a man with a wooden leg. Nature may have made the procreative instinct strong, but she has evidently not safeguarded it against distortion.

In some of these cases the object of sexual desire may be normal, namely towards those of the opposite sex, but the *activity* is of a perverted nature, e.g. a man beating a woman or exposing himself to her without any desire to have sexual intercourse with her. In other cases the activity may be relatively normal but the object abnormal, as in homosexual sodomy, where there is a desire for sexual penetration, but per anum and with one of the same sex. But in most cases both the object and the activity are abnormal, as in the case of the woman who had the sadistic desire to overcome, sexually expose and murder another woman; or the man who desired only to expose himself to boys; or to parade himself in women's clothing; or in the case of the sexual attachment of the fetichist to patent leather shoes.

Apart from these perversions and aberrations there are numerous sexual abnormalities such as impotence, premature ejaculation or split libido in the male, frigidity and vaginismus in the female, which completely wreck the marital life and happiness of numbers of people.

Biologically we regard the sex perversions as abnormal because they pervert the ends of reproduction; psychologically, because they are due to repression with arrest of development of a function which should find natural expression in adult life.

Biological considerations. The sexual "instinct" differs from others like fear and aggression in that it is not necessary to the preservation of the individual. But just because it is not essential to the individual, it is necessary that the pleasure associated with it must be proportionately greater if the instinct is to find expression and the race perpetuated. That puts sex in a different category from the other urges. It is therefore not surprising that it gives rise to problems of a more acute nature, as it does in the psychoneuroses and in social life. Another important consideration is that other functions like fear and assertiveness are operative in childhood and serve their biological functions from birth onwards, whereas the sexual activities whilst capable of arousal in infancy, serve no such purpose, and do not do so until maturity. This makes them more liable to perversion than the other instinctual activities. Indeed, if these infantile sex tendencies are exaggerated they tend to be fixated, resulting in arrest of adult sexuality and the development of perversions. There is some biological justification therefore for the discouragement of sexual activities in early childhood, which have been regarded by mothers as morally wrong.

The sociological and legal implications of sex perversions are also important. They differ from the other psychoneuroses, for a man with an hysteric paralysed arm and a woman with fear of close spaces are a nuisance to themselves and to some extent to others, but the homosexual apart from the fact that he is incapable of reproducing his species, is capable of perverting others, and the exhibitionist, by exposing himself to young girls, may precipitate in them a fear of sex, frigidity and neurosis. It is not surprising, therefore, that society regards the pervert as vicious and ostracizes him, while the law regards him as a criminal and punishes him. Yet this is unjust, for whether we regard such perversions as innate, or as due to complexes formed in early childhood, the sexual pervert is a victim of tendencies for which he is no more responsible than the man with a phobia: indeed he is no more responsible for his sadistic or fetichistic impulses than the ordinary person for his attraction to the opposite sex. It is true that to some extent the pervert can restrain his perverted impulses from overt acts, just as the normal person is expected to control his passions, and so far he is responsible for his actions when he is not responsible for his propensities. But the pervert is in a worse state than the normal person, for his propensities emerge from complexes that are dissociated, and therefore less under the control of the will than is normal sex desire.

Sexual perversions must, therefore, be distinguished from sexual vices, for a man may commit rape because he is a low-grade character and without morals, in which case punishment may deter him from future crimes; or he may be a man of the highest character who is the victim of sadistic impulses as horrible to himself as they are terrifying to others. One man may expose himself to little girls simply because he has no sense of decency; or he may do so because he is a sexual exhibitionist, whose perversion excludes all normal sex desire. It is most necessary in the legal interest as well as for medical treatment that these two conditions should be distinguished; fortunately the diagnosis in any particular case is not very difficult for an expert. But as psychopathologists we are here concerned not with a social evil, but with the sex perversion as an individual disorder.

But before discussing the nature and causes of sex perversions we must consider what we mean by normal sexuality, and its relation to love.

The difficulty some authors have had in defining love is that they have failed to recognize that *love is a sentiment*, that is to say, a *group of tendencies centred round some object, idea or person*. The most important components of love are dependence, devotion, tenderness, protectiveness, friendship, loyalty, possessiveness, sexuality, self-regard, pride, admiration, affection and respect.

In any particular case several of these may be attached to the object of our love, so that love takes on a different aspect according to the specific components which are called into play. In films and novels it is the sexual component which predominates, so that love is made almost synonymous with sex. But "love" has a very different meaning when used by an Archbishop. In the most primitive form of love, namely the love of the mother for her infant, the main feature is that of tenderness and protectiveness, the associated sensuous pleasure encouraging the biological function of motherhood. In the sentiment of patriotism, or love for one's country, the aggressive element may be strong, or pride in its achievements and culture. In true philanthropy self-sacrifice is an important component; in false philanthropy it may be *self-regard* and the desire for praise and gratitude which are the dominant factors. Love is therefore a sentiment whose specific nature depends on the components which happen to be predominant.

Hate also is a sentiment consisting of many components. The difference between love and hate is that love is a sentiment in which there is *attraction* towards the object of our love whereas in hate there is *repulsion* from the object of our hate: for even if we go towards the object of our hate, it is in order to attack and destroy it, and get it out of our sight. To say, as some do, that "love and hate are the same thing" is absurd; they are *opposite* sentiments, but it is true to say that frustrated love often *turns* to hate against the one who refuses to give us the love we desire, and attraction then turns into repulsion as in so many love affairs. In sadistic love, however, the two are combined (though still not "the same"), as in the case of the animal who destroys what it would devour, the infant who bites the breast whose milk it craves, or the man who has the impulse to strangle the girl he loves. Freud identifies love with sex. "We call by that name (i.e. Libido, sexual hunger) the energy of those instincts which have to do with all that may be comprised under the word 'love.'

The nucleus of what we mean by love actually consists . . . in sexual love with sexual union as its aim."[1] He regards conditions like admiration and respect as "aim restricted," that is to say sexual activities bereft of their sexual aim. Again, "Psychoanalysis then gives these love instincts the name of sexual instincts."[2] This view is not only contrary to popular usage and to the view of love which we have just outlined, but is contradicted by anthropological findings. Briffault[3] has brought ample evidence to prove that "tenderness and affection between the sexes are not originally connected with the sexual impulse," whether amongst animals or in primitive human life. For instance, "South American Indians are said to have no love for their wives." Again, "I have never witnessed any display of tenderness between man and wife," says Dr. Ward, of the Congo tribes. Devotion between husband and wife is absent in many primitive tribes, although of course sex relations exist. The apparent devotion between man and wife lies in their common interest in the offspring, not affection to the mate.[4] *The original springs of love lie not in sex but in the tenderness and devotion of a mother to her offspring*, which are to be found amongst the most primitive humans, and amongst the higher animals, the mothers of which will give their lives for their young.

Freud also appears to make sex synonymous not only with love but with the sensuous. He says, "we describe the pleasure derived from sucking as a *sexual* one,"[5] and regards the breast as a sex object.[6] Again, he "extends the designation sexual to include these activities of early infancy which aim at pleasure."[7] With these views of Freud we have always disagreed.[8]

---

[1] *Group Psychology*, p. 37. [2] *Ibid.*, p. 39.
[3] *The Mothers.* [4] This applies for instance to birds.
[5] *Introd. Lect.*, p. 261. [6] *Ibid.*, p. 264. [7] *Ibid.*, p. 273.
[8] Freud's classification of the instinct into the sex instincts, the ego instincts, and the aggressive instincts were devised for clinical purposes, and are useful, but the classification is nevertheless illogical. This is obvious when we inquire upon what criterion they are based. The ego instincts at first being merely the group of tendencies which stand in opposition to sex instincts and repress them (*Introd. Lect.*, p. 294), appear to be transformed into self-preservation instincts and concerned with reality (pp. 298-9); whereas the sex instincts appear to be defined in that they are being desired for their erotic pleasure alone, that is to say as a purely subjective experience. Freud "extends the designation 'sexual' to include those activities of early infancy which aim at 'organ pleasure' " (p. 273). According to such definitions, to which group of instincts does the activity of sucking belong? According to the first criterion it obviously belongs to the ego instincts, as subserving self-preservation; according to the second it is sexual, as Freud maintains, for "The gratification obtained (in sucking) can only relate to the region of the mouth and lips; we therefore call these areas of the body erotogenic zones, and describe their pleasures derived from sucking as a *sexual* one." Another corrective may be suggested. It is often said that the

There are many forms of love, like tenderness and affection towards a sick child, in which sex plays no part. There are many other activities, like eating or swimming, which give sensuous pleasure but are not sexual.

We shall therefore use the term "sensuous" as a general term for all pleasurable physical sensations, normal as well as abnormal, and whether associated with egoistic functions like eating or with distinctively sexual functions. We shall use "sensual" of those sensuous activities which are specifically abnormal like thumb sucking or masturbation.

Normal sexuality consists in the sensuous attraction of one person for an appropriate person of the opposite sex, culminating in sexual union. *Sexuality may therefore be described as that group of tendencies whose natural end is procreation.* This does not mean, of course, that it always culminates in procreation, nor even in sexual union; there are many sexual activities which go no further than sexual "play" like embracing, kissing and stimulation of the genitals which have no object or purpose other than the sensuous pleasure enjoyed; but in so far as they arouse impulses and desires whose natural end is reproduction, they fall within the scope of our definition. Kissing therefore may be sexual in that it arouses genital stimulation; but it may be non-sexual as in the tender kiss of the mother for her ailing child which gives the child assurance of *protective* love. Similarly there are the perversions, like sadism or fetishism, which do not in fact lead to sexual union, but on the contrary exclude it: nevertheless they arouse feelings, sensations and tendencies whose *natural* end is reproduction, although in these cases these tendencies have in fact been perverted to *un*-natural ends; and that is why we give them the name of "perversions." The definition we have suggested has the advantage that it finds a place for both the biological and the psychological aspects of sexuality.

Normal sexuality may be exaggerated constitutionally because of physiological causes such as endocrine development. Sex may also be exaggerated by the *encouragement* of sensuous and sexual stimulation in childhood, by fondling and petting, or by more

---

infant is entirely *auto-erotic*, in contrast with having *object love*. This is not the case. The infant's first love is object love, namely the breast, which is the first love object. It is only after it receives the breast that it experiences the pleasure. The reflex action of sucking came before the pleasure derived from it, and is a biological response to a need rather than to a pleasure. Once the sensuous pleasure is associated with the activity, whether sucking defection or urination, it continues to encourage the biological functions. This symbiosis of sensuous pleasure and biological function is the normal process of life.

direct forms of stimulation. Sex may also be exaggerated by *frustration*. For this reason the girl too strictly brought up and without the opportuntiy to sublimate in friendships with boy friends, is often the one to get into trouble: and it is often the man with the inferiority complex and who feels unattractive who compensates by becoming the philanderer.

Sex perversions are the persistence of infantile sensuous activities to the exclusion of normal sexuality.

The *mechanism of sex perversions* may be explained in this way. Sex activities may be reactions to the feeling of deprivation of love, the sensuous pleasure being resorted to as a solace for the loss of love. It is then accepted as a substitute for love, and *represses the love craving*. But the sexual indulgence does not give him the love he really wants and causes disappointment and depression. It is also liable to be punished by threats from the mother. Therefore the sensuous pleasure activity has itself to be repressed in favour of the super-ego, usually of asceticism or aestheticism. This repression of sex means that it is arrested in development, and fails to assume adult forms, so that when it naturally emerges in puberty, it appears in the form in which it was originally repressed, that is to say in an infantile form. This constitutes the perversion. There is, as in most psychoneuroses, a double repression, one of the love craving, one of the sex.

Since sex perversion is the emergence of infantile sexuality to the exclusion of normal adult sexuality, we must direct our attention in the first place to a study of these infantile sensuous and sexual activities.

Infantile sensuousness. Every child has a number of biological reflex functions such as sucking, defecation, urination and movements of the limbs, each of which is necessary to the life and well-being of the organism. *These functions of the body are then associated with sensuous pleasure*: sucking is pleasant, defecation and urination give sensuous gratification (as we may observe from the smile of pleasure on the face of the infant after passing a successful motion), and the child likes kicking its limbs and having its body naked to the air. The manifestation of sensuous pleasure in these activities is observed in the behaviour of the infant and is amply confirmed in the analysis of the adult patients; indeed it often persists in adult life. The first year of life is therefore characterized by the enjoyment of sensuous pleasure; it is the golden age, the age of bliss in which there are no taboos, no inhibitions, no shame; it is the garden of paradise in which it is no sin to enjoy oneself, and in which the infant "knew not that it was naked," gives full and free play to all its activities and finds exquisite pleasure in the healthy performance of all its natural functions.

The value of this sensuous pleasure is not far to seek: *it serves the function of encouraging the biological activity.* It is pleasant for the child to suck and the pleasure of sucking encourages the activity. If sucking were unpleasant (as, indeed, it sometimes is when the food is distasteful or difficult to get), the child would cease to take its food. It is pleasant for the child to defecate; the child is, therefore, encouraged in the performance of this necessary function by the pleasure associated with it. It is of value for the child to have its skin exposed to the air, to exercise its limbs, to urinate, and the pleasure accompanying these activities encourages the infant in the healthy performance of these functions. Healthy activity of whatever kind, in childhood as in adult life, consists in the pleasurable performance of our biological functions; and the pleasure associated with these functions encourages adaptation to reality. The mother's sensuous pleasure in suckling the infant is shown in the erection of the nipple which in turn facilitates the function of sucking.

Obviously *these early sensuous activities like sucking are primarily egotistic and not sexual* in their nature; that is to say, they subserve the biological needs of the individual as such, his well-being and self-preservation, and not those of reproduction. The fact that the function of sucking, urination and defecation are associated with pleasure does not justify us in calling them sexual: they are sensuous but not sexual since the sensuous pleasure is attached to functions entirely devoted to the well-being of the child himself. It is to be observed in fact that the biological activity came before the sensuous pleasure associated with its successful performance and therefore the anticipated pleasure encourages the activity.

Nor are these infantile activities "perverse," as Freud calls them; they are primarily healthy and natural tendencies subserving and encouraging the normal biological functions of life.

There is, therefore, no fundamental incompatibility between the pleasure principle and the reality principle; for the pleasure principle serves the functions of reality and encourages adaptation to life. Pleasure, indeed, in its sublimated form as joy in activity, is necessary to the highest achievement.

The biological significance of pleasure has never been fully appreciated, for it is either condemned by the moralist as merely hedonistic, or it has been indulged in by the epicure quite apart from its association with the natural functions of life. Pleasure has its importance for life, and not for gratification only. Even feelings of displeasure like pain and hunger have, like pleasure, their biological functions and act now as a stimulus of activity and now as a means of avoidance of danger. This conception therefore gives to sensuousness a biological significance, which differs alike from that of the epicure who divorces pleasure from its natural functions for reality, and that of the ascetic who deprives the functions of life of the stimulus of joy.

The sensuous pleasure therefore tends to encourage these infantile biological activities, *until they become established as habits*, after which their pleasurable tone tends to pass; so defecation and urination give but the mildest pleasure, if any at all, to the ordinary adult.

Infantile sensuous activities then take four directions: (*a*) some are transferred into pleasure in other forms of activity; (*b*) some develop into higher forms of specific character traits; (*c*) some are transferred to the uses of adult sexuality as wooing activities, thus following the biological path; (*d*) and some are arrested in development to become the sex aberrations and (*e*) perversions.

(*a*) In general some of the *sensuous* physical pleasure of infantile life becomes transferred into the *joy in activity and achievement*, and ultimately into *happiness* which is the affective tone accompanying the full expression of the whole personality, and is a sign of mental health. Thus pleasure continues to serve the functions of life. (*b*) Some of these early tendencies develop into higher forms of *character traits* of later life, normal and abnormal. The pleasure in talking for its own sake often traces itself back to an oral erotism or love of "mouthing it." Parsimony, which the Freudians ascribe to anal-erotic activities,[1] are more correctly referred to infantile breast activities, holding on to what one has, which is a natural reflex in the infant. But of course such characteristics may come from other sources such as identification. The tendency to manipulate the breast in infantile life (a native reflex movement to squeeze out milk) is associated with great sensuous pleasure, and is then transferred into pleasure in the manipulation of other material, especially of clay, mud and other material of the same texture, and is sublimated in the plastic arts and the desire to make things. This tendency to manipulate is also regarded by the Freudians as anal-erotic, originating in the pleasure of playing with one's faeces,[2] but this is only a later manifestation of the earlier pleasurable activity at the breast, not the origin. There is no specific reason why a child should play with its faeces. But there is a definite biological reason why it manipulates the breast

[1] E. Jones, *Psychoanalysis*, pp. 665–683.   [2] *Ibid.*, p. 634.

in infancy, an activity which may be observed in most infants who make these squeezing movements with the hand while sucking: and it is when the child is deprived of this that it takes to plastic substitutes, like the faeces, and to stroking soft material like silk.

The following quotation, taken from a woman who was sadistic and also had a horror of brown shoes and brown bags, illustrates the true origin of such activities in the breast, its transfer to faeces, and its development, by repression, into the obsession.

"I emptied the chamber with faeces on the floor and liked messing about with it like plasticine . . . I had that same feeling of something giving way to my hand against my mother's breast, all soft and warm; and it gives me a sense of power. It is the joy of making something *give* under your hand. Eating a banana, it sometimes becomes squashy and then I want to throw it all away (due to a later disgust and rejection of the breast). I now hate to be alone because I feel I might do those things" (the fear of the repressed desire). The horror of brown shoes represented the thwarted desire to manipulate the faeces, but the function of manipulation itself goes back to the earlier breast phase.

The pleasure in feeding is also transferred to higher activities and gives rise to many expressions which revive the sense of the original pleasure. In literature, for instance, we "browse" amongst our books, we "digest" a book, we "thirst" for knowledge, we "absorb" information and we "devour" a novel with the same zest as an infant does his milk; in fact, we may observe people reading a book with zest, making movements with the mouth as of sucking, whilst others cannot enjoy reading unless they are sucking a pipe. If it is said that these are only symbols it may be replied that most symbols are in the first place derived from facts of experience and get their feeling tone from that experience and its revival in memory.

Another of the most primitive reactions of the infant is that of putting everything it holds into its mouth, and this turns into the fascination of pushing things into holes and fitting one thing into another (characteristic of the child of ten months), and leads to later ingenuity in fitting together mechanical toys. This tendency to fit one thing into another is interpreted by some as a sexual activity representing coitus, and one cannot exclude the possibility of a tropistic urge of this kind. But it is obvious that an infant has had no experience of coitus whereas it has had an actual experience of pushing things into a hole, namely its mouth, from which it derives this sensuous pleasure and naturally seeks for a symbolic repetition of the experience. The law of parsimony of hypothesis, as well as our experience in analysing these character traits to their source, compels us to accept the simpler explanation.

So these physiological functions associated with the mouth, anus, penis, or urethra, are transformed into later activities and help to determine and colour some of our character traits.

But are we to regard these character traits as *originating* in these activities as the Freudians appear to do; or merely as expressing themselves *through* these activities? Obstinacy is often said to be an anal character trait,[1] as though it is derived from anal activities, but a child may express its obstinacy with its mouth, its penis or its anus, or for that matter with its arms and legs or vocal cords. It is the child *itself* who is obstinate, and it expresses its obstinacy by any means available. We are therefore no more justified in calling obstinacy an anal-erotic character trait than we are in calling it a vocal-erotic or pedal-erotic trait. In our experience the only reason why obstinacy is found to be more associated with anal activities is because the most effective method a child has of showing its obstinacy is in refusing to defecate, and wild horses cannot make him. But that is an accidental not an essential association.

(c) When these early sensuous activities have served the purpose of establishing the biological functions as habits they tend to pass but become *transferred to the uses of sexuality*. These later constitute the *wooing tendencies*, which are *the persistence of infantile sensuous activities for the uses of normal adult sexuality*. Normal sexuality, as Freud has pointed out, is of two types, the preliminary or wooing activities, like kissing, fondling, exposing and admiring beauty of form, voice and gesture: and secondly, the act of coitus or sexual intercourse. The wooing activities are largely derived from infantile sensuous experiences transferred to the uses of sexuality. An instance of this transference is the stereotropic tendency to keep close to another, originally for protection, but later used for sex as expressed in the lovers' embrace. Kissing is another instance; kissing is obviously little else than sucking, whether in the movements or in the noise produced; and the parts of the body chosen for kissing are the soft rounded parts like the cheeks, reminiscent of the breast, or the mucous membrane of the lips which is reminiscent of the nipple. That appears to be why a kiss on the lips is more sensuous than one on the cheeks, just as the nipple is a more sensuous object to the infant than the breast itself, and many a girl who will allow a kiss on the cheeks

[1] E. Jones, *Psychoanalysis*, p. 665.

would forbid it on the lips. To those who are sceptical of the possibility of such transferences from one biological function to another, we may point to a physiological analogy to this transference of functions in the use of teeth which, it is supposed, were originally devised for attack, but later became the instrument of eating and chewing; or in the Eustachian tube (the passage from the mouth to the ear), originally a gill for breathing, now used for hearing. The pleasure most lovers have in fondling the cheek, the hair on the head, the rounded parts of the body, possibly originates in pleasure experienced by the infant in fondling the round soft contours of its mother's breast, and the pleasure many people have in stroking soft, smooth things, like silk or velvet, appear to be derived from the same experiences. A similar pleasure is shown in the pathologic sensation in fetichism, the fetichistic object being found to be almost universally a substitute for the breast. On the other hand, many people dislike kissing, finding it repugnant and disgusting, and when that is so we can usually trace the disgust back to the definite experiences in early childhood in which sucking was regarded with repugnance; such as being sick at the breast through having been suffocated with too much milk. But kissing is not merely a sensuous feeling transferred to adult sexuality; it also retains its original self-preservation significance as a symbol of protection and security. The child taken to hospital wants his mother to kiss him, not to give him sensuous pleasure, but to give him the assurance of her protective love and care. To regard protective love as "aim-restricted" (i.e. a sexual activity robbed of its aim) is to reverse the true order; the biological reflex and function of sucking came first, the pleasure was secondary. It would be truer to say that sex pleasure sought for its own sake is robbed of its real aim.

As with kissing and close contact so with other sensuous activities of infancy. The sensuous aggressiveness of the infant persists in the normal aggressiveness of male sexuality, as it does in the perversion of sadism. "I could eat you," says the passionate lover in the novel, "devouring her with his eyes," while the perverted sadist would make short work of her by strangling her. The sensuous passivity of the infant persists in female sexual passivity and in the masochism of the male pervert. The excitement in seeing someone of the other sex undressing (more exciting to most than seeing them completely naked) is often found to be derived from the excitement which one may observe in the infant as the mother is preparing to feed him. So with exhibition and observationism which play so important a part in infantile and later in social life. It is interesting to note that the varying fashions in women's clothes in civilized communities ring the changes on the various sexually attractive features of the female form—at one time the bust, at another the hips, legs, neck, hair. In the 1930's it was the whole personality, for a change.

When, however, we say that the wooing tendencies are the transference of infantile sensuous activities into adult life, we do not, of course, deny that there are other and specifically adult modes of sexual stimulus. The observation of the sex organs which stimulate sex desire is not wholly derived from observation in infancy, but may be a direct stimulus in itself quite apart from any infantile experiences. But where these activities are strongly marked in infancy, this exaggeration determines which wooing tendency is preferred and which perversion is dominant. In some of these activities, such as kissing, the infantile features are obvious; and when we analyse out the perversions we invariably find their roots in such fixations of infantile experiences.

So close is the correspondence between the infantile sensuous activities and wooing tendencies of adult sexuality that it is not surprising that Freud has regarded these infantile activities as themselves sexual; but neither the fact that they both give rise to sensuous pleasure, nor the fact that we may demonstrate a continuity between them and the sex perversions, justifies us in regarding them as themselves sexual, since their primary functions are obviously egoistic in origin. But the sensuous pleasure associated with these infantile experiences makes their transference to the biological uses of later sexuality an easy and natural one.

The particular wooing activities chosen are those which in early years have given particular gratification, and so continue to do so in the service of normal sexuality. Thus the stimulation of this or that infantile activity by indulgence determines the preference for this or that form of wooing. So some people tend to be more exhibitionist, some more sadistic or masochistic in their wooing and such preference may be regarded as normal, especially when the wooing tendencies of both parties happen to correspond; indeed, there is little doubt that many marriages are brought about by such mutual attraction. So the man's observationism may not be unwelcome to the woman who takes a particular delight in exhibitionism. But whereas one man is more stimulated by nudity, to another it makes no appeal whatsoever; some women whose aggressiveness and obstinacy has been developed in infantile life are not in the least aroused by the idea of being overmastered, and this may make it impossible for them to have an orgasm; whereas to others this is the most exciting form of sexual stimulation.

The function of the wooing activities is obvious; it arouses sexual interest and enhances sexual desire. Indeed there are some, particularly women, who would not have their sexual desires aroused at all, were it not for the preliminary stimulus of being wooed. But with the stimulus of kissing, touching, fondling and embracing, there is an accumulation of sexual libido which creates a desire so strong that it becomes almost compulsive. So does nature encourage the process of reproduction, providing for the perpetuation of the species and the fulfilment of its ends; or, if we are to be strictly scientific and avoid anthropomorphism, it is those species in which this occurs which survive.

But wooing serves another function than that of stimulating sexual feelings; *it enhances the value of the person loved*, and gives lovers the opportunity to develop qualities of admiration, respect and affection for each other such as existed in the original relationships in infancy between mother and child. This is particularly encouraged by the custom in higher civilizations of a period of engagement in which sex intercourse is denied, for the very fact that sex is restrained means that the effect so produced is *transferred to other components of love*, such as tenderness, by means of which the sentiment of love is more strongly developed towards the loved person. This helps to make the bond of marriage stronger and to establish a more lasting relationship. The custom of continence before marriage, not confined to Christian countries— Tacitus mentions it of the ancient Germans—also has the same biological value. So these infantile sensuous tendencies are not only transferred to the uses of adult sexuality, but sublimated in the service of adult love, and help to establish a firmer family relationship.

Wooing therefore is the persistence of infantile sensuous activities to the encouragement of normal sexuality, in which there is no repression and no perversity; the infantile sensuous tendency is naturally used for the enhancement of adult sexuality.

Unfortunately, things do not always develop so happily: and these infantile sensuous activities, instead of being transferred to the uses of adult sexuality may be repressed, arrested and fixated, in which case *they persist as aberrations and perversions*.

(d) *Sex aberrations* are those activities in which the persisting infantile traits are *preferred* to, but not to the exclusion of, normal sexuality. They may exist side by side with normal desires for sexual intercourse. They are sometimes described as an "undue" concentration upon the perverse tendency, whether sadistic, exhibitionist or fetichistic, to the detriment of normal sexuality. But as it is difficult to determine what we should call "undue," we may give the name aberrations to those perverse tendencies which are *preferred* to normal sexuality, though not to its exclusion, as in the case of the homosexual who is a married man and the father of a family, but prefers to go with boys, or the married woman who gets her orgasm with stimulation of the clitoris and regards complete intercourse with comparative indifference. Many an exhibitionist prefers to expose himself but is at the same time capable of ordinary sexuality; many a woman would be frigid were it not for the phantasies of being beaten. Whilst such reactions do not exclude normal sexuality, they detract from the full functioning of sex relations and being preferred to the latter they must be regarded as abnormal.

These aberrations are often a disturbing factor in married life, since one partner in the marriage may be preoccupied with a form of perverse desire which may be repugnant to the other partner, which is detrimental to normal love relations. If a sadistic husband has a masochistic wife, all may go well; but even so their preoccupation with their own gratification rather than with love for the other makes the relations unsatisfactory. The situation is worse when one partner is normal and the other prefers some aberration. This may cause discord in married life since what is ardently desired by one partner is disliked by the other; though mutual understanding and affection will lead to an accommodation to the other's idiosyncrasies.

The aberrations seem to arise from two sets of circumstances. In some cases there has been the repression of the need for love in favour of the perverse tendency as a solace which is therefore exaggerated and persists as an abnormal reaction trait. In other cases this perverse tendency is subsequently repressed, but only partially, so that it may persist side by side with a certain amount of ordinary sexuality and not to its complete exclusion. There are these two types of aberration.

(e) *Sex perversions*. Whilst the wooing activities normally encourage and enhance normal sex relations, and the aberrations are detrimental to sex relations in that they are preferred to them, the sex perversions are the persistence of infantile sensuous and sexual desires to the *exclusion* of normal sexuality; there is such a complete preoccupation with the perverse desire that the pervert is completely indifferent to normal sex relations and may hold it in the same abhorrence that the ordinary individual regards the perversion.

Infantile perversity.[1] The beginning of perversity is to be found in earliest infancy. We have observed that normally the infant's sensuous pleasure is associated with biological functions like sucking and defecation. The first stage in the perversity occurs when the child, once having experienced the pleasure, may seek the pleasurable activity for its own sake, *apart from the biological function*. In this case the pleasure becomes the principle and even the sole motive of these activities, and instead of subserving the biological functions, the pleasure principle may become a rival to the reality principle of biological needs, and may therefore be regarded as perverse.

The mucous membrane of the various orifices of the body, as we have seen, give sensuous gratification when stimulated by their appropriate objects, such as taking food in the mouth, the expulsion of faeces from the rectum, and urination. These activities are both pleasurable and biologically valuable. But obviously other than these natural functions can stimulate the pleasurable sensations, and the child may gratify its sensuous pleasure in sucking its thumb, frequency of micturation, or putting things into the anus. Says one patient, reverting to infancy, "Putting something in my anus is analogous to putting something in the mouth as a baby, and produces the same feeling of gratification and comfort. It keeps me quiet, solaces me. The rectum is like a mouth, a part of me and yet separate from me—as though I have two personalities, one at the mouth, one at the anus, both giving pleasure."

Such sensuous activities, being dissociated from the biological functions must be regarded as perverse, and this is our criterion of perversity. But these activities are not necessarily to the exclusion of normal activities, and probably all children indulge in them. They are the beginning of perversity, but of so innocent a type that little harm comes of them unless indulged in excessively or unless they are repressed; indeed, more harm may come through taking these things too seriously and checking them unduly, so that by being repressed they are arrested in development, than in allowing them ordinary expression in which case they will probably give place to the natural processes of sexuality. It is the same with the stimulation of the genital organs, whose biological functions do not emerge till years later, but the pleasure of which may be indulged in at an early age in masturbation. This too is a perverse

[1] We distinguish perversity from perversions proper.

tendency, in that the pleasure is divorced from any biological function, but as long as it remains a simple sensuous pleasure it is of no great consequence and usually transfers itself to adult sexuality. There are reasons why it is undesirable, as we shall see later, but it can usually be corrected by counter-attractions and activities: these simple sensual pleasures, though perverse, are not themselves true perversions.

A stage further is reached in the production of a perversion when the sensuous pleasure is indulged in not only apart from the biological function, but *to the detriment of the biological function*. The function of pleasure, as we have said, is to encourage the biological function, so that the pleasure in defecation, for instance, encourages evacuation. But supposing the child discovers, perhaps because he has been punished for dirtying himself, that holding in his motions itself produces a sensuous pleasure, he may continue to retain his faeces for the pleasure alone, which is of course detrimental to the healthy functioning of his body. Moreover, the cure of it by an enema increases the pleasure and so perpetuates the perversion and is commonly found to be the predisposing cause both of chronic constipation and of sodomy.

But *the main reason for perverse sexual activities is the feeling of deprivation of love*. A child suffering from loneliness and depression, commonly resorts to sensuous gratification as a solace and then clings to this gratification as a substitute for the love he has lost. This substitute is a very natural one, since in infancy the love relation to the mother is so closely associated with sensuous pleasure that the child, seeking to recover the lost relationship, resorts to the sensuous pleasure with which it was originally associated. Thus he masturbates when feeling lonely, sucks his thumb when feeling the sense of insecurity, becomes exhibitionist in order to recover the attention he has lost, reacts sadistically against the mother who has deprived him of his sensuous pleasures, and indulges in masochistic phantasies in his desire to return to the passivity of his infantile state. These sensuous reactions are always exaggerated.[1]

These sensuous and sexual activities are *definitely perverse*, for (a) they are *auto-erotic*, being directed to the child's own body instead of the object love for the mother; (b) they are *perverse*, being turned from their true aim, and indulged in apart from the biological functions which they serve; (c) they are *opposed to the demands*

---

[1] Many girls become "mistresses" not from excess of sex, indeed many of them have no pleasure in sex as such, but from want of affection, which makes them give in return for what they get.

of reality so that there now exists a conflict between the pleasure principle and the reality principle. Indeed the child will suck its thumb, masturbate, or indulge in phantasy as an escape from reality. (*d*) They are *exaggerated* because the whole of love is now concentrated upon its sensuous aspect, which becomes the one solace in life; and (*e*) they lead to *arrest of sexual development*, since these earlier activities become fixated, and fail to develop into more mature forms of sexuality. Such a child clings to his auto-erotic activites like a dog to his bone, and since he has found in it his sole joy in life, is reluctant to surrender it for the more uncertain joys of adult love. In milder cases he may get married and have sex relations, but his sadism or exhibitionism always retains an undue place in the shrine of his devotions, and he is liable to revert to them especially if his marriage is in any way unhappy. This is one type of aberration, as we have observed.

But even these perverse reactions are of little importance provided they exist side by side with the desire for love, for when opportunity arises the child returns to normal love. That is why so many children, while indulging in these perversities, grow out of them.

The danger point comes when the child definitely *represses the love craving* in favour of the perverse activity and says, "I don't want anyone's love, now that I have this pleasure which I can have whenever I want!" This is not merely apart from, but contrary to, the biological functions of love which are for protection and security. *Sex has now become a substitute for the whole of love.* In such cases there is not only an over-accentuation of sex, but an inhibition of love, so that in adult life these people are sex-ridden, but devoid of affection. They have numerous "love affairs" but they never love, for they are cynical about love; they may even become nymphomaniacs. The sensual or sexual becomes the one absorbing pursuit in their lives. But they also suffer from depression, disappointment and disillusion for they are denied and refuse the love they really desire, so that those who live a gay life not uncommonly end in suicide.

So far these various forms of sexual perversity are reaction character traits, which may persist through life. But even they are not true perversions.

For the development of true sex perversions these sexual and sensuous reactions are not only exaggerated, but must themselves in turn be repressed. It is this repression which completely arrests and fixates them.

Before proceeding further let us consider a case of sex perversion as illustrating the mechanism and the psychopathology of those conditions.

The case is of a young man, Clarence, who had a fourfold form of perversion, first of having his hands tied behind his back (masochism), of wearing a girl's waterproof cape (a fetichism, and a transvestism), and of parading in this at night (exhibitionism). Tracing his symptoms back by free association we discovered the following facts relating to his perversions. His mother had fed him very successfully in his infancy and then become a chronic invalid. The child was suddenly deprived of both protecting love and sensuous pleasure. He then became depressed; but his sexual feelings were then accidentally but constantly stimulated by his napkin being put on too tightly, which gave him sex pleasure of a *masochistic* type. This became a solace for the loss of love and a substitute for it. Stimulated by the napkin he also took *to masturbation*, and to cure him of this his hands were tied behind his back, a punishment which was therefore associated with sexual pleasure and accentuated the masochism. But at the same time it filled him with resentment and with humiliation, which led to the *repression of sex*. This punishment "cured" him of his habits, and he thereafter became a "good boy." But buried beneath was the longing for affection of which he had been deprived, and also the sexual craving had been adopted as a solace and a substitute for love, and had become the symbol of the lost love.

The symptom of wearing *the girl's waterproof cape* originated when as a small boy at school he was sent out of class, again as a punishment, and made to stand in the hall. The headmistress came along and seeing him cold, put her waterproof cape over his shoulders. This kindly act revived his old longing for motherly love repressed long since; the cape was a protection, the headmistress a mother substitute. There was in itself nothing sexual about this, and nothing in itself to produce a perversion. But the contact of the cape also revived an attraction to india-rubber (a common object in fetichism) which came from a waterproof used in childhood because of his bed-wetting, which was itself associated with urethral erotism. Not only so, but the attraction to rubber was in this case, as in so many other fetichisms, associated in its soft smoothness with his mother's breast, and with the body smell which was not unlike that of rubber. The reason why it had to be a *girl's* cape was not only that it was a woman's cape thrown over him by the headmistress, but that because of the deprivation of his mother's protective love in infancy, he would secretly like to be a girl like his sister because for him it meant a life of freedom from responsibility and a return to the dependent life of infancy. Not only so, but in childhood he was given a long cape, like that of his older sister, of which he was inordinately proud and *showed off*. But unfortunately he was jeered at by the other boys for wearing a girl's cape: that is why his parading had to be at night. Thus all the factors of the fetichism, masochism, transvestism and exhibitionism were accounted for. The repressed feelings were released and sublimated, and the patient was cured, and married.

The psychopathology and mechanism of sex perversion is well illustrated in this case. There is the initial feeling of deprivation of love, through the loss of his mother; then the repression of the love craving in favour of the perverse activity, especially masochistic phantasies associated with masturbation. This perverse activity might have persisted and become merely an aberration; but in the perversions it is itself repressed, in favour of a super-ego usually of the moral ascetic or aesthetic type. The sexual development is therefore arrested, and later emerges in its infantile perverse form to the exclusion of normal sexuality which has never had the opportunity to develop.

What distinguishes the sex perversion from the hysteric or obsession is, as we have seen, the specific reactions to the deprivation of love which determines the form of the psychoneurosis. In some cases the reaction is one of self-pity and dependence leading to hysteria, in other cases of rebelliousness and self-will leading to the obsessions. In the case of sex perversion the reaction to the deprivation of love is a resort to sensuous pleasure as a substitute for the loss of affection.

This occurs most frequently when the love originally given by the mother was of a very sensuous form, as in our illustrative case; or when sex pleasure was accidentally discovered as a solace when the child felt deprived of love. It is such conditions which both exaggerate and fixate the infantile activities. The child who has its sensuousness over-stimulated, fondled, cossetted, petted and otherwise sensuously stimulated by a mother or nurse is likely to become excessively preoccupied with the sensuous aspect of love. This sensuous fondling may go a step further and become definitely genital, either deliberately as in some cases, or unintentionally as in most. This attachment of the mother to the child occurs especially where the mother has little affection from her husband, or is not sexually satisfied by him, so that she has a surplus of libido: also if she is frigid and dislikes the sexual attentions of her husband, but finds sensual gratification in fondling her son; or again in the case of a widow who substitutes her son for her husband in her sensuous affections. By such means the child may become sexually bound to the mother.

But when the love is withdrawn it determines that the child resorts to this sensuousness as a solace and substitute. The age of the child is another factor, for the first year of life is the sensuous phase of childhood. That is why we nearly always find that the sex perversions relate back to the first year of life. Phobias and depressions also go back to the first year of life, for these three are the characteristic reactions of the year-old infant to the deprivation of love; so that sex perversions are often associated with anxiety and with depression.

The choice of the *specific type of sexual perversion* depends on the specific form of sensuous pleasure in which the child finds solace, whether sadistic, exhibitionist, masochistic, fetichistic, or narcissistic, and this may depend on a number of accidental circumstances, as in this case the napkin, and the hands being tied producing masochism. In other cases if the deprivation of love, say at the breast, is associated with rage and anger, it conduces to sadism. Or it may depend on whatever type of sensuous pleasure, say exhibitionism, was previously encouraged, or in which the child has previously found particular pleasure and to which it therefore naturally resorts if it is depressed from lack of affection.

Repression is an essential factor in the production of complete perversion, for it is this which by fixating the infantile perverse activity prevents its further development into adult sexuality, so that when it emerges later it appears in this arrested form as a perversion. We cannot, therefore, agree with those who maintain that there is no repression in sexual perversions; or regard them as the mere persistence of these infantile traits. In every case of true sex perversion we have analysed, we have found repression to be a vital factor in its production.

There are biological reasons for this repression, for as we have seen, whereas other tendencies like assertiveness and fear find some normal outlet in the child's activities, sexuality is immature and serves no biological function, so that if it is aroused, as in masturbation, it is bound to be perverse, and more liable to be repressed, being out of keeping with both biological and sociological demands.

The most common *cause of repression* of the sex activities is fear, and this may come from various sources: (a) Fear of the mother's disapproval, or loss of love: or of threatened consequences· of punishment by castration or of being ill. The child is therefore placed in this peculiar situation, that it is usually on account of the deprivation of love that the auto-erotic reaction is resorted to, but it is because of the *need* of love that it then has to be repressed. Or the sex may be repressed by feelings of shame, disgust, humiliation or guilt, such feelings being induced by the attitudes of others. These forms of repression require no further comment, except that it lays a considerable responsibility upon parents and others who regard ordinary and quite innocent sensuous activities of the child with horror (often owing to their own repressed complexes); or who more frequently fail to realize the significance of masturbation in the child as commonly due to frustration or the deprivation of love, and therefore treat it by punishment which increases the sense of deprivation. (*b*) Sometimes the sex is *repressed by a stronger emotion, such as anger and hate.*

The following is a case. "I was furious with nurse because she gave me food instead of having my mother's breast. But the only way I could show my antagonism was by messing myself in bed, and I took pleasure in making her clean it up. But I hated her cleaning me up because it began to make me feel sensuous with her powdering me and I began to like it; but I hated liking it because it meant that my anger would be dispelled. She tickled me and I laughed, and that is just what I didn't want to do, because it took away my feeling of supremacy over her."

So pleasure in sex gave place to hate, a not uncommon condition found in adult women who are therefore frigid when they wish to be sexual. (*c*) *Repression by the actual physical consequences of sex experienced by the child.* Sexual excitement even in a small child sometimes ends in orgasm, and this may produce fatigue, nausea, actual sickness, trembling, weakness in the legs, palpitation, suffocating feeling, and other physiological conditions, all of which may be in the child, the *natural* consequences of a sex orgasm. *Psychosomatic conditions* such as these may therefore be *the direct results of repressed sex emotion.* To quote a case: "The orgasm is followed by the nausea and shame and dislike and wishing it had never happened. I must have it, but it is very horrible for me to do so. It made me sick literally and sick with myself, and that is a phrase I have often used of myself." The idea that sex is "disgusting" often arises from these feelings of physical nausea so often accompanying early sexuality and not always from teaching. The orgasm experienced by the infant may also be so overwhelming as itself to be terrifying, for the sexual emotions possessing the child are felt to be stronger than itself and threatens to overpower it. (*d*) These overwhelming emotions are often reproduced in *nightmares* and projected in the form of hideous monsters, vampires, spiders, crabs, or some great overwhelming and overpowering force suffocating their life. These creatures are the projection and personification of the child's organic sensations. Such nightmares are far more terrifying, and therefore produce far more complete repression, than any of the consequences of sex already mentioned, and are likely to result either in sex impotence, sex perversions or anxiety states. The nightmare of being pursued, but being rooted to the spot with terror, weakness and palpitation are often traced to infantile masturbation with its accompanying orgasm of which these are the associated sensations. *Thus sex becomes the natural cause of its own repression.*

These results of sex, physiological and psychological, are particularly interesting because they show that irrespective of morals sexual feelings become repressed by the organic results of their own excitation. Nature itself has her methods of repressing the sexual indulgence of infancy, more drastic than the threats of moral teaching of those around. For an infant to have a sex orgasm is often more dangerous than preventing it indulging in sex.

This may account for the common taboo against sex in primitive as well as civilized people. It may also explain why, as we have said, an instinct so natural and necessary for the reproduction of the race is so universally associated with guilt; and why it is so commonly repressed and therefore subject to aberration and perversions.[1]

Super-ego in sex perversions. The first result of this repression of the sensual and sexual desires, whether by fear, disappointment or disapproval, is that a new standard, a new ego ideal, is set up, one that is in conformity with the demands of others, and one that is opposed in every way to these indulgences and designed to keep them repressed. The nature of the super-ego is often determined by identification with the attitude of those who condemn the sexual activities: but it is also determined by the nature of the tendencies repressed, by way of contrast and compensation. Therefore the super-ego of the sexual pervert is usually either *ascetic* or *aesthetic*, by contrast in the one case to the indulgent, or to the nasty and disgusting. Whether the super-ego takes an ascetic or aesthetic form also depends upon the amount of the sensuous feeling which has escaped repression and been sublimated. It is ascetic when the sensuous tendency is so deeply repressed and condemned that the super-ego must take an extreme form in the opposite direction. It is aesthetic when some of the condemned sensuous feeling is utilized as part of the super-ego.

It is therefore a recognized fact that many sexual perverts are men of the highest *moral character and idealism*, and this makes

[1] The "castration fear" is therefore by no means the only form of repression of infantile sexuality, although this is often the case in boys who require a circumcision, which is interpreted as a punishment of sex. It is of course accentuated when nurses and mothers actually make it as threat that if he masturbates he will have his penis cut off.

their perversions the more distressing. Paradoxically enough, it is the maintenance of this excessively rigid standard of morality or aesthetics which keeps the sexuality arrested in development, and so perpetuates the very perversion it condemns. Clinical evidence for the association of perversions with idealism, ascetic and aesthetic, is not far to seek. The man with a fetichism for shoes became a lecturer in moral philosophy; the strangling sadist became a magistrate (who was, on his own showing, excessively severe on those convicted of offences with violence); the sadist who had the impulse to cut off the hair of girls was a clergyman; the exhibitionist was a social worker amongst boys in a settlement; the anal-erotic was a musician, and the woman who had a violent impulse to murder and sexually violate anyone she met in a lonely place was matron of a girls' school. The super-ego is thus an over-compensation to the impulse it represses. Because of the early repression of love in favour of the sexual reaction, the super-ego often takes the form of a *rigid morality devoid of love*, and hardness of character, which keeps itself from a breakdown at the expense of others. In others it takes on a *religious* and ascetic form which despises, if it does not condemn, sexuality as lustful, and discourages marriage for those who would reach the highest spirituality. Such is the case of the man whose wife refused to have more children, but whose religion forbad him to have sex relations with preventatives. The result was a perpetual psychosomatic headache due to the frustration, and a hatred of his wife which was hardly in keeping with his religion.

As with the ascetic so with the *aesthetic super-ego*. It is a well-known fact that many homosexuals and other perverts are conspicuous for their aesthetic taste in music, painting and literature. To the uninitiated it seems incredible that men of otherwise refined aesthetic taste can resort to practices, say of a sodomistic nature, which are to others of so revolting a nature; indeed, it is often a matter of astonishment to the pervert himself to find within himself tendencies so alien to his refinement of character and taste. But the reason is that whereas part of his original sensuous nature has become sublimated into these higher forms of artistic feeling and literary appreciation, another and a large part has been repressed and arrested, and therefore appears in its primitive form. The two are related: the more exaggerated is his sensuous nature, the more refined must be his aesthetic nature to keep sexuality repressed; the more refined the super-ego the cruder will be the forms of sexuality manifesting themselves.

Those acquainted with the perversions can also detect morbid perverse tendencies in the work of some artists, whose sadism, masochism, anal-erotic or exhibitionist tendencies are freely displayed in their work. But that is not to say that art is merely a sublimation of sex: Romanesque or Byzantine architecture, for instance, is far more than a sublimation of sex; it is manifestation and expression of the spirit of man and of the age. The same applies to religion.

For the repressed sexuality may emerge in sublimated form as in *aesthetic forms of worship* which however appeal to the senses, and are often associated with ceremonial rituals which are little else than obsessional acts, designed as a propitiation for these forbidden desires, and at the same time, like most obsessional acts, giving a symbolic satisfaction to these sensuous feelings. Such a religion too often evades the moral issue by circumventing it, and uses ritual as a substitute instead of an aid to spiritual life. It provides a temporary peace, but as in all obsessional acts, the propitiation has to be repeated constantly to give the necessary assurance. From the psychopathological angle, ceremonial is an attempt to solve the moral problem. Thus some religions emphasize morality, some are sensuous in nature, some are condemnatory, some are propitiatory, some are terrifying and threatening, whilst others, which strive after "personal holiness," may be a sublimated form of narcissism in which there is little real love for others, but only self-absorption in the desire for personal "perfection." In most of these the love for others which is characteristic of the mentally healthy adult, and of true morality, is absent.

These ascetic forms of worship are often found to co-exist with sexual perversions, a combination which appears strange until we understand that they arise from the same basic cause; the asceticism representing the over-compensating super-ego, the perversion representing the arrested sexuality it represses. This is no argument against religion and morals, but only against false religion and false morality: but even this false religion must be regarded with toleration, because it is after all the attempt of the individual to solve a problem which was none of his making, and which is in fact insoluble without treatment and for which for the time being he has found the only solace.

There are, however, other modes of religion which accord with the fundamental longing for affection and find in the love of a "Heavenly Father" as in the Protestant Faith, or in the "Virgin Mother" as in the Catholic Faith, the satisfaction of the needs for tenderness and affection of which they felt themselves denied in infancy. Such religion is no doubt often infantile and self-centred in form, but in so far as it supplies them with the sense of protective love it is capable of producing what should have been provided in early childhood, namely the sense of security, and therefore confidence to face life. By providing the individual with love it is capable of developing love, confidence and even self-sacrifice for others. Religion therefore may prove to be of great therapeutic value, a real stimulus to life, a means of allaying anxiety, a source of courage.[1]

To the psychologist, religion is a fact of experience, whether or not it corresponds to objective reality: it cannot be excluded from scientific investigation. But modern psychology is somewhat sceptical of the older methods of scientific procedure which rejects what it cannot scientifically prove. There are other ways than empirical science of arriving at the truth; one is intuition, another is faith. The *faith* in the possibility of something can often bring it about when it would not otherwise have happened.[2] *Intuition* is *subconscious inference*; and the subconscious or intuitive appreciation of the meaning of events, whether in politics, in science, in the Stock Exchange or in our judgment of persons, is often a far surer guide than judgment based on "scientific facts." Even a medical diagnosis based on intuition sometimes proves to be more correct than that based on laboratory tests in so far as it takes cognisance of the behaviour of the whole person. Religious truth is admittedly a matter of faith and intuition (as in mysticism), not of proved fact.

The precipitation of the sex perversions is often quite early, and the patient can often recall having his first perverted exhibitionist, sadistic or homosexual impulses perhaps at the age of six to eight. But it more frequently occurs in puberty or adolescence when sex is biologically aroused.

(a) The precipitating cause is often the excitation of the genital organs by some objective experience, as in the case of the boy whose fetichism for patent leather shoes was precipitated by finding comfort in his nurse's shoes under the table, the shape of the shoes, their smell and their soft round contour being a symbol and substitute for the breast, and of the mother love he had lost. Any external genital stimulus—tight foreskin, accidental discovery of masturbation, climbing ropes in the gymnasium, sliding down bannisters, riding bicycles, romping or wrestling with others is enough to rouse the sex feelings. But these experiences happen to everyone, and usually pass without untoward effect: it is only when there has been a previous repression and fixation of the

¹ See Suttie, *The Origins of Love and Hate.*   ² See p. 52.

infantile sensuous and sexual tendencies, that it emerges in the form of a perversion. The earlier fixation and not merely the stimulation is an essential factor in the perversion. For that reason we cannot say that a perversion originates in such experiences, but is only precipitated by them. The later factors only become operative when related to an early infantile predisposition.

(b) In many cases the precipitating cause of the perversions is the onset of adolescence itself, with the physiological stimulus of *internal* sex functions. The sexuality that has been successfully repressed during the earlier years cannot withstand such physiological stimulus, and surges up. But instead of coming out in the natural forms of sexuality characteristic of adolescence, it emerges in arrested forms stunted by long years of repression. In many such cases the stimulus at adolescence is of a perfectly normal kind, whereas the impulses it arouses are perverted and abnormal because of such fixation; so the youth in whom the normal desire is to make love to the girl, has aroused in him the morbid impulse to strangle her, or the desire to cut off her hair, or to be beaten by her, which are obviously derived from earlier impulses.

(c) It is, however, not invariable that the precipitating cause is sexual, for frequently it is the sense of loneliness, depression, a feeling of inferiority or lack of affection which drives him to seek consolation in sexual gratification, as it did in the original reaction in infancy. A great deal of masturbation in puberty and adolescence is due to such loneliness, or to inability to keep up with work, a sense of social inferiority, or to a feeling of unpopularity at school, and not primarily to any desire for masturbation itself, which is felt to be unsatisfactory. It is obvious that to blame or disapprove such masturbation is to accentuate the trouble by increasing the sense of ostracism and condemnation. In one case of homosexuality, for instance, the boy had lost his mother who was devoted to him, and was lonely at school, until an old boy coming to the school was attracted to him and seduced him. It was not the sexual experience that impressed him so much, but the fact that somebody important had taken notice of him and given him affection in his loneliness. It then became the symbol of affection and regard.

It is similar with schoolgirl "affairs" or "pashes" which are of four types: there are those in which the loved girl is a substitute for a man in the Adamless Eden of a girls' boarding school, in which case she is usually an older girl, captain of games, or gymnastic mistress or other substitute for the male. There is nothing particularly abnormal in such passions, which are later transferred to the man when opportunity arises. In the second case there is the simple indulgence in sexual pleasure with another girl by mutual masturbation, a simple character trait in which there is no repression and which later develops into normal channels, though with an accentuation on the sex side of love. In the third group is the girl who has had a repressed craving for affection which now emerges more strongly with the onset of puberty. This kind is not so much sexual as a sentimental yearning for affection, or a craving for someone in whom to confide, in which case sympathy and affection will ease the situation. A fourth type is definitely homosexual, due to repressed sexuality of a perverse and auto-erotic type in early childhood. These are psychoneurotic; more difficult to deal with and requiring expert treatment.

(d) In other cases the precipitation of the sex perversion is associated with a rebuff in hetero-sexual interests, which brings about a *regression* to an earlier mode of sexuality. We have frequently found that homosexuality started when the boy was "put off" girls. But we find this to occur only when there have been earlier fixations, so that when the forward moving impulse is rebuffed it reverts to its former mode of pleasure.

The specific symptom. (a) When the symptom is precipitated in later life, *it emerges in the form in which it was originally repressed.* The reasons for these specific forms of reaction we have already discussed. So one child deprived of affection displays exhibitionistic tendencies if by exhibitionism it previously got attention; another indulges in sadistic anger which was what it experienced against the mother when it was deprived of its sensuous pleasures; another who has found its solace in an enema becomes anal-erotic. These experiences, if they are repressed, therefore provide the specific forms of perversion from which the individual later suffers. The particular form the symptom takes therefore depends to a large extent on the original reaction to the deprivation of love, which is largely accidental.

There are, however, *later contributory factors* which contribute to the form of the later symptom. The waterproof cape for instance, in the case quoted, which was a later addition. But even these as we discover from deeper investigation are often linked with infantile sensuous experiences, as in his case the waterproof of his cot and the body smell of his mother. But the fact that it was a cape came from the experiences at school and his earlier desire to be a girl to escape the responsibilities of life. The relation between the later precipitating experiences and repressed infantile experiences and desires is illustrated in the case of the man who had the sex perversion to cut off girl's hair. This specific symptom arose in adolescence; but it related to the feeling of his mother's hair which fell over her shoulders as she fed him at the breast. On one occasion he got a strand of the hair down his throat which choked him so that he fought against it and thereafter was afraid of the breast and repressed its sensuous pleasure. His rage and hatred of the sensuous loved object was the source of his sadism, which was aroused again in adolescence when he saw girls bathing, and took the form of wanting to cut off their hair. In such cases we find infantile roots for the perversion, but also contributions from later experiences which are often taken for the sole cause. The fetichism for trousers did not appear till the age of six, and it was aroused by riding on the back of a boy with a corduroy coat. The trousers represented an attraction to the buttocks, and this reverted back to the breasts of the mother. The corduroy came from later life, the urge to the buttocks from infantile life. The sodomy which was said to have been caused by a sodomistic assault by a bigger boy, was in fact only precipitated by it: the basis of the sodomy was in repeated enemas given in early childhood which produced passive sexual stimulation. The assault alone would not have made him a sodomist: nor probably would his early experiences but for the assault: both factors were required. The form of the perversion is also affected by the process of maturation, the most obvious instance being that whilst an earlier masochistic desire to be beaten may in the girl persist at puberty in a natural though exaggerated desire to be beaten, in the boy it may be transformed into a sadistic desire to beat, as this is more in keeping with the development of male aggressiveness; the pleasure in the *idea* of beating remained, its *form* changed. Thus the later perversion may often be a projection on to others of an earlier personal experience. For instance, a man has the sexual phantasies of getting hold of girls, stripping them, humiliating them with shame, and then beating them. This was derived from an experience when he himself was treated in this way by his mother who took off his clothes and smacked him, producing sex feelings. The pleasure was repressed by the pain and humiliation. About the age of nine it came out as a masochistic phantasy, himself suffering the humiliation; but still later in adolescence, as his sexual assertiveness developed, it became sadistic. In this phantasy he was also inflicting humiliation and so vicariously getting his own back on his mother through the female sex, as well as gratifying his desire. Incidentally, a good deal of sex impotence is an unconscious desire to revenge the woman by depriving her of what she desires.

In other cases, *the super-ego comes into the symptom*, as in the case of the young man who to punish himself for his masturbation would periodically have himself beaten by a prostitute, by which means he surreptitiously gratified both his sexual desires and his moral disapprobation of it.

Sex perversions are closely associated with other forms of psycho-neuroses. Persistent sex desires which are disapproved cuts a child off from those upon whom his security depends, and so he falls into a state of *hysterical anxiety*. Loss of love also leads to depression which is a very common accompaniment of sex perversion. This "well of loneliness" is often ascribed to social ostracism, but the real cause of the depression of homosexuals and other perverts is inherent in the sex perversion itself, being bound up with the original longing for affection. Both the depression and the perversion are reactions to the same deprivation of love.

The sense of guilt associated with sex may also lead a child to resort to a *conversion hysteria* in order to win back the sympathy of those on whom he depends, and whose love he has forfeited by his forbidden desires. The patient develops an hysterical pain not merely as self-punishment, but in order to turn away the wrath of the parent by an appeal for sympathy and so avert the consequences of his forbidden sexual desires. Thus many hysterias are based on repressed sex, but the dependence and need for protective love is the dominant factor in hysteria.

Sex repression may also, as we have seen, produce *psychosomatic* disorders like sickness, palpitation or headache. In other of these cases, the sex appears as such in the symptom, though not in the form of a perversion. This is particularly so in the *sex obsessions*, such as a fear of raping, calling out obscene words, of exposing oneself, in which a self-willed persistence in the forbidden desire perpetuates the obsession. In sex obsessions, such as the fear of raping, the sexuality appears in consciousness as part of the symptom. *As we have seen, the difference between sex perversions and sex obsessions is that whilst in sex perversions the act is desired* though it may be disapproved, *in the sex obsession it is loathed and feared*, though there is a compulsion towards committing the act.

In other cases, the sexuality is completely unconscious, but is the motive force of the symptom. This is particularly the case in the *propitiatory obsessions, most of which in our experience have a sexual basis*. The sense of guilt gives rise to hand-washing rituals and over-conscientiousness. But the sense of guilt may take on a particular turn, and the very self-accusation may, as we have seen, be an invitation say to be punished and beaten to gratify one's masochistic desires. In such cases, the repression is so complete that sexuality does not appear at all in the symptom, but the shame and disgust as such may emerge as the dominant symptom whenever the sex is unconsciously aroused. So we get not only anxiety states, but states of inferiority, self-consciousness, guilt and shame, the basis of which is sexual, but of which the individual may be quite unaware. In those cases, because the individual is unaware of the true cause, the fear or shame or guilt may be attached to other objects, such as the fear of knives (phallic as well as an aggressive symbol), or of suffocation (representing the suffocation felt in the orgasm), or shame that one's body smells (in anal-erotic cases).

Whether the complex emerges as a sex perversion, an obsessional anxiety, sex obsession or a compulsive ritual depends on the relative strength of the repressed sex, the repressed self-will and the super-ego respectively.

Before discussing clinical types, we may side-track for a moment to consider the idea that *sex perversions originate in conditioned reflexes*. The mere association of the sexual impulses with some object or activity has much to be said for it, and *association* undoubtedly explains a great deal. The observationist originally had his sexual feelings aroused by seeing a girl undressing; the homosexual by being seduced by another boy.

But this theory, while it may be an important factor in causation, and may help to explain the *form* of the perversion, is inadequate to account for the existence of perversions as such. For if early associations of this kind were sufficient to produce lasting perversions, we should all be perverts, for probably none of us had his or her sexual feelings aroused in the first instance by a normal sexual desire towards one of the opposite sex, but usually in association with some other object or experience in early childhood. Or if it is said that we are heterosexual because our mothers were our first sex objects, this might account for the heterosexuality of men, but on that showing all women should be homosexual. Since the first deliberate sexual acts of so many boys are concerned with other boys, why are not all boys homosexual? Yet these accidental occurrences are often given as the sole and effective causes of sex perversion. Even McDougall seems to fall into that error in ascribing a fetishism for hair to the fact that the schoolboy indulged in sex talk while looking at the long hair of schoolgirls sitting in front in a trolly-car. That may have been the precipitating cause: but obviously other predisposing factors are involved, which determined that this boy and not the other developed the perversion.

These deeper factors usually need to be discovered to produce a radical cure: they will be referred to later. In a case of the fetichism for corsets it was not merely the accidental contact, but that the corsets represented the unconscious and repressed desire for the breast of which the child was deprived, and which represented both sensuousness and security.

Again, were these conditions due to conditioned reflexes alone, it should be possible, by means of reconditioning, to inhibit these abnormal responses, and restore or replace them by advocating sexual relations: but actually we do not know of a single case of true perversion which has been cured by reconditioning, or in which the morbid response had been abolished and the original and natural response restored. The nearest approach is to be found in treatment by *suggestion* which is an attempt to break the association between, say, cutting off of hair and the sexual feelings, and re-establishing new and healthy associations. But the favourable results in suggestion we have met with have been in the treatment of impotence, by the removal of the inhibitions to sex, and not of the positive perversions.

Investigation into the actual cause of these conditions by free association proves their origin to be more complex than these theories would suggest, and they can only be dealt with by the discovery of the whole chain of associations, conscious and unconscious, which is done in analysis.

CHAPTER XV

CLINICAL TYPES OF SEX DISORDER

(A) *Sex disorders*

We must first make mention of one or two disorders which are not necessarily perversions but have serious consequences in marital life.

Sexual impotence appears to be far more often due to psychological than to physical causes, although impotence of physical origin, such as endocrine deficiency, whether pituitary or gonodal, is not uncommon as in the case of the long and lanky youth. But it is not, in the vast number of cases, that these people are physiologically abnormal, for the seminal capacity of such men and the reproductive functions of such women are adequate. The disturbance appears to be in the psychological sphere.

Impotence in the sense of failure to effect coitus is of course a common accompaniment of all perversions, but the pervert is in no sense impotent towards the object of his perversion and is capable of complete orgasm: men are capable of emissions in relation to their fetichistic objects, and women homosexuals are quite capable of bearing children, although they may have a loathing for sex relations. Impotence and frigidity may also be due to general and not to specifically sexual causes, especially where there is a lack of love for his partner. Many men are potent only with women they love, but impotent with those whom they do not love, however sexually attractive. For where sex is an expression of love, the sex functions without love refuse to function, in spite of conscious desire. Another is impotent with his mistress but not with his wife, because of an unconscious sense of guilt. We have also mentioned the case is which the impotence is an unconscious revenge against the wife, as it may be against women in general. In other cases a man is impotent with his wife and not with his mistress because his wife stands for his mother. The worse cases of impotence are probably those in which there is a devotion to the mother, with a fear of facing life and responsibility, combined with a sexual fixation upon the mother about which the child is made to feel guilty. The mother remains his first and only love, and to break away from her would be disloyalty, whereas sex feelings towards anyone else is regarded as guilty. Such simple impotence differs from the perversions in that *the desire may be quite normal but the execution inadequate.*

The difference between impotence and sex perversion depends on both the previous stimulation and on the degree and nature of the repression. If the sex desire is not particularly strong before its repression by fear or shame, it may simply result in *impotence.* So the child who is exhibiting himself, or innocently playing with himself, and is severely rebuked may for ever after feel shame about sex which makes it impossible for him to consummate his marriage. The little girl who is sexually assaulted may suffer fear of sex and become frigid. But impotence is also commonly caused by the sex feelings being fixated upon the mother as sex object, or upon oneself (narcissism), which are thereafter repressed and prevent the expression of sexuality to a mate however much desired. But if the infantile sexuality is exaggerated in any of its perverse forms and then repressed, it is more likely to emerge as a true *sex perversion,* or in less marked cases as an *aberration of* the second type mentioned.

Ejaculatio praecox (premature ejaculation in the male) is a distressing symptom to the newly married and is usually found to be due, not to excessive desire, but to inhibition. It is in fact a form of sexual impotence, and having the same motives. In this case, however, the sex function is not checked altogether as in impotence, but the inhibition achieves its aim of avoiding intercourse by making the ejaculation premature. A mother fixation, fear of life, sexual guilt and other conditions are common causes.

The man who marries his mother is a common and tragic type. Due in the first place to a mother fixation, often due to a sense of deprivation, the condition is one in which the lost mother is sought and found in an older woman, a stronger and more capable woman, such as a nurse, career woman or a widow. Such marriages often end in disaster because the man after marriage grows up and then no longer wants his "mother," but someone of his own age. The unsuspecting wife, on the other hand, who had no knowledge of his marrying her as a mother-substitute, naturally suffers grievous injury at the break-up of the marriage. In other cases when a man marries a nurse or a widow as a mother-substitute, he looks forward to being cared for, whereas the wife in getting married feels that at last she has someone to look after her instead of her being independent and looking after others. They are both disillusioned; when she finds she has a dependent husband incapable of making his own decisions she despises him: the weakling husband, instead of finding in her the mother, finds her "bossy," and the marriage ends in failure and disappointment.

Split libido. In this condition, instead of the *whole* of love being directed towards one person, it is split, so that devotion, respect and admiration are felt towards women of one type (usually one of one's own social class and culture) whom he would wish to marry, but towards whom he has no sexual feelings at all; whereas his sexual feeling is aroused only towards women of another type, often of a lower social status, but for whom he has no respect and whom he would not think of marrying. "Nowadays," says one such patient, "I like being with working-class girls with a human smell, as compared with my mother who was fragile and delicate and clean." Extreme forms of this may prevent a man marrying at all; and when he does there is often a breakdown from "incompatability of temperament," for whichever "side" of him marries, the crude or the cultured, the other side is repelled by the wife chosen.

It is usually found on analysis that split libido originates in early childhood, when devotion and love were attached to his mother, who, however, condemns any expression of sensuous feeling, whereas his sex feelings were aroused by a maid or other less inhibited person for whom he had no love or respect. So his devotion has a different love object from his sexual feelings, and his libido is split. Indeed, he comes to regard love as "pure" and sex as "impure," and divides women into the "pure" whom he must not (and afterwards cannot) "defile"; and the "impure" who exist for that purpose alone. Normally in infancy love and sensuous feelings are both combined and associated with the mother, and this combination is later normally directed towards the mate which appears to be the ideal in marriage.

Frigidity in women occurs more frequently than impotence in men, partly because of the lesser physiological sex urge in women (which we maintain is the case, in spite of the view that "women are just as sexual as men"), partly because women more often marry someone with whom they are not completely in love, and partly because the sex urge in women is modified by the accompanying responsibilities or fear of child-bearing. Indeed, the fear of getting a child is itself enough to inhibit an orgasm. Thus a woman may be frigid towards one person and not to another, towards the husband she does not love, but not towards her lover or a second husband whom she does love; for love is a function of the whole personality. Other women have pleasure in sex relations but never get an orgasm which may be because of physiological incapacity or because of an unconscious fear, shame, guilt or humiliation. A terror of sex may come from an early assault, and disgust from sickness following an early orgasm. Like impotence, frigidity is often associated with perversion, which should be looked for. The woman who had a sex attraction only to a man's hairy wrist, or the other who could get an orgasm only when she was in a rage, is not likely to be responsive to normal sex relations. Such incapacity in the woman varies from mere indifference and boredom to positive loathing and disgust. Frigidity does not prevent a woman having children; but it does mean that an act which should be an expression of love between husband and wife becomes an occasion for discord which is almost bound, ultimately, to give rise to unhappiness and recrimination. Probably more unhappiness in married life is caused by the lack of sexuality than its excess, for sexual intercourse is the symbol of love, and where both partners are normally sexed they find satisfaction in one another; whereas the lack of sexual response in the husband is taken by the wife to signify a lack of affection even when this is not the case, and the frigidity of the wife is interpreted as indicating lack of interest or response to the husband's love. Sexual frigidity is amongst the commonest causes of the infidelity of husbands and waywardness of wives. Thus harmonious family relationships in marriage are extremely difficult and sometimes impossible in the absence of happy sex relations. Such sexual disharmony often passes under the name of "incompatibility of temperament," which is a real enough condition and sufficiently distressing to wreck marriages.

Vaginismus is a condition in which the woman may desire intercourse, but when it is attempted there is such a painful contracture that intercourse is made difficult and sometimes impossible. It may have a physiological origin such as a partially ruptured and painful hymen; but it is usually psychological, the cause of which is commonly found to be an early assault of some kind which was fraught with pain, contracture and fear, but at the same time aroused sex feelings. The arousal of these sex feelings is thereafter associated with fear and produces contracture.

(B) Sex perversions

Exhibitionism is not primarily sexual: it is originally a method of the child for calling attention to itself, and is particularly evident in the latter half of the first year of life when the cessation of weaning makes the mother less physically attached to the child, and so makes it the more necessary for the child to call attention to itself to keep within the notice of the mother. In other words, it is primarily an egotistic *biological function* serving the process of self-preservation. When it is exaggerated we have the "limelight" child whose showing-off tendencies are usually the result of anxiety and insecurity, and not necessarily a sexual exhibitionism. Such a tendency may be *sublimated* in dress, acting, writing and public speaking. The more encouraged is the tendency in early childhood, the more prominent will such character traits be later, providing they are not repressed.

Apart from the need to call attention to itself, the exhibitionist tendency is encouraged by the pleasure a child experiences in having the air playing upon its naked body, a biologically healthy activity, which most people enjoy at the seaside. So the infant loves to kick off its bedclothes, and leave itself naked to the open air.

It takes a sexual form when the child, feeling left out and wanting to call attention to itself, naturally assumes that the part of the body in which it finds so much pleasure will be attractive to others, and will secure their attention and affection: so it calls attention to itself by exposing its sex organs. Later on, this tendency is transferred to the uses of adult sexuality as a *wooing* tendency the main function of which is to arouse sex feelings in the person desired.

But if a little girl, feeling the loss of affection, exposes herself in this way and is then made to feel shame and humiliation, she may repress her sexuality and later suffer from feelings of shame, disgust, blushing and self-consciousness; or she may suffer from frigidity, or later on the exhibitionist tendency may emerge as a perversion. It is a notable fact that many beautiful women with strong exhibitionist tendencies are sexually frigid.

Masochism. Sensuous dependence and passivity is also a normal characteristic of infancy: it persists in the female whose sexuality is passive or receptive and who loves to be overmastered; indeed, she will run away so that when captured she will be the more strongly overmastered. So she unconsciously secures that she breeds only from the strongest males. It is a perversion when the pleasure is experienced to the exclusion of normal sexuality as in cases when the one desire is to be beaten, to be tied up, or even to be scolded or bullied. Masochism is often defined as pleasure in having pain inflicted on one by the sexually loved person: but there are masochistic tendencies like the sex pleasure in being bound which are not associated with pain. It is not the pain which is the crucial factor, but sexual pleasure in submission and dependence. So we prefer to define masochism as the sex pleasure in being overmastered, even to the extent of suffering pain.

Hysteria is also a craving for dependence, passivity, security and freedom from responsibility: masochism is where this passivity is associated with sex feelings and indulged in for their gratification.

The character traits of such people are often of the same nature, apologetic, cringing, ingratiating, self-depreciating, all of which may be, though they are not necessarily, sexual masochisms. But because the passivity is repressed, these people are often self-willed and must have everybody doing what they want. Beating phantasies often originate in a child's being beaten for "playing with himself" for then the beating is associated with the sex stimulation; not only so, but the beating itself on the buttocks reflexly arouses sex feelings, which is a strong reason against caning boys and, still more, girls.

Finally we have had cases in which the desire to be beaten arose from the sensuous excitement produced in infancy when the mother embraces the child and gently pats the buttocks, a practice the child finds soothing and sensuously comforting. Such a harmless practice cannot itself cause a perversion, but it may determine the nature of the perversion. The particular circumstance colours the particular form the masochism takes.

Another case was that in which sex feelings were aroused by the phantasy of being "squeezed or pressed against somebody and at the same time being smacked."

"I felt that I ought not to want love and affection, because I was told I musn't be a baby. But I felt sexual feelings in being held tight between my nurse's knee and being helpless; that gave me some satisfaction when I couldn't get affection." Another patient had phantasies of annoying people so that they turned on him and beat him. He carried this into practice by constantly having argumentations with masters at school and the family at home, which was regarded as mere aggressiveness, but was primarily designed to make them beat him. The masochism traced itself back to his being smacked by the nurse over her knee which stimulated him sexually, and seeing this she hurriedly put him to bed as the father was coming into the room which produced in him the feeling of guilt. "After that I continued masturbating secretly, thinking about being beaten. Eventually she caught me masturbating and she started beating me again very hard and frightened me: and that stops me. I forgot it for a time—in fact, until I was eight or nine at kindergarten school, when beatings reminded me of it again; it revived the feelings in me when I got beaten there." This case shows the cause of the original perverse reaction, the subsequent repression and the precipitating cause of the perversion.

We have met adolescent girls who persistently committed delinquencies in order to be beaten and experience the sex pleasure.

Sadism on the other hand is the sexual pleasure in overmastering the loved object even to the extent of inflicting pain. It is typical of the male whose sexuality is active. All bullying and pleasure in inflicting pain is not necessarily sadistic: it may be mere cruelty, a manifestation of aggressiveness not of sex: even the fact that the cruelty is enjoyed does not make it sexual, for all successful activity is pleasurable. Perverted sadism originates in infancy. An infant may be observed to get excited and "attack" the breast in feeding: if the breast fails the child feels anger and resentment against the loved object so that he bites, hits or "strangles" the breast. This behaviour is resented by the mother and the child is punished and therefore represses its sadistic impulses and regards all sensuous pleasure as wrong. When sexuality later matures it emerges in this arrested form in which it was originally repressed. There was the case of the magistrate already mentioned who had the impulse to strangle any girl towards whom he was sexually aroused. In reviving the original experience he said: "That breast is not giving me what I want so I bash it and bump on it, prod my finger into it, grip at it, smear it with its own milk, squash it out, bite it, kick it, stamp on it. I battered it, strangle it, go for it—anything you like—I can almost bite the nipple off, very hard—and take a delight in making that person squirm." This picture of infantile sadistic tendencies is very reminiscent of some recent brutal murders. In another case of sadism in which there was a sexual attraction to *dead bodies* with a desire to mutilate them, the analysis revealed in infancy a thwarted desire to kill the mother and mutilate the breast and have it dead, so as to have complete control over it, like killing a prey, but in this case associated with a sensuous loved object.

Anal erotism. A case showing repression and its multiple consequences may be quoted. It follows the giving of an enema which successively produces rage, indigestion, psychosomatic disorders, shame, guilt and propitiation.

"The effects of the enema were to produce wild feelings and sex feelings which are mutually antagonistic. I want to fight and be violent: I don't feel furious *about* anything or *with* anybody but just furious, as if I wanted to fight. Then the sex side made me all limp and give in—it was a kind of thrill—it produced a pleasant sensation. (Sex repressing rage.) Then I want to pass water and that makes me ashamed and hide. (Sex repressed by shame.) Afterwards it gives me a horrid indigestion feeling (psychosomatic), uncomfortable, upset and bad. Then I let go and forgot about being afraid. (Sex repressing fear.) I let go because the feeling made me, and it overcame all the fear. Then I felt miserable and frightfully afraid (obsessional anxiety), and frightfully ashamed like a dog going to be beaten; I felt all guilty and wanted to propitiate (propitiatory obsession) and frightfully wanted to be loved and forgiven."

A case of homosexuality, sadism and sodomy may be given in greater detail as it illustrates several points in the development of perversion.

"My attraction has always been to the buttocks because I have always felt that the sex organs are filthy; that is why the idea of intercourse is always loathsome to me. It all goes to my mother: she humiliated me, laughed at me, and mocked me when I was feeding at the breast. At first I got pleasure in revelling at the breasts: then in hitting them. The sensuousness got associated with hate (sadism). I was angry with them. The buttocks fit because they are the same shape as the breast. I got my sensuousness there (sodomy). It was the same with the boys (homosexuality)—I hated them but I got sensuous feelings in hurting them. When did I change over and think the breasts were filthy and change to buttocks? That was when I got sick with feeding too greedily. I felt it was nasty and filthy and yet attractive. I feel the same contradiction about buttocks now. I feel ashamed at my filthy indulgence because it made me sick: and never again would I have anything to do with a sensuous attraction that makes her laugh at me. I push the whole filthy creature away altogether: I'd kick her. I don't think I would hit the breasts—or would I? No! I pushed her away and got into a rage with her. The immediate reaction was masturbation when I felt dull and lost all interest in life. But that turned filthy too (because of nightmares of spiders and crabs) so I pushed that away and later turned to buttocks." The sensuous pleasure of the breasts was repressed because of the mother's mocking: the genital pleasure was repressed because of the nightmares so the buttocks were chosen as a substitute for the breast and because of their proximity to the genitals: the homosexuality was due to the hate of the woman, his mother, and the resort to autoerotism to himself the male.

Fetichism as we have seen is the sexual attachment to an inanimate object, often to the exclusion of normal sexuality. (Some, however, would include animate objects like ankles, hair or hand, but even they are objects and not persons.) In all cases of fetichisms we have analysed, *the fetichistic object proved to be a breast substitute:* for the breast is the first loved object of the infant, even before the mother herself becomes so. This is obvious in the common fetichism for corsets which is a natural substitute; the fetichism for shoes is because of their duality, shape and body smell; for the hood of a perambulator because it is round and shiny; waterproof rubber coats are attractive like shoes because of the body smell and shiny smooth surface. The beginning of fetichism may be observed in a child of one or two years of age who sucks its thumb (in place of the nipple), and at the same time fondles a quilt, silk handkerchief, or anything soft, like the breast. Apart from the infantile association there is usually the occasion later when these fetichistic objects are associated with genital stimulation which fixates the perversion. The fetichism for boys' corduroy trousers commenced at the age of six. But this mere association was not enough to explain the case. Why corduroy *trousers* and not the coat? It was their round shape and soft, warm, smooth feeling which took the patient immediately back to infancy, the buttocks representing the lost breast attraction. A fetichism for hair combined with the impulse to cut off girls' hair, originated with the soft feeling of her mother's long hair which he fondled as he fed at the breast in infancy. Choking and suffocation caused by a hair getting in his throat enraged him against the loved object, and later love objects, but the original repressed desire emerged as the fetichism. In wooing, many like to stroke the hair or soft rounded parts of the body because of this substitution.[1]

Homosexuality or Inversion, the sexual attraction to the same ($\delta\mu o$) sex (Lesbianism in women), has been variously explained as an anthropological, physiological and psychological phenomenon.

The essence of homosexuality on the *psychological* side is that it is a development of narcissism or self-love: homosexuality we may therefore describe as "self-love once removed": the individual is in love with himself, and then falls in love with another like himself, one of the same sex, a mirror of himself. But there are a number of contributory factors.

An illustration showing such reactions and their repression is that of the homosexual who revives the following early experience after weaning:

"That makes me think of the first time I discovered self-abuse. I had a hot-water bottle in bed and pulled it between my legs and felt the pleasant feelings (autoerotic). The first thought is of interest and then the feeling that I no longer need my mother—whom I had needed up till now. (Repression of the need for object love.) I wanted to get rid of her so that I can get on with my pleasure. (Opposed to biological function of protective love.) It gives me the *feeling* of self-sufficiency, security and fulfilment. I was perfectly contented with myself.

---

[1] It is interesting to note that we have never found a case of true fetichism in a woman. The reason is obscure unless we may assume that it has to do with the fact that she has breasts of her own, which are always accessible.

(Narcissistic, instead of object, love.) But there is a certain amount of guilt about it, because it is connected with other excretory functions—I feel that it is dirty and not to be public." (Repression of the perverse tendency.) The homosexuality was a development of this narcissism.

But homosexuality in the male is frequently found in those who have a strong attachment, both sexual and dependent, to a mother who is sexually loving, dotes over them, and at the same time domineers over them, so that they become narcissistic and at the same time the passive female partners to the dominant mother. This partly accounts for the feminine characteristics of so many male homosexuals. This is accentuated if the mother wanted a girl, and so brings up the boy in a girlish fashion, which he in turn responds to as a means of getting her love, instead of being the disappointment he is made to feel that he is for not being a girl. In the female there is the resort to one of the same sex who represents both her own narcissism and the need of the mother-love. If the feeling of loss of love was because the mother wanted a boy, the girl also impersonates a boy as a further means of recovering the lost love.

We have not found that identification with the parent of the same sex is a common source of homosexuality, but there are a number of homosexuals whom we have failed to cure, so that we cannot exclude factors which others claim to have found.

A case of homosexuality who was cured was that of a man whose mother was very sensuously attached to him and then died. He was then brought up rigidly by his father with no affection, and suffered from depression. (Depression and homosexuality often go together because they are both reactions to the loss of affection.) Then an "old boy" at school gave him the attention and stimulated him sexually when he was about thirteen, and this awakened in him the old longing for affection; which however must now be from a male. In later life the male partner (like the old boy) must be bigger than himself, to whom he desired to play the female rôle; but as he himself was fourteen stone, such a partner was difficult to find! He married, but preferred boy friends. The release of these complexes cured him, and the last we heard of him was a press report of his being divorced from his wife for running off with another woman with whom he had fallen in love!

In another case, an early circumcision made a boy feel he was defective as a male, and therefore consorted with males to give himself the sense of male uplift. Apart from this motive was fear of sex from the circumcision, a strong sensuous attraction to his mother, who aroused these feelings in him because she was sexually frustrated, and arrest of physiological development. The attachment to the mother not only fixated the affection and encouraged narcissism, but discouraged any normal heterosexual tendencies, as did his fear of sex in general. He had no alternative but to be homosexual. The patient also was cured, which we mention simply because some people say that homosexuality is incurable. Sometimes it is.

Homosexuality is often associated with other forms of perversion like fetichism, and when that is the case we find the prognosis of cure better than when it is pure homosexuality. In other cases it is associated with anxiety which is also promising, but we have had a case in which the anxiety was cured, but the patient continued to be homosexual without anxiety, which is hardly desirable!

The constitutional factor in sex disorders. It is often maintained that the sex perversions, like homosexuality and exhibitionism, are constitutional and innate; that just as an ordinary man and woman are constituted so that they are attracted to the opposite sex so it is in the nature of the homosexual or other pervert to be attracted by those of their own sex, or constitutionally predisposed to exhibitionism.

Predisposed they certainly are, but the question is whether this predisposition is part of their physiological constitution, or whether they are predisposed by conditions and experiences in earlier years. In our opinion, temperamental and physiological factors are an important contributing factor in some sexual disorders since the sexual functions and desires depend to a large extent upon physiological conditions like the endocrine glands, rendering some highly sexed and some feebly sexed, and upon changes of the organism like fatigue or the state of tumescence. It is also true that some conditions of impotence can be helped by drugs, and some by endocrine gland extracts; a moderate amount of alcohol which removes psychological inhibitions or an aphrodisiac which temporarily stimulates sexual functions may break a vicious circle so that coitus is effected. But that throws very little light on the nature and causes of those disorders.

On the *physiological* side, everyone is a mixture of male and female, both physically (the male has non-functioning breasts and a minute uterus; the woman has the clitoris representing the penis) and mentally. Some are well differentiated, such as males of the Herculean type, women with the typical female contour and broad hips; others like the Adonis type of man and the boy-like girl are less differentiated. It seems probable that there are some in whom the constitutional factor predisposes to homosexuality. But that homosexuality is not purely constitutional is

evidenced by the fact that they can sometimes be cured by psychotherapy.

Against the exclusive constitutional theory is also the fact that
some of the most notorious homosexuals have been men of
exceptional virility and manliness, without the slightest trace
either of effeminacy or of immaturity. The same is true of women
with the typical womanly contours, some of whom are homosexual. In these particular cases we can only conclude that the
condition is psychological and not constitutional, as far as can be
judged.[1]

Even if we conceived that a condition like homosexuality may
be physiologically determined, it is difficult to explain how a
fetichism for the hood of a perambulator can be inborn; or the
sex instincts constitutionally aroused only by the thought of a
horse vomiting (which was in fact due to an identification of himself with the horse—ride a cock horse—whilst his vomiting was
associated with sex feelings). Such conditions must surely be
derived from individual experience.

But while we reject the constitutional theory as adequate to
explain the sex perversions, that is not to say that constitutional
factors do not play a part in many cases of homosexuality, and
even of other perversions.

We cannot have much contact with homosexuals without
realizing that there are often constitutional differences which
encourage the view that the homosexual male is "feminine" and
the female homosexual "masculine." As it stands, however, this
statement is incorrect, and requires modification. For it is not in
fact the masculinoid woman with the male physical characteristics who is the typical Lesbian, although homosexual women
may be attracted to her as to a male. It is truer to say that both
male and female homosexuals are often *physiologically immature*;
they are both adolescent. It is true, as is pointed out, that the
homosexual woman often has the "boy-like figure," flat chest and
narrow hips. But this is the *boy*-like figure, not the masculine
figure; it is the immature figure. Such a woman is deficient not
only in masculine but in female characteristics such as breast
development; she is *sexually undifferentiated*. Some Lesbians may

[1] Havelock Ellis maintained that conditions like homosexuality are constitutional, but admitted to me in conversation, when I pointed out the fact that
some homosexuals are cured by psychological means, that he had overstressed
the constitutional aspect in his anxiety to impress upon the public that these
persons were not responsible for their propensities: but of course the same lack
of responsibility equally applies if we regard them as acquired and due to infantile experiences.

appear masculine because of their make-up and dress and their liking to masquerade as males, but these characteristics are assumed and not physiologically conditioned, and are usually due to the *desire* to be a male which may be either because the mother wanted a boy or because of jealousy of boys. It is so with the homosexual male; true, he is often not of the well-differentiated masculine type, but neither is he feminine, as is so often asserted; he has not the typical *female* contour which is one of curves, large hips and breast development, although he might like to have them in his desire to be feminine. These may be typical of the hermaphrodite type of male, but the hermaphrodite is not the typical homosexual. The homosexual male, like the Lesbian, is commonly adolescent, physiologically immature, and sexually undifferentiated. He is called "effeminate" because he has not developed a man's form, not because he has developed a woman's; and because, in some cases, of his psychological attitude, his mannerisms and the dress he adopts.

How, then, does the constitutional factor function in the development of a homosexual? Every youth and girl probably goes through a phase of homosexuality during adolescence: boys at puberty mix with the gang of boys and have a scorn of girls; and girls though to a less extent have similar attractions to girls and regard boys with distrust. They then normally become sexually differentiated into the manly man and the womanly woman, with corresponding secondary sexual characteristics. But where there is an arrest of physiological development in the adolescent period, they tend to remain in this undifferentiated state instead of their sexuality being differentiated into the typical male and female adult types. This means that they remain immature and therefore there is less urge towards heterosexuality and more tendency to remain homosexual.

In some such cases of homosexuality, the individual may be so arrested in physiological development as to remain in the homosexual phase of puberty, without ever developing into adult life. In the nature of things we do not often see these in the consulting room since they do not regard their condition as an abnormality; they are merely adolescents and do not want treatment.[1]

On the other hand, there are many men of this "immature type," always remaining boy-like in appearance, build, and even

---

[1] The few male "homosexual" prostitutes we have met appear to be of this juvenile type, playing the female rôle; but we are informed that such prostitutes are not themselves homosexual as a rule, any more than the woman prostitute who caters for men's perversions is herself a pervert. It is merely their business.

interests, who are not homosexual but have developed a satisfactory degree of heterosexuality. They ought to be homosexual, but they are not!

Now it stands to reason that if the constitutionally immature person is subjected to morbid psychological complexes from early childhood, these factors will have much more effect upon such an individual than on one who is sexually well differentiated. The physiologically highly sexed and well differentiated individual will force his way through almost any psychological difficulty in early childhood, and emerge a true heterosexual: his sex is so strong that it will refuse to be side-tracked by any adverse psychological conditions. But the man who is already constitutionally immature or sexually weak will more easily succumb to adverse circumstances than those not constitutionally predisposed, and is more likely to develop a homosexual perversion.[1]

There are at the same time a few men and women who are sexually well differentiated and in whom there is no physiological immaturity, but who become homosexual. Those are the ones in whom conditions are so adverse in early childhood that they come to grief even without any constitutional predisposition. Such are the male homosexuals who are typically masculine in form and build, and Lesbians who are typically women in contour with normal secondary female characteristics, but who become homosexual because of psychological factors alone. Indeed there are some Lesbians who are so not because of any constitutional predisposition nor even from sexual fixation, but because of frustration of love. They form these attachments not from the sex it gratifies, but from the love it provides. They are not genuinely homosexual, and if they marry, they cease to be homosexual. Men are not denied the possibility of marriage as are so many women and therefore this type is less frequently found in men. Men may practice homosexuality simply because of the customs of the country, as in some places in the Middle East, where it is considered the right and proper thing; but these people also are not true perverts and are quite potent heterosexually.

This emotional arrest in adolescence coupled with intellectual maturity may account for the oft-quoted statement that *the homosexual often shows signs of genius especially in artistic and literary interests*. Adolescence is the age of spontaneity and creativeness

---

[1] Such immaturity is more liable to produce homosexuality than other perversions because arrest of development means that these people remain in the homosexual phase of adolescence: and that is also why the constitutional factor is more relevant in the production of homosexuality than of other perversions.

which naturally finds its expression in creative art. If this creative spontaneity persists and is combined with the intellectual maturity and technical skill of adult life, one gets a combination likely to be most productive of works of genius. But it is precisely such a person, who because of his arrest and lack of sex differentiation is constitutionally predisposed to homosexuality. It is not that homosexuality produces genius; it is that both depend upon a prolongation of adolescence, an age most fertile in creative ideas.

Treating the homosexual is difficult, first, because he desires his symptom and so far does not wish to get well. He may come for treatment because he knows it is an abnormality and would like to be like other people, or because it is opposed to his ascetic or aesthetic character, or because of the fear of discovery, or because of the depression and anxiety associated with it. But the symptom as such like all sex perversions is desirable, and most homosexuals would no more thank you for getting rid of their homosexuality than the ordinary individual for getting rid of his normal heterosexuality. Secondly, homosexual activities are more natural than say a fetichist or sadist, because there is at least the attraction to another *person*, with the expression of love as well as sex towards them. In sodomy especially, the act is very like the normal and is towards a loved person; therefore they desire nothing further. Thirdly, the constitutional factor may be a barrier to complete cure. If therefore we meet with a man who is of the juvenile nancy-boy type, and is a practising homosexual, we have little hope of curing him, for the odds are too strong against us: in our experience, though possibly not in the experience of others, it is a hopeless case. But we should not despair if the patient is physically well differentiated, is not a practising homosexual, is anxious for cure, and will co-operate in treatment.

Mental hygiene. Keeping in mind the biological function of infantile sensuous pleasure, namely, the encouragement of biological activities, the first principle of mental hygiene should be that we should, as far as possible, keep the sensuousness of early childhood associated with their corresponding biological functions. As long as they are associated with such activities, there should be no suppression of natural sensuous enjoyment, for this not merely encourages the biological functions but give the fullest opportunity for the development of this healthy pleasure into adult sexuality and its sublimation as joy in activity and achievement. A happy child is usually a good child, nor resents necessary discipline.

But there are very cogent reasons why excessive perverse stimulation should be avoided, (*a*) for if these feelings are over-stimulated this in itself tends to wrest them from their natural biological functions and encourages the cleavage between pleasure and reality which may persist throughout life. They constitute a definite danger point and their persistence is quite rightly discouraged as abnormal by mothers and nurses. Indulgence in them encourages sensuous gratification at the expense of finding one's joy in meeting the biological demands of life; it encourages lethargy instead of activity, phantasy rather than reality. (b) By encouraging auto-erotism it discourages love for others which is essential to happy married life and the basis for social relationships. (c) Not only so, but the persistence of the habit of masturbation produces over-excitation of the nervous system, and therefore anxiety. The most anxiety ridden child we have ever seen was one whose parents permitted him on principle to masturbate as much as he liked. (d) The very exaggeration of these functions often leads to their repression and neurosis. In analysis we have several times found instances such as where the mother sensuously stimulates the small boy, and as soon as he gets an erection she is shocked, frightened or scolds him, and the child adopts the same attitude towards himself with subsequent repression and neurosis.

But apart from inhibitions and threats from parents and others, there are, as we have seen, those repressions which come within the child himself, such as nightmares of ogres and witches which are the natural consequences of the sexual orgasm which overwhelms the child, and makes it terrified of its own impulses. Masturbation in early childhood is therefore not a matter of such indifference as some psychologists maintain, nor can we agree with those who maintain that even simple and "innocent" masturbation should be permitted, because of these possible consequences.

It is true that provided it remains a simple sensuous pleasure it is of little importance. But if sensuous activity like thumb-sucking or masturbation is over-stimulated, and especially if it is a perverse reaction to the lack of affection, it is more serious. One may be sure that if a child persistently takes refuge in masturbation on which scolding, tying up and smacking has little or no deterrent effect, it is because it is suffering from a definite complex probably involving both the need for affection and also resentment at the denial of affection and at being thwarted in its pleasure. It is obvious that such treatment as scolding and punishing will drive him further into the very conditions which made him resort to auto-erotism, so that instead of curing him it makes him worse, which is what the distracted mother finds to be the fact. In other cases the punishment frequently stops the child's "bad habit," but in doing so we may be predisposing the child to impotence, fear of sex, or perversion because of the repression. The proper treatment is to discover the cause of it, and provide the specific remedy. In such cases where the complex is more fixed and has become a psychoneurosis, play diagnosis to discover the cause and play therapy to redirect the energies may be required.

Sex is only one function or activity in the whole personality, and no amount of effort to prevent sexual disorders will be of avail unless opportunity is given to the child to develop its *whole personality* by the encouragement of love, of interests in life, of joy in activities and the pursuit of aims and achievements, so that sex falls into place as one of the functions of the personality, subject to the demands and under the control of the personality as a whole. Given the healthy development of the whole personality, one need not as a rule trouble about a child's sexual life.

NOTE ON THE OEDIPUS COMPLEX

We are now in a position to assess the Oedipus complex, which Freud interprets as the incestuous wishes of the infant for the opposite parent which becomes repressed by fear of castration. This is regarded as the "nuclear complex" of the psychoneuroses by the psychoanalysts who, we understand, maintain that the preference of the child for the opposite parent is inevitable though not necessarily innate.

There are however other interpretations of the facts.

That infants have sexual feelings is now generally recognized, and that they may be aroused towards a parent, as indeed towards others like a nurse, is also accepted.

Whether there is an elemental and perhaps tropistic tendency which makes a child innately attracted to the parent of the opposite sex it is too early to say. But there is no doubt that most parents are more attracted to the child of the opposite sex, the mother being devoted to the son, and the father's favourite being the little girl whom he likes to fondle and pet. Naturally the child responds to the parent who gives it most attention and pleasure. The sexual selection, therefore, is primarily on the part of the parent and only secondarily on the part of the child, the attachment of the child to the opposite parent being for no other reason than that it is usually from the opposite parent that the child gets most affection.

This situation often gives rise to jealousy which is a common experience of everyday family life; the father being jealous of the son who has taken some of the mother's love, and the mother feeling left out, being jealous of the daughter who now plays up to the father. This jealousy is often manifested as a harshness towards the child.

This attachment may go a stage further if the sex feelings of the child are aroused by the artificial though not necessarily intentional stimulation of the child's genital organs, by the girl being given "rides" on her father's knee, or the little boy "romping" with his mother in bed. This is more likely, for the reasons given, to be towards the opposite parent, and may produce a sexual fixation on to the opposite parent, preventing the child from growing up sexually, and frustrating the development of adult love. This results in a "father complex" in the girl and a "mother complex" in the boy.

These infantile sexual experiences commonly lead to repression, for the child, being innocent of any wrong in them, resorts to overt manifestations of the activities—the little girl, for instance, being stimulated by the ride on her father's knee wanting him to see or touch her sex organs, and the boy, innocently fondled by his mother in bed, getting an erection. This shocks the parents and results in disapproval, guilt and repression, and the repression further arrests sexual development.

These early experiences are of a sensuous and sexual type but are not usually a desire for sex intercourse with the parents, although they may be later interpreted as such. When, however, adolescence arrives with the desire for sex intercourse, these feelings being arrested by the fixation are thrown back to the original sexual object and so take the form, as Sophocles remarks, of dreams of sexual intercourse with a parent, which are not uncommon in puberty. That is why these dreams emerge in puberty and usually not before. So too the patient, free associating in analysis, visualizes himself or herself in childhood having sex relations with the opposite parent. These dreams and visualizations are *a composite of early genital stimulation interpreted in the light of later sexual feelings*, a reading back of adult sex feeling into the early childhood experience. It does not imply a desire on the infant's part for sexual intercourse with the opposite parent.

This explains also the visualizations of the patient who sees himself as a child being seduced or raped by an adult person. Freud found that these imagined assaults as they stood were fantasies, and he made the false deduction that as the assaults were untrue, they must refer to infantile *desires* for sex intercourse. Upon this his theory of the infantilism of sexuality and the Oedipus complex is based, although "recollections" of infantile sexual desires for intercourse with the opposite parent may be just as unreliable as recollections of the assaults. Our experience suggests that these visualizations are not as imaginary and baseless as Freud suggests, but they originate in an actual and often innocent sexual stimulation by the parent as in the instances mentioned above, upon which later sexual interpretations have been superimposed. The patient's adult desires are for sex intercourse; but if the sex feelings were originally aroused and fixated upon a parent, what is more natural than that the two shall be combined and the picture presented of the child having sex intercourse with a parent. These imagined assaults, like the imagined sexual desires of the child for intercourse, are a mixture of infantile sex experiences and later interpretations; it is the interpretation of infantile experiences in terms of later sexuality.

The typical Oedipus complex therefore occurs at the age of adolescence as Sophocles implies, when the desire for sex is frustrated in its normal development by its early fixation to the parent, so that the youth has incestuous desires towards the opposite parent. The Oedipus complex in our opinion is therefore neither innate nor inevitable, but the result of such early experiences and fixation: it is in fact a complex. It is commonly found as a cause of neurosis, but not universally; nor is it the essential feature in the neurosis. This in our experience is the feeling of insecurity and the need for protective love.

This indeed is confirmed by reference to Sophocles' tragedy. It was a Laius complex not an Oedipus complex. The trouble started with Laius, King of Thebes, and father of Oedipus, whose jealousy of his son (whom the fates said would kill his father and marry his mother) led him to have his son exposed on the hills to die. The shepherd instead hung him up on a tree by his foot (Oedipus = swollen foot).

What produced Oedipus' neurosis and breakdown was the insecurity and anxiety occasioned by this brutal treatment with its complete lack of protective love and security when he was thus exposed and deserted, which is precisely the type of experience to produce a neurosis. It was natural that when Oedipus arrived at adolescence he failed to grow up owing to this fear of facing life; he developed a "mother fixation," the need of a mother for protection and security, and became a neurotic. Many youths of this anxious type "marry their mother," such as an older woman, because they want to be cared for. The myth therefore demonstrates the fact that the psychoneuroses are due to infantile insecurity and the deprivation of protective love which arrests development and renders the individual incapable of facing life and brings all sorts of disaster upon him. The later sexual fixation, the Oedipus complex, is a result not a cause of the neurosis.

We may contrast this story with the parallel myth of Perseus; he had a jealous grandfather, Acrisius, who, under the same threat of the fates as was Laius, put both son and mother in a chest and set them adrift at sea, surely an ideal situation for the development of an incestuous complex! But Perseus did not become a neurotic; he proved himself a real man in love and war: he showed his heroism in slaying the Medusa, rescued Andromeda and married the girl! Why the difference in the fortunes of Oedipus and Perseus? Because, whilst Oedipus was abandoned and deserted by his parents and so became neurotic, Perseus, even when cast away in the barrel, had the comfort and protection of his mother, and therefore developed confidence to face life.

Incidentally, Freud's choice of Electra as representing the female counterpart of the Oedipus complex is equally unfortunate; for not only was her devotion to her father, Agamemnon, whose wife was philandering while he was at the wars, quite natural; but it was the son, Orestes, whose hatred of the mother for the same cause was equally strong, who in fact slew his mother, surely a parody of the Oedipus complex! If Electra was in love with her father she should have welcomed the defection of her mother. One wonders why Freud did not stand by his story of Oedipus and take Antigone as the female counterpart since in her devotion to her father, Oedipus, she wandered the earth with him in poverty when the fates turned against them. Antigone was certainly a better example of such devotion to the father than Electra.

We have, however, found the Oedipus complex in the Freudian sense (a sexual attachment of the boy to the mother and fear of the father) very common in our Jewish patients; but this is not surprising when the Jewish boy is brought up with the idea of an awe-inspiring Jehovah, who demands castration, in the form of circumcision, of the infant son.

PART III

TECHNIQUE AND TREATMENT

CHAPTER XVI

TECHNIQUE AND TREATMENT

IT has so often been objected that medical psychologists discuss the causes of the neuroses, but rarely give away the process of treatment and cure, that we may be forgiven for going into this matter with as much detail as space will allow.

But before discussing analytic technique we must say something of the principles underlying Persuasion and Suggestion, since these are not as alien to analysis as some suppose, and indeed may be used in analysis.

PERSUASION

Treatment by persuasion is an appeal to reason: it is designed to convince the patient of the irrationality of his symptoms with a view to countering the forces which make for the illness. It consists largely in getting rid of false intellectual difficulties and preconceptions: it sets out to explain to the patient how his symptoms arose, and the motives for them; how his headaches are an escape from responsibility; how his fears are a means of getting his own way; how his obsessions imply a sense of guilt for which he must propitiate; that his sex impotence is due to a latent fear, or to an unconscious antagonism towards women. It instructs him in the exercise of his will, and in the release of his emotions. It sets out to convince the person with an inferiority complex that he is capable, and so gives him confidence to assert himself.[1]

[1] In the hands of Dubois (*Psychic Treatment of Nervous Disorders*) such treatment consists in explaining to the patient the causes of his disorder (as far as these are known), and thereby encouraging him to the *exercise of his will*. In the hands of others like Dejerine (*Psychoneuroses*), it is an appeal to the reason, but with a view to affecting the *emotional life* of the individual. Adler's system is in practice a method of persuasion, which explains to the patient the origins of the disorder in his "organ inferiority," his lack of co-operation with others, and his fictitious goals to counteract this inferiority. The patient is encouraged no longer to take refuge in fictions and symptoms to excuse from failure, but to find satisfaction in objective achievement.

It was also used with great effect by Hurst and his colleagues at Seale Hayne Hospital during the war of 1914–18, where many cases of paralysis were cured at one sitting, by demonstrating to the patients that there was nothing organically wrong, and that they could move their limbs, thus overcoming the morbid autosuggestion that they couldn't. Many such cases were permanently cured

A patient had a fear that she would do an injury to the children she taught: she also found she could not discipline them. It was explained to her that her fear was due to an unconscious aggressiveness; and to our surprise she immediately lost both symptoms. Asked how this had occurred she explained that the idea that she was really assertive instead of the feeble creature she thought she was, gave her such a new confidence in herself that the aggressiveness released itself in normal ways, including good discipline of the children; and the fear of hurting, having lost its unconscious motive, disappeared. But such results are unusual.

Persuasion treatment has its uses. (*a*) In mild cases it may cure: indeed every day we use it on one another to correct minor abnormalities of behaviour, to convince one another of the error of our ways, or the absurdity of our ideas, by an appeal to reasonableness. (*b*) In more serious cases the cure takes place by the breaking of a vicious circle. When the Seale Hayne cases who were convinced that their arms were paralysed were shown that they could move the paralysed arm, however slightly, it broke the idea that they could not do so, and by such demonstration the patient got well. (*c*) In other cases it helps a patient to see the reason for his symptom; and to realize that there is a reason for it is considerable comfort: and even if the patient cannot get rid of the symptom he can accommodate himself to it. (*d*) Such treatment is also of value in getting rid of intellectual difficulties and preconceptions and so paves the way to analysis. A common idea is that these morbid fears, impulses or peculiar sensations are a sign of insanity, since the layman's idea of insanity is that he has ideas and emotions that he cannot control. Such a belief makes the patient worse and its correction is a great relief. It is true that in insanity we do lose control, but having such symptoms is not necessarily a sign of insanity. Again, most patients fear that analysis will make them worse; it may be explained to them that this is only temporary.

Every psycho-physician, therefore, finds that even in a single interview conducted sympathetically, the patient goes away feeling greatly relieved that there is someone who understands, and does not think him a fool; that there is a "reason for his madness," and

because the vicious circle was broken: others relapsed because the basic cause of the trouble was not removed. There is also some doubt whether morbid fears and anxieties were as effectively cured by this method as were hysterical paralyses. It is questionable how far this process of persuasion is really an appeal to reason, or how far its success depends on suggestion and on other personal factors, the care, interest or forceful personality of the doctor overcoming the resistance of the patient rather than persuading his reason.

that it is something for which he cannot be held altogether responsible.

But these methods are necessarily superficial in that they do not deal with the deep-seated causes of the disorder which is necessary to the radical treatment of any disease, physical or mental. It is not much good explaining to a mother that her dislike of her child is activated by jealousy if this jealousy is rooted in something in the past of which she is quite unconscious. A patient with a morbid sense of guilt may be comforted by our reassurance for a time, but the treatment gives only temporary relief; he is as bad as ever the next day and more hopeless. Such patients know that their symptoms are irrational as well as we do; that is why they come for treatment. What they want to know is how to get rid of them. "What is consolation for the mind is not consolation for the heart."

In any case, for persuasion to be effective it should be used in conjunction with a knowledge of psychopathology. If such a person has a sense of guilt about something quite irrational, it is probable that he *is* guilty although unconsciously. To try to persuade him that it is irrational and that he is not guilty goes counter to his conviction—and to the truth. It is more to the point to persuade him that he *is* guilty, find out what is the guilt and make him willing to face up to it. These short methods of treatment should therefore be used only by those who have had a training in the fundamental principles of psychopathology and who have mastered the technique of analytic treatment of whatever school of thought. Otherwise what appears to be common-sense treatment is often entirely wrong in any individual case. Especially must the physician remember that the symptom is due to a repression of part of our personality, and an attempt to restore the personality to health. Merely to abolish the symptom is not to cure the personality: but the symptom should be abolished by the cure of the personality.

Occupational therapy may relieve the patient in making him forget his worrying problems, and in canalizing and directing his energies to progressive ends helps to sublimate some of the energy now being discharged in neurosis. It also has the advantage that if the work undertaken is successful it restores to the patient the confidence he lacks. But it may only succeed in side-tracking the patient from facing the real issue. It is therefore of greater value in the psychoses in turning the patient's mind to the objective world, than in the psychoneuroses where the mind should be turned to solve the inner problem.

SUGGESTION

The essence of suggestion treatment is the implanting in the mind some idea, and evoking an emotional response, whilst the mind is in an acquiescent, non-critical and receptive state.

A distinction must here be made between suggestion and suggestibility. *Suggestion* is the process of transmission and acceptance of an idea: *suggestibility* is the state of mind which makes such acceptance possible. The technique of suggestion treatment is the production of a state of suggestibility. When the mind is sufficiently suggestible there is an abolition of the critical function so that the individual accepts without question whatever is suggested. Coué failed to make this distinction: he said people cured themselves by "auto-suggestion," but they did so only after they had been worked by him to a state of heightened suggestibility. The success of suggestion depends fundamentally upon a condition of suggestibility, that is to say, of passivity.

Suggestibility is a state of psychic dependence. Just as an infant in the first year is in a state of *physical* dependence upon others, so suggestibility is a state of *psychic* dependence in which the individual takes over the ideas, feelings and moods of another person. In such a state of passivity the individual is non-critical and accepts without question what is suggested to him.

This conception of suggestion corresponds with the commonplace use of the word. When we say that a person is very suggestible we mean that he accepts ideas without question and is more than usually responsive to emotional situations: he is non-critical. When in ordinary language we "make a suggestion" we mean that we offer the idea without expecting it to be too critically handled: we merely "offer it as a suggestion." When we speak of a joke or wisecrack being "suggestive" we mean that while it suggests something illicit, it is put in such a way as to evade criticism; that is the function of the *double entendre*.

Certain conditions and situations conduce to a suggestible state of mind. (a) Suggestibility is common in people who are constitutionally dependent; or in those in whom a dependent disposition has been developed. This is irrespective of whether the person is intelligent or unintelligent. (b) The person persistently *under authority* like the soldier or sailor is more obedient and submissive to command and therefore more suggestible, and is found to be more easily hypnotized than the average individual. (c) A state of *heightened emotion* makes a person suggestible, for emotion checks critical thinking. Therefore the person in a panic will accept suggestions given him however unreasonable; the man in a rage will believe everything that is foul about a man whom he till recently respected: and the girl who is in love is ready to believe him endowed with the beauty of Apollo, the strength of Hercules and the wisdom of Solomon. (d) A *crowd* is suggestible because in a crowd the individual identifies himself with the group and so yields his private judgment to the will of the herd. He behaves very differently because his identification makes him ready to think or do whatever the crowd says. He is functioning with a part of his personality and indeed with the part of his brain (the granular layer of the cortex) in which reason and criticism are in abeyance. (e) The use of *drugs* like cocaine produce a state of suggestibility, possibly for the same reason.

Therapeutic suggestion depends upon the abolition of criticism and the production of a condition of mental passivity in which the patient accepts the healthful suggestions of the physician. All the conditions just mentioned may be used in inducing suggestibility, whether by hypnosis or otherwise, and are designed to this end.

In suggestion treatment apart from hypnosis, the subject is put into a state of passivity, dependence and receptivity, with his criticism temporarily in abeyance: but he is not so completely dissociated that he is unaware of what the physician is saying, although too lethargic to criticize. Some physicians consider that this conscious realization of what is being said is more effective than if the patient is deeply hypnotized, in that it carries the conscious as well as the subconscious mind with it.

The technique of inducing suggestibility can be most simply described as that which we should use in quietening down a frightened, nervous, anxious child, by getting him to lie down, relax his body, to be calm and quiescent.

One method is by *progressive relaxation* of body and mind into a sleepy and drowsy state, which abolishes criticism and renders the patient passive to suggestion. Another is by the *concentration on a light* or some other object. This method of heightened attention appears the exact opposite of the last method, but in point of fact achieves the same purpose. For attention is, at any rate partly, a process of inhibition as Pavlov says. In concentration we inhibit all extraneous stimuli except the light and the voice of the hypnotist: and then by closing the eyes of the patient he is made attentive to our voice and that alone, to which he is now exclusively responsive. All criticism of what we are saying is in abeyance and therefore the patient is obedient to our commands and dependent on our will, there being no rival thought in the mind. Hypnosis (as its name implies) is near akin to sleep, not so much in its inactivity, for a hypnotized person may be very active, but whereas in hypnosis the patient is attentive to one stimulus only, namely the voice of the hypnotizer, and is asleep to all else, in deep sleep *all* extraneous stimuli are cut off. This is supported by the fact that if we leave a hypnotized person to himself the *rapport* will cease, and the hypnosis will pass into normal sleep. We agree with Bernheim of Nancy (Du Sommeil) that hypnotism is sleep plus *rapport*. Even in sleep a mother may be *en rapport* with her child, and a doctor with his telephone, and most people have experienced that a determination to wake at a certain time will persist in sleep all through the night, so that we wake precisely then.

The *concentration upon a monotonous sound* like that of a metronome appears to combine both the relaxation and the attentive methods: for monotonous sounds produce a state of lethargy (as with some sermons); but also the attention to the sound during treatment distracts the mind from what is being said, and therefore from criticism of it, so that the patient is passively receptive of what is being said.

Another factor influencing suggestion is the *prestige of the physician* which renders the patient more dependent and submissive. Suggestibility to authority is an experience of everyday life and is valuable, for we cannot "prove all things" and must accept the verdict of experts and those in authority. But an absurd perversion of such suggestibility to authority is that because a person is an authority on one subject, we submissively accept his views on other subjects. Because he is an authority on the drama we accept his views on vivisection; another, who is a capable novelist, we accept on matters of religion and the existence of God: and because a man is a psychiatrist and an expert on insanity, we accept his advice on the bringing up of children. Instead of the injunction to prove all things, we should first prove all men.

The identification of the physician with either father or mother is also conducive to a state of dependence and therefore of suggestibility. Ferenczi has pointed out that the methods of inducing hypnosis are those of authority, like the father, or those of tenderness, like the mother. This does not necessarily imply a sexual fixation: it may simply mean that as children we are biologically submissive to both influences of tenderness and authority.

Certain misconceptions regarding suggestion need to be corrected. A popular idea of suggestion is that it consists in making a person believe what is not true. That of course can be done, such as making a person believe that he is paddling, or sees a ghost: and some would say it is the same when we tell him that he has not a headache when he has, and not paralysed when he is. That, however, is not necessarily so. *The function of therapeutic suggestion is rather to disabuse the mind of a false belief.* The hysteric believes that he cannot walk, and as long as he believes that, he cannot do so; it is only his false belief, and perhaps his wish, that makes him unable to do so. He *can* walk except for the belief that he cannot: and the fact that he can is proved by the fact that when he gets rid of the false idea, he does. Suggestion does not consist in making an individual believe what is not true: *suggestion consists in making something come true by making him believe in its possibility.* By giving him the belief that he can walk we are making come true something which would not have occurred, had it not been for the belief. Faith plays a great part in treatment, as it does in business, in science and in social life. The belief of a patient that he can walk, makes him walk. The belief in analysis that the doctor can cure him is of great assistance in the analysis, because it wins the co-operation of the patient, whereas the patient who refuses to believe he can get well is a great burden. Not only so, but the belief of the doctor in the patient, who sees in the patient not what he is, but what he may become, is a most important factor in the cure. The doctor who does not think he can make much of a patient is not likely to. The employer of labour, the officer in the Army who expects most of his men is likely to get the most out of them.

Suggestion treatment is therefore rational in ridding a patient of false ideas.

A further function of suggestion is to *reinforce healthy ideas.* A man is inferior because he believes he is so, and he believes he is so because he wishes to be excused from responsibility. But the patient also wishes to be well, although this wish is temporarily in abeyance, overwhelmed by the morbid desire to be ill. Suggestion not only counteracts the false belief and wish, but encourages the healthy desire to be well, reinforces his will and confidence to face life and makes him well.

Suggestion in fact can only operate if there is something which responds to it in the personality. In other words, suggestion treatment is not so much putting ideas in from without, but reinforcing and bringing to the surface something already there but at present inactive. When it is said, for instance, that the patient takes up some medical suggestion that he has a pain in his arm, it is only because there already exists a wish for such a pain. On the other hand, when we suggest to a patient who has a hysterical paralysis that he will be able to walk, we are merely reinforcing that in him which wants to be well, but which for the time being is overcome by a fear of life: we are reawakening and making effective these healthy desires, by adding the force of our suggestion to his desire to be well. From this point of view suggestion fulfils the same function as analytic treatment in that it *releases latent desires* and so restores the patient to health. The timid patient requires courage, and we can give him this either by inspiring him with courage and confidence as by suggestion, or by discovering and removing the basic fear which saps his courage, as in analysis. The latter is certainly the more effective and radical, but one must not ignore the possibilities of the former, especially in mild cases and in cases of present strain and difficulty.

Again it is often said that suggestion treatment is opposed to analytic treatment in that it is supposed merely to bolster up the super-ego. It may be false treatment if it encourages his morbid super-ego of achievement or over-conscientiousness against which he is rebelling by his breakdown. But that may not be the course or purpose of our suggestion, which may be directed towards debunking the false super-ego, encouraging the patient to take things easier and not be so strained and thus be more efficient, or to be less over-conscientious and not be so hard on himself, with the result that he will be more human. Suggestion may rid him of an exaggerated notion of his piety or self-importance and to be more affectionate to others. But it is hard going, since these are the things which the patient believes in, and he will not accept what is morally repugnant to him. It is, however, very effective where a patient is beginning to realize the falsity of his ways, and helps him to a proper readjustment. After all, the overstrained man is wanting ease and relaxation from the tyranny of his super-ego, and if by suggestion we can induce him to a greater tranquillity it may save a breakdown.

Thus suggestion is not necessarily a repressive measure bolstering up the demands of the super-ego against the needs of the ego which are expressing themselves in the symptoms, but may be used to encourage the expression of those impulses which because they are repressed, produce the symptoms.

The aim of therapeutic suggestion is therefore (a) to get rid of morbid autosuggestions, and replace them with healthy ideas and desires, (b) to arouse new emotions, confidence instead of fear, quietness instead of anxiety, (c) to break morbid associations between emotions like fear and the objects to which they have become attached, such as open spaces, which are, however, not the real but only the projected causes of fear, (d) to break down a vicious circle; for if by suggestion we can once make him walk, or talk, or see, or be assertive, or control his temper, the vicious circle is broken and a complete and permanent cure may take place. This is especially the case if, as in war-shock cases, the motive for the symptom has passed, or when the symptom fails of its purpose, in that the patient does not get the sympathy for her headaches but is regarded as a nuisance. In such a case the patient is ripe for cure, and seizes the opportunity to get rid of a symptom which no longer serves any purpose, but has let her down.

The weakness of suggestion treatment lies in the fact that whilst the patient wants to be well he has an unconscious wish to be ill. There is a fight therefore between the physician's suggestions of well-being and the much older and firmly established *auto*suggestion of the patient that he is ill: for if he loses his symptom he no longer gets the sympathy he desires and which his symptom was designed to secure. That is why the suggestion may temporarily cure the patient, but he relapses under the influence of this unconscious urge. A patient wishes to be rid of his obsessions but he will not willingly release his forbidden impulses because the fear of consequences still remains: it is only by discovering the cause of the fear that we can effectively explode it. If it is a sex perversion, whilst the patient may want to be rid of it, he is also reluctant to give up what is his one solace in life. In most cases of impotence, however, there is often not an unconscious wish but only a fear, so that these conditions are more effectively treated by suggestion.

The indications for suggestion treatment are therefore fairly clear.

(a) It is of great value in *milder cases* where the complex is not too deep rooted.

(b) It is of particular value when it is a *present-day difficulty* which is causing the anxiety, depression or sleeplessness, and which the patient finds himself incapable of dealing with. He needs support, and suggestion provides the temporary splint he requires by giving him confidence and courage to carry on till he *tides over the difficulty* and can carry on for himself. Ordinary encouragement does a lot, as we know in everyday life, but such encouragement given him in the quiet relaxation of a suggestible state of mind is doubly effective.

(c) Suggestion is also useful in those who are *constitutionally* anxious, nervous, highly strung and over-sensitive to the rebuffs of life: it helps to brace them and reinforce their feeble courage.

(d) Suggestion is also indicated when the patient comes in a state of such *anxiety and distress* that immediate analysis is impossible, which is particularly the case where there is a psychotic element. Calm and quietening suggestion is often more effective than sedentary drugs. It is also of value during the course of analysis when, as not infrequently happens, the patient gets into a state of such unbearable distress that he feels he cannot go on. This, however, is hardly feasible unless we have previously given him suggestion treatment; and we must be careful that this suggestion is an encouragement and confidence to continue, not a substitute for the analysis.

(e) Suggestion is also of great effect in *simple psychosomatic disorders*, because many of these are based on simple worries and anxieties of the present time which may be allayed by suggestion. Where that is the case, a "nervous headache" from worry may often be cured in a few minutes by quiet relaxation and suggestion of peace and tranquillity. By quietening the emotion we relieve the congestion in the head which is causing the headache; by getting rid of the anxiety we relieve the indigestion, palpitation, trembling or sickness.

(f) Suggestion is also of value when there is some specific habit like alcoholism, drug taking or bad temper to be overcome. Such habits are often the result of a vicious circle, the worry causing the alcoholism, the alcohol making it impossible to deal with the worry. Once the habit is broken the patient may then manage for himself, but he needs help to break it.

(g) Suggestion is also of value in *older people* for whom analysis is too drastic and in whom the process of cure may be worse than the disease: it brings comfort to the sick, solace to the aged, and peace to the dying. Analysis is no more difficult in the old than in the young, but the old cannot readjust themselves so easily. It is a simple matter for younger persons to discover that they have been living on a wrong principle, and change: but it is little consolation to older people to discover they have lived their whole life wrongly, for they cannot start afresh so readily. Nevertheless we have had patients over sixty who would rather see the truth at last than never!

(h) Suggestion can very effectively be given by *a mother to a sleeping child*; quietly, so that the child does not wake, repeatedly, so that the ideas are absorbed. But let it be remembered that positive suggestions of confidence, reassurance, calmness are much more effective than negative ones that the child "will not be afraid." To suggest that he will "wake up and get up when he wants to pass water" is more effective than that he "will not wet his bed." The "subconscious mind" does not deal in negatives. It is true that his bed-wetting may be a desire to return to infantile life, but it is also true that it humiliates him in making him feel a baby: so that if he breaks the habit by suggestion, it gives him confidence and encourages him to be grown up. By breaking the vicious circle it produces a permanent cure.

ANALYSIS

One of the most important discoveries in psychopathology in recent years is that the underlying causes of the psychoneuroses are to be found in experiences in early childhood. The predisposing causes are usually of far greater importance than the precipitating causes; but long since forgotten, they cannot be revived by any effort of memory.

Another important discovery of Freud is that neuroses are the result of repression; therefore special measures are necessary to remove the resistance so as to discover the unconscious and hidden sources of the neuroses. Taking a case history, however thorough, will never provide a complete picture of the causes of the neuroses. Nor is dealing with the conscious causes of the disorder an adequate form of cure.

Every science, bacteriology, astronomy or chemistry has its particular methods of discovering the causes of the phenomena it studies; in psychology it has been found necessary to devise special means for recovering these early experiences since they cannot be recalled by ordinary efforts of memory. This recovery is made more difficult by the fact that these original experiences are of a painful nature, or incompatible with the aims of the personality as a whole, and that is why they have been actively repressed. There is, therefore, always a resistance to their recall, and this resistance has to be overcome before the memory of the experience will return to consciousness. Forgetting, as Freud has told us, is an active process.

The original method of recalling such experiences was by hypnosis, which is sometimes still used. The history of this process is interesting. The mesmerists had cured people by what we should now call hypnotic suggestion, though following the theory of "animal magnetism" they ascribed it to a magnetic fluid, a physical agency foreshadowing modern treatment by rays. It was probably to the Abbé Faria that is due the credit of recognizing that the neurosis was psychogenetic and that "all was subjective"; and to James Braid, that the treatment and cure were also subjective and psychologically akin to sleep to which he therefore gave the name "hypnosis" as contrasted with animal magnetism. Liébeault and Bernheim of Nancy used hypnosis for curative suggestion, and the latter regarded suggestion as a normal function in life, maintaining that hypnosis was simply a phenomenon of sleep plus *rapport*. Charcot went a stage further by using hypnosis for experimental purposes, and producing hysterical symptoms under hypnosis, thereby proving by experiment the psychogenetic nature of these disorders, and suggesting the lines of treatment. "We have here," he writes, "a psychical affection; it is therefore by mental treatment that we may hope to modify it." But he regarded hypnosis as a morbid condition; which is not surprising as he used only pathological subjects for his experiments! Janet went a stage still further, and used hypnosis as means of recovering forgotten memories and so the causes of neurotic disorders, especially in cases of dissociation and dual personality. It does not appear, however, that in Janet's hands this revival of the original experience under hypnosis necessarily led to curative results. Later on, as we know, Breuer used the same method of hypnosis for reviving the original cause of hysterical conditions, but in his hands, and those of Freud who worked with him and extended his work, the reproduction of the original experience led to the disappearance of the symptom.

The secret of this success seems to be due to two circumstances of the Breuer-Freud technique, namely (a) that the original experience had to be relived with emotional tone ("affectless memories are almost utterly useless"), and (b) that the dissociated and forgotten states revived under hypnosis had to be remembered afterwards in the waking state, and "talked out" in consciousness; that is to say, they were reassociated with the rest of the personality. Janet did the former, but does not seem to have exploited the latter; with the result that the revived experiences remained dissociated and the patient uncured. Freud at first termed this method of cure "catharsis," the purging of the personality of the noxious experiences which constitutes the disease; and indeed this release makes the patient feel "spring-cleaned." But by a more apt and accurate metaphor it was also called "abreaction" reacting to the original experience as one should have reacted, and with the emotion which was previously denied expression, and so releasing the "strangulated affect."

Hypno-analysis. Hypnosis still remains an effective means of recovering lost memories in traumatic cases, or where people suffer from loss of memory. It is also of value in cases of conversion hysteria—pain, headache, indigestion, paralysis, since such patients are comparatively easily hypnotized: but it is of little use in the obsessions, since these patients are not hypnotizable or only with the greatest difficulty owing to their obstinate and aggressive nature.[1] In any case the physician skilled in the use of free association can recover experiences almost as readily by association as by hypnotism.

War cases are easier to hypnotize, particularly those suffering from conversion hysteria, for the soldier and the sailor are notoriously suggestible owing to the training in discipline and the attitude of dependence to authority, and dependence is the basis both of hypnosis and hysteria. Indeed in the first World War we used to hypnotize twenty at a time each morning for treatment by suggestion, treating them individually afterwards, and we found that on an average seventeen out of twenty were hypnotized to the extent of being anaesthetic to pain, a pin being put through a fold of skin.

The method of "hypno-analysis," as the author originally called it,[2] combined the use of hypnosis for the recovery of forgotten experiences, with suggestion to help the patient to readjust himself to the situation when the causes have been discovered. This combination of suggestion with analysis can, as we have seen, be effectively used with free association apart from hypnosis, and also with narco-analysis, the patient being given suggestion treatment as he emerges from the drug.

If hypnosis were more generally possible, hypno-analysis would be the simplest, most direct and quickest form of analysis and therefore the method of choice. Unfortunately we can deeply hypnotize only a small proportion of our patients, chiefly the traumatic and conversion hysteric patients, whereas (apart from psychosomatic disorders) by far the majority of patients in civilian practice are cases of anxiety, obsession and obsessional anxiety. This practical difficulty puts a limitation on the use of hypnosis, and is in our opinion the only objection to its use.[3]

[1] But all conversion hysterics are not easy to hypnotize, for there are those cases we have called "resistive hysterics" in whom aggressive tendencies are strong, though not dominant, and in these hypnosis is very difficult.

[2] *Functional Nervous Disorders.* Ed. H. C. Miller, 1920.

[3] We have never been able to appreciate the objections apart from the practical one already mentioned, raised by Freud to the use of hypnosis in treatment, namely that hypnosis is a form of sexual transference to the physician, who

The discovery of a simple method of inducing hypnosis would be one of the greatest benefits to mankind not only for suggestion treatment and hypno-analysis, but for producing surgical anaesthesia for major and minor operations; for hypnosis takes first place as a form of anaesthetic not only ridding the patient of pain at the time of the operation but afterwards, abolishing the sickness and apparently producing a far less degree of shock. Indeed an effective method of producing hypnosis would have no less effect than *the abolition of all pain*, a boon of inestimable value to suffering humanity.

In skilled hands the danger of hypnosis is non-existent. The most common objection to hypnosis on the part of the patient is that he gives up his will to the hypnotizer, but it is an exploded fallacy that the physician can make a person do what is morally repugnant to him, or what is wrong, although recent attempts have been made to revive the idea.

This was humorously illustrated in a patient of ours during the war who had paralysed legs and to whom under deep hypnosis we were suggesting that he would be able to walk "With a long, strong stride." "No, sir!" he protested under hypnosis. "Yes!" we insisted (thinking his protest was merely motivated by unbelief). "No, sir!" he replied with even greater vehemence. "Why not " we said. "Because," he replied, "my regiment has the shortest step in the British Army!" It was a matter of honour with him, so that even under hypnosis we were able to shift this deep-rooted conviction only with difficulty.

Narco-analysis. Because of the difficulty in inducing hypnosis, it has been largely superseded by the use of Nembutal, Evipan, Pentothal or other hypnotic drugs, under which, as in alcohol (which is, however, uncertain in its effects!), inhibitions are removed and the patient gives vent to his feelings. This has been

stands in the place of father; and that so long as the hypnotic relationship persists it means that the patient still has this transference to the physician, which prevents the patient from getting down to the deepest levels of the mind (Freud, *Introd. Lectures*, Chap. 28). Transference is itself a morbid process, as Freud insists (*op. cit.*, p. 371), and yet is definitely used by the psychoanalysts as a means of liberating affect, so that the objection hardly holds. If it be argued that the psychoanalysts proceed to get rid of the transference we may point to the fact that in actual practice as the patient being treated by hypnotic suggestion gets better, he in fact becomes less hypnotizable, which means that the "transference" situation is spontaneously passing away—even under hypnotic treatment. The diminishing hypnotizability as treatment proceeds is to be explained by the fact that as the patient ceases to be ill he becomes less dependent and therefore less hypnotizable. In any case we do not agree with Freud that hypnosis is fundamentally a sexual transference, but like hysteria it is based on an attitude of dependence, which is more deep-rooted than a sexual relation.

given the name of Narco-analysis, by which means repressed and
forgotten experiences may be restored to memory.[1] These drugs
have the advantage of rapidity and can be easily and almost
universally applied. They are therefore of great value in hospital
treatment where pressure of work makes short treatment necessary. But they have their limitations. For one thing they cannot
be used too frequently because of their toxic effects which are
cumulative, whereas hypnosis can be. Moreover, whilst these drugs
are useful in breaking down the resistance, they fail to elicit the
more subtle feelings and emotions of the patient and the more
deep-seated causes of the disorder. Sometimes they fail altogether
to elicit a response, as in the woman whose repressed hate we
hoped to release, but in whom the drug produced such a pleasant
effect that she was at peace with the whole world and could hate
nobody! The main objection to the method of narco-analysis as
the sole means of analysis is that while it may release the repressed
emotions, it does not touch the super-ego, which is a more static
attitude of mind, and is the real obstruction to analysis. We
therefore use these drugs, but only when we get stuck in free
association and when we find it too difficult otherwise to break
down the resistance. Even so we follow up the narco-analysis with
free association after the resistance has been broken. Narco-
analysis is therefore best used as an adjunct to free association,
not as a substitute.

Dream analysis is perhaps the most commonly used form of
analytic treatment; but while years of experience has modified,
it has not radically changed our view previously expressed
(*Psychology and Morals*) that valuable as it is as an adjunct to
reductive analysis, it remains unsatisfactory as the only means
of unfathoming unconscious problems. No doubt dreams have
a meaning, but dreams are mainly symbolic and the interpretations
given are at present too subject to the idiosyncrasies of the
analyst; and as long as the schools of psychology vary as much
as they do over the interpretation of a single dream, it cannot
be taken as scientifically established however much it may be
clinically useful. (Freud himself says that in interpretating dreams
he had to "draw upon his own resources.") Symbols need to be
interpreted, and whilst some symbols are so apt that they are
almost, but not entirely, universal, as in the symbol of the tree
meaning life, and the snake a phallus, there are others that have
quite a different significance for different persons—so water may
imply purity, it may mean birth, it may mean the unconscious,

[1] Horsley—*Narcoanalysis*.

or it may refer to the fact that the patient once tried to drown himself, as in one of our patients. For those who are dogmatic as regards their theories dream analysis is a simple matter. But like surrealist pictures, they are fascinating because we can read into them what we will! Yet a wrong interpretation can obviously misdirect the whole analysis and lead to confusion, and therefore dream interpretation must be used with caution. Dreams are not, as is often remarked, the royal road to the unconscious, they are an indirect and often very tortuous road; their very symbolism makes them uncertain. The direct road to the origin of the psychoneurotic disorder is by means of the symptom, which is the precipitate and epitome in consciousness of the underlying complexes, a direct representation of the unconscious wish. But obviously the more open-minded and skilled we are in our interpretation of dreams, the more they will reveal to us. But arbitrary interpretations should give place to those based on the free associations of the patients. We therefore do not discard the use of dreams: but we do not rely upon them as our mainstay. As an adjunct to the more direct method of analysis they are most useful.

Some dreams are obvious. In analysing a married woman we had reason to touch on her relations with her father whom she adored. She protested that she was completely in love with her husband; but she had a dream that they had bought a dilapidated house, renovated it, filled it with beautiful furniture, but then it became in a worse state of dilapidation than it was to begin with, and they sold it. The manifest content of the dream was that she and her husband were in fact looking for a house. The latent content of the dream helped to convince her of what the analysis was leading up to, namely that she and her husband had made a gallant effort to build up their marriage to something successful but she was refusing to face the fact that it was a failure. Her *symptom*, which was a fear that her husband would meet with an accident, revealed the same conclusion. It was necessary for her to face up to the situation if she was to solve either the objective situation of her marriage or the subjective problem of her neurosis. Such a dream is the more convincing in that the interpretation comes from the patient, and the more so that it was confirmed by corresponding with the reductive analysis.

Nightmares are particularly important for showing the nature of the problem, whilst ordinary dreams suggest a solution. For as we go to sleep to escape the problems of the day, so we wake up to escape the unsolved problems of the night. Dreams, by reproducing in vivid form the unsolved problems of the day help us to solve them.

Word association. It is a curious fact that in lay books on psychotherapy it is often assumed that the method of investigation most commonly employed is that of word-association tests, the method in which a test word is given by the examiner and the response reveals the nature of the complex. We do not know of a single medical psychologist who uses this as a routine, but it is a very useful method in delinquency, and in other cases in which we have to deal with an unwilling patient. These patients will refuse to be communicative, but they may consent to the word-association tests, since they are only required to give the first word which comes to the mind, not realizing that they will thereby give themselves away and reveal their guilt.

Word-association tests are also of value in proving the *innocence* of a person wrongly charged with a delinquency or crime, an instance of which is the following:

A senior boy at a boarding school was accused of writing indecent letters to another boy, one of which was found in his pocket; and he was expelled from school. As he intended becoming a medical missionary and had already won a scholarship to Oxford, this expulsion meant abandoning his prospects and career. We put him under word-association tests which, while they revealed complexes of other kinds, failed to give any complex indication whatever, relative to the crime, which proved his innocence; and this was confirmed by a handwriting expert. He was taken back to school and his complete innocence later proved when the real culprit was accidentally discovered and confessed, namely the boy to whom the letters were addressed who used this method to get our patient into trouble.

Free association. The method almost invariably used now in medical psychology is that of free association devised by Freud, as a result of his observations of some experiments made by Bernheim, who demonstrated that a patient could be made to recall experiences he has had in the hypnotic state and which he had forgotten, by being pressed to remember. Freud argued (did not James say that genius is the capacity to see analogies?) that if this could be done in hypnotic amnesia, why should it not be done in hysteric amnesia, with those forgotten experiences which were the cause of the hysterical symptoms. He found that by pressing the patient and getting him to concentrate, such experience could be recalled without the use of hypnosis. Free association has thus become one of the greatest discoveries in the technique of psychological medicine; for the method could be universally applicable, whereas hypnosis could not, and it is the use of this method which has made modern psychotherapy what it is. Free association is the gateway to the forgotten past.

The *data* of free association are of various kinds; first by getting the patient to concentrate upon some definite experience; secondly, by taking a certain symptom or dream as a starting point, and then allowing the mind to associate freely upon that; or thirdly, without taking a theme at all, to instruct the patient to tell whatever comes into his mind apropos of nothing. It is found that the patient associates most freely when he is in a state of relaxation, as on a couch, as he then is less likely to be critical or cautious, and his associations are more likely to be free: also when he is free from distraction, so that a quiet room is desirable. The patient is asked to visualize and as far as possible to relive the original source of his symptom. When free association is in full swing he often goes off into a semi-dissociated hypnoidal state, detached from his present surroundings and living in the original experience with all its emotional force.

These visualizations sometimes come out merely as emotionless objective pictures without personal reference. It is more satisfactory if the patient visualizes *himself* experiencing them. But it is most satisfactory if the patient not only visualizes, but experiences and *feels* himself undergoing them, for in analysis it is the release and reassociation of emotion which is the essential factor. We feel now as Freud did originally, that the emotional release in some form or another is necessary to a successful cure, whether the release is effected in relation to the original experience, in transference, or in relation to present-day situations.[1]

In many cases the imagined picture is an elaboration based on actual experience. Many of the imagined sexual assaults of early childhood are not true to fact, as Freud said: nevertheless that

[1] Freud insisted that the patient should say whatever comes into his mind, however insignificant, however repugnant and unpleasant, and however untrue it may appear to be. It is this last which we always find it necessary to emphasize, for the patient will inevitably try to *remember* what happened and the more he tries the more the memory eludes him—like trying to catch a pigeon—whereas if the imagination is given free rein without our bothering whether the experiences are true or not, the complexes will of themselves be released into consciousness, and the memories of the real experiences will emerge. It may be objected that as we do not stress the truth of these imaginations they may be quite fictitious. Sometimes they are and this is a matter that must be cleared up later; but even so there must be some reason why these specific imaginations came to mind; they probably reveal some complex, even if it does not represent some objective experience. There must be some reason why a patient sees herself being thrashed by her father, if in fact she never was thrashed: the imagination obviously refers to some complex within her, perhaps a masochism, perhaps self-pity. The visualization is a psychological fact, even if it is not an objective fact.

does not mean they are pure imagination, for they are often found to be partly based on fact, and later elaborated. We are not, therefore, justified in jumping to the conclusion as Freud did that these were simply infantile sexual wishes. As we have already said, a little girl who has a "ride" on her father's knee will be sexually aroused towards him, and in adolescence when her sexuality matures this can easily be interpreted in analysis or in dreams as sexual intercourse with her father. A combination of early fact and later interpretation account for many an Oedipus or Electra myth.

On the other hand, what appears as a memory of some past experience may be discredited by the patient as absurd and impossible, and later turn out to be quite true. It is natural that the patient should regard as incredible what he has previously repressed as unpleasant and refused to acknowledge.

Free association works on the principle that if you give a man enough rope he will hang himself; if you give his thoughts free play, it will inevitably lead to his complexes. In brief, *the chief value of free association is that it is not free!* It is free in the sense that it is not consciously directed as in ordinary thinking; but it is not free in that it is fatally determined by the underlying and often unconscious complex.

In an attempt to recover the repressed and forgotten experiences there are factors working for and others against the emergence of these repressed complexes.[1]

Modern psychopathology can never be sufficiently grateful to Freud for the discovery of the method of free association and of the mechanisms such as conflict, repression, unconscious motivation and symptom formation as the expression of a repressed wish. But that does not necessarily mean that, with further investigation, we need accept all his theories and interpretations as to the origins of psychopathic states. Freud, like a truly scientific investigator,

---

[1] *In favour* of bringing these complexes into consciousness is the fact (a) that the patient wants to get well, and must therefore be prepared to meet the unpleasant in himself and make sacrifices; (b) there is also the fact already mentioned that these complexes are all emotionally charged, though under repression, and therefore contain in themselves the urge to expression, even against the repression which keeps them down. *Against* the emergence of these complexes is the fact (a) that the patient does not like to face unpleasant experiences, or to be made to recognize his vanity, egotism or sensuality, or sense of guilt. (b) More unconsciously he is unwilling to lose the advantage which the symptoms themselves bring, the sympathy which he gets for his nervous headache, the relief from responsibility which the anxiety attack gives him, the self-pity he derives from his sense of grievance. Like the man possessed of devils in the Gospels he says, "Let us alone! What have we to do with Thee!" It is this resistance which free association is designed to overcome.

changed his own views in the light of further fact, as when he accepted aggression as well as sex as a primary factor.

There are, therefore, many who starting off with the methods of Freud have not followed him either in his later methods or in his theories. Historically these have included Jung, Adler, Stekel and others. These psychologists are therefore not psychoanalysts, nor would they be accredited as such by the psychoanalysts themselves; but most of them are analysts.

The term *analysis*, as used in psychological medicine, is a term particularly applied to the investigation of the *unconscious causes of a neurosis*, especially the predisposing causes in early childhood, but also as in Jung's analytical psychology, of the present-day unconscious problems.

Psychoanalysis is one form of analysis specific to the Freudian discipline. It is used, now of a technique or method of investigation, now of a form of treatment of the psychoneuroses, now of a body of knowledge as discovered by that method; so we speak of psychoanalytic methods; of a person being cured by psychoanalysis, and we read that "psychoanalysis teaches" us certain truths. As a technique *psychoanalysis may be described as the use of free association to overcome the resistance by means of the transference*. But whereas the use of free association is the classical method of the Freudians, we gather that their method has become in practice more and more an interpretive one, the analyst suggesting to the patient the interpretation of his symptoms, dreams and behaviour. This is justifiable if one is sure of one's ground.

As we have stated, our own position is that we accept in the main Freud's mechanisms as providing the most convenient explanation of mental processes found in the psychoneuroses, such as conflict, repression and projection; and we use free association on his lines. But our use of these methods has led us to conclusions regarding the psychopathology of the neuroses different from Freud's, as set out in the previous chapters. Our methods also differ from his in that we do not analyse by means of the transference, and use dreams only as a second line of interpretation, preferring to discover the actual incidents and experiences, especially in early childhood, which caused the disorder. This method we call direct reductive analysis.

DIRECT REDUCTIVE ANALYSIS

It is no part of our purpose to give a detailed account of our technique, but some description is necessary of the methods by which we have arrived at the psychopathology described in the preceding chapters, and to indicate the process of cure. We style our method direct reductive analysis: it is *reductive* in that we analyse back to the deep-seated and predisposing causes as well as the more recent precipitating causes; and it is *direct* in that we deal directly with those experiences and not primarily by the symbolic interpretation of dreams, nor by means of the "transference."

Almost all psychopathologists are agreed that the psychoneuroses date back to experiences in early childhood. Our aim in direct reductive analysis is first by means of free association *to discover the experiences which originated the psychoneurotic disorders*; secondly, to break up the complexes then formed; thirdly, to release the repressed emotional tendencies; and fourthly, to direct them to the higher uses of the personality. Reductive analysis therefore is not merely diagnostic, it is at the same time therapeutic; it aims not merely to abolish the symptom, but by releasing repressed emotions, to permit them to develop and so to restore the whole personality to health and happiness.

The whole skill in analytic treatment is the skill with which we are able to get free associations from our patients. Once this is secured it is possible to bring all these earlier experiences to light. The student should therefore study the technique of free association as assiduously and as carefully as he does his operative technique in surgery. By means of free association, experiences of infancy, even in the first year of life, may be revived. We say "revived" advisedly and not "remembered," for the patient does not remember the happening as we remember what occurred yesterday, but they are *relived*, and sometimes with such vividness that the patient cannot doubt that the reproduction is the revival of a real experience.[1] Moreover such emotional revival often brings about a sense of relief, which confirms its authenticity.

The starting point of our analysis is the symptom. It is the symptom of which the patient complains; it is the symptom he wants cured; it is by dealing with the symptom therefore that we shall best secure his co-operation in analysis. *The symptom is the royal road to the deep-seated causes of the disorder; the epitome of the disorder in the personality.* It is not that we consider the symptom to be the real disease, nor its abolition the complete cure, for the patient is not cured until his whole personality is restored to health. But the symptom is the end product of more deep-seated disturbances, the resultant of the underlying com-

[1] See "The Reliability of Infantile Memories," *Lancet*, June 16, 1928.

plexes which beset the personality, the manifestation in conscious life of unconscious disturbances, and, like the bubbles on the surface of the ocean, direct us to the wreckage below. Not only so but the symptom is a reflection of the complexities of the disturbances in the personality itself, and gives us a clue to their nature and to the experiences which gave rise to them.

A man, for instance, has a sexual fetishism for boots: but they must be button boots, or military lace-up boots, and black of the Derby pattern, and rough such as a chauffeur wears, but not too rough, and of a certain texture, with hooks for lacing. These characteristics do not come, as one might imagine, from one experience in which such a boot figured, but each feature goes back to a different sensuous experience in childhood, which it symbolizes, and all of which contribute to his present symptom. In one he had a ride on his father's boot, which stimulated his sex feelings to which he resorted when he was in a mood of loneliness; the blackness related to the black nipple of his feeding bottle from which he got sensuous comfort; the buttons of the boots and the hooks of the lace boots were also symbols of the nipple; the round shape and texture of the boots, especially the calf of the high boots, were reminiscent of his mother's breast in infancy, and the smell of the leather reminiscent of the body smell. On the other hand, the roughness and the military nature of the boots related to a manliness which was lacking in his personality repressed by his sensuousness. All these were related to emotional experience, and all were revealed by free association from the patient and by no interpretation from the analyst. The symptom, therefore, apart from symbolizing sensual objects, epitomizes this basic conflict in his personality, between his infantile sensuousness and his need to grow up.

The cure of the symptom is valuable as an index of cure; for although it is true you may cure the symptom (as by suggestion) without solving the basic personality problem, you may be sure that if the symptom or any part of it is not cured, you have not solved the problem.

Further, *we take only the symptoms of which the patient complains*, and not what we may see to be his symptom. If he comes complaining of an inferiority complex, it is for that we treat him although it may be obvious that he really has an enormous conceit of himself; he will discover this for himself during analysis and be the more convinced. If the patient suffers from the feeling that people dislike him, we do not try to convince him to the contrary by bringing evidence of his obvious popularity, but accept his symptom, and leave it to the analysis to discover whether it is in fact so, and if so why, or whether his feeling of being disliked may be based on the fact that he expects to be universally loved. Though moral considerations play a large part in mental health and in mental disease, the physician's attitude during analysis should be one of moral detachment, lest he be identified with the patient's super-ego. So when a man complains that he is impotent with his mistress, though not with his wife, we pass no moral judgment, which it may be the function of the priest to do, but treat him for the impotence of which he complains, which ultimately, however, proves to be due to an unconscious sense of guilt, which he has refused to acknowledge till now. He is thus led to face the moral issue, which is perhaps more effective than passing moral judgment on him.

Starting with the symptom, then, we carry the patient back by free association to the *precipitating cause*, that is to say, to the moment when the symptom first emerged; it may be a month ago, it may be fifty years. The patient may not remember this, in which case we start on the first time which comes to his mind and associate back till he discovers the original precipitation of the symptom. The precipitating experience is always important because *it contains the elements of the basic conflict* which produced the symptom, such as the conflict between anger and fear, or sex and shame. The girl who has the panic of leaving home discovers that it appeared for the first time in adolescence when she was away for a week and alone for the first time, but recovering the experience she realizes that she then had a guilty sex desire, which was fraught with dread and made her fear the consequences of leaving home. The patient who had a headache at 11 o'clock each morning discovered it originated when it was announced to his regiment that they were to go overseas to France, when fear struggled with his sense of duty. The conflict comes to a head in the precipitating experience, and it is there that we shall best discover the nature of the conflict.

The analysis of the precipitating cause may be enough to reveal the basic personality problem and cure the patient. But in most cases it is necessary to trace it further back to its *predisposing* cause in early childhood, and it is here that memory particularly fails and resort must be had to real skill in free association.

Predisposing causes may go right back to infancy, and experiences even in the first few months may be revived in free association. But the causes of any neurotic condition may be indefinite in number, and it is impossible to analyse them all out. Fortunately this is not necessary. For therapeutic purposes we aim particularly at discovering and analysing what we have termed *Nuclear incidents,* that is to say those experiences in which the individual makes a complete change in his attitude of mind; from being aggressive, he becomes docile; from being full of hate, he becomes afraid; from having a craving for love, he becomes embittered, from being emotional he becomes stoic and indifferent. Those experiences are the turning points of his life; for therein he represses one attitude and adopts another and different one. Many instances of such a change have been mentioned. The nuclear incident itself is usually of causal significance, and is of importance in producing this change of attitude. In other cases it is only the last straw, the culmination of a series of experiences; but even so it is of significance in revealing the basic conflict and in giving the key to the patient's complexes.

The value of concentrating on the nuclear incident is that it reveals (a) what was repressed, (b) why it was repressed, (c) by what it was repressed, and (d) in favour of what attitude it was repressed. But most important of all, it brings about a therapeutic result; for the result of reliving the nuclear experiences is that the emotions which were there repressed are released, and so bring about the cure we desire.

We may discover the nuclear incident either by tracing a symptom or attitude of mind backwards to its origin; or by tracing forward a known earlier attitude. The patient may, for instance, know that he was natural and spontaneous at about three, but moody with a serious sense of responsibility say at five, in which case we may trace the former forwards or the latter backwards to discover the moment at which the change took place and why.

In analysis, therefore, we spend a great deal of time upon the nuclear incident considering that it is the key to the change in our personality, the discovery of the causes of repression and the means of liberating repressed complexes.

When we have discovered a nuclear incident it is necessary that the whole of the experience should be revived, both of the repressed emotion and of the resulting attitude of mind. Many a failure in analysis has been due to leaving behind some part of the complex, with the result that the patient improves but does not get completely well. A patient, for instance, had the whole experience of being blown up except the awful moment when he lay on the ground not daring to move because he thought his neck was broken. When the last bit was recovered, he immediately and completely recovered. It is like getting bits of shrapnel out of a wound which cannot heal until the last bit is removed. It is necessary therefore to go through the nuclear incident a number of times in analysis, partly because on different occasions different emotional attitudes are experienced: but also to make sure that all the emotions and reactions have been released. These changing attitudes towards the incidents and the changing stories of the patient make it appear that the incident cannot be true; but the fact that a patient one day feels hatred for the mother and the next day a deep yearning for her does not prove that either is false: he may have felt them consecutively or even both at the same time.

The analysis of the actual experience in early life is a more effective method of releasing the repressed emotions than by means of the transference, and *this revival of the actual emotion is necessary to the process of reconditioning it*. The release of the emotion may be slight, and is certainly not always as dramatic as some of the illustrations quoted in this and other books, but it must take place, however mildly, if a new orientation is to take place. It is therefore very necessary that in reproducing these experiences the patient should not only visualize them, but be made to feel them. It is one thing for the woman patient suffering from sickness to know the fact that she was disgusted with sex on an occasion when she was assaulted by an older brother, but it is necessary for her to revive and relive not only those feelings of disgust and nausea, before she can readjust herself to the whole incident and experience the sense of relief which this brings, but also the repressed feelings of sexual pleasure which she experienced and which unconsciously perpetuates the symptom. These sex feelings now being released from repression will then develop into normal sexuality.

The results of analysing out the nuclear incidents are varied.

(a) By analysing the nuclear incident the symptom may disappear. The headache vanishes, the fear disappears, and the patient finds the strain is relieved, he is sleeping better and has more confidence. Explain it as we will, the relief which results from the abreaction of the original experience as described by Breuer and Freud is a fact too frequently experienced to be set down to chance. This is the more surprising as we should have expected that this raking up of the past would only make the patient worse, which indeed sometimes occurs. But when the man with paralysis and headache relives the *whole* experience of being blown up his symptoms usually disappear.

(b) But instead of making him better the analysis of the nuclear incidents may make him temporarily worse. Indeed he usually gets worse before he gets better: he is thrown into a greater state of distress, his anxiety becomes more overwhelming, he becomes more truculent, selfish, irritable, defiant and rebellious; the compulsions to obsessional acts grow more active, the headaches more acute. If it is depression, he feels everything is going wrong, life is not worth living (although in fact it is no different from yesterday) and everything is overcast with gloom: he bemoans the degradation of world politics, the decadence of sport, the futility of marriage.

It is not surprising that at this point in the analysis the friends and relatives of the patient point out the harm that analysis has done: "they told him so"; and the patient himself complains that he is feeling worse. This sudden change in his character surprises the patient and his friends more than it does the analyst who has come to expect it.

The reasons are obvious: we have aroused up emotional conflicts, which have previously been repressed; and as they were repressed because they were distressing we must expect them to be distressing when they are revived. These changes in analysis are in fact a good sign; it means that things are moving, that we are touching on important conflicts. We do not mind whether the patient is getting better or getting worse; what we do dislike is when nothing happens! But if the patient is left in that disturbed state, or gives up analysis at this point, he remains, for some time at least, worse than when he started. A patient having an abdominal operation is worse than before it started, and we do not stop half-way through with his abdomen open. Analytic work is more akin to surgery, whilst suggestion is more akin to medicine.

During the release of these repressed tendencies the analyst is in the paradoxical position of having to encourage the expression of tendencies and feelings like self-pity, bitterness and hatred, which are certainly not ultimately desirable; but it is disastrous for the physician to disapprove these feelings for it is necessary that the patient should give expression to them. But this does not mean that the patient need give expression to them in common life; indeed this would only give rise to further complications. What is necessary is *psychological* expression during analysis and in relation to the original experience, not objective expression in present-day life, nor even to the analyst.

(c) As we proceed with the analysis *new symptoms emerge*; the indigestion goes but the repressed anxiety which caused it comes, depression is cured, but abnormal sex emerges, the ingratiating person becomes bitter, and the arrogant person full of self-pity. Instead of being the clinging, helpless, fear-ridden object, acquiescent and amenable person, the patient begins to be obstinate, rebellious, domineering, selfish, impatient, sulky, hateful, irritable and querulous. He sees himself in his true colours and does not like it. These new symptoms arise from various sources:

(i) They may arise from the complex itself which we are analysing, feelings which have been repressed but which are being released now that the repressing force has been removed. For instance, in the case of the girl assaulted by her brother; first she experienced the sickness, then the fear, then the sex feelings which this fear was repressing with disgust, then finally the anger she felt towards him. It is like peeling off the layers of an onion.

(ii) But very commonly the new symptom *anticipates the analysis*. Symptoms cast their shadows before, and we experience between treatments what is going to emerge in the following treatment. It is an almost invariable rule, corroborated in most cases of analysis, that the new symptom that appears between two sessions of analysis corresponds to the next phase in the nuclear incident we are analysing out. All we need to do, therefore, is to continue with the analysis of the original nuclear experience and we shall almost always discover the source of the new symptom.

(iii) In other cases the patient may lose his symptom of sickness or fear, feels well and says he requires no more treatment; for this newly released assertiveness fills him with confidence. But this may only be temporary, a phase of the liberation. It may leave him over-confident, but after a few days new symptoms arise and he feels himself too sensitive to people's criticism, too anxious to get their approval, and unreasonably depressed if he feels that people are against him. This relates to deeper layers as yet unanalysed, and further analysis is therefore called for. It is a warning not to break off the analysis too soon even if the patient feels fit.

(iv) When during analysis of the nuclear incidents experiences of the past are revived, the liberated emotions, such as repressed love, cravings, depression, self-pity, jealousy, sex feelings, hate and bitterness, are naturally apt to be *transferred to people and situations of the present*. The patient becomes truculent with his employer or irritable with his wife, rude to the analyst, antagonistic towards his children, towards God, and even towards himself. If it is love that is emerging he craves for affection from the analyst, wants to be his only care, jealous of other patients, feels that his own family do not care for him, is filled with self-pity. If he is feeling elation he feels "on top of the world" and nothing can go wrong. The absurdity of these feelings may be realized by the patient, but he cannot help it: but in other cases the feelings may be so real and overwhelming that for the time being his life is entirely coloured and dominated by them, and he believes in their reality; he has in fact become temporarily "psychotic" in the sense that he is dominated by these morbid emotions, lacks insight, and cannot distinguish fantasy from reality. This creates a serious difficulty in treatment.[1]

[1] *Transference.* When the need for love, the anger, obstinacy, and hate direct themselves against the physician himself, this is the "transference" which according to Freud is the displacement of affect on to a person to whom it does not properly belong. In the course of the analysis the patient is indifferent to the analyst, then hates him, then loves him, then feels he is callous, then tries to dominate him. In cases of *positive* transference the patient is irrationally attached to the physician, feels that there is nobody like him in skill, in understanding, in sympathy, and has towards him a feeling of dependence, of admiration, of love and like Titania, being given the love potion, feels amorous towards the most unattractive and endows him with the most godlike qualities. In *negative* transference no words can express her loathing for him, her desire to revenge herself on him. She snubs him, expresses her hate of him, tries to humiliate him, and threatens him. All this is due to the liberation of emotions from complexes which belong to early childhood. This obstinacy was expressed by one patient, who, when asked to associate on a certain symptom, said, "The first words that come to my mind are 'Be damned if I do!' "

Owing to the nature of the disorders a "positive transference" is more liable to occur in conversion hysteria, since dependence and the personal need for love are more characteristic of this condition; whilst a "negative transference" is particularly liable to happen in obsessional states, since self-will and obstinacy are characteristic features of the obsessions.

Transference is important not only as a phenomenon affecting analysis, but because it is used by the psychoanalysts as a means of liberating the repressed affect: they analyse "by means of the transference," that is to say by encouraging the patient to let off these feelings towards the physician.

Freud's attitude to the transference may be summarized in these quotations. He says in his *Autobiography* (p. 74) that "In every analytic treatment there arises an intense emotional relationship between the patient and the physician." "An analysis without transference is an impossibility" (p. 75. See also *Introd. Lectures,* p. 372). "Nevertheless its handling remains the most difficult part of the technique of analysis."

The difficulty arises whether the transference is positive or negative. If it is a positive love transference the patient may claim a superabundance of attention which the physician cannot give and feels slighted at the most trifling signs of disapproval and indifference, real or imaginary. Or, wanting the love of the physician, the patient will be unwilling to reveal the things about himself which are unpleasant or shameful for fear of losing his approval, so that free association is hindered and analysis prolonged. If the transference is negative the patient is rebellious, antagonistic, obstinate against the analyst, and may refuse to continue the analysis. If you press him to go on with the analysis, he will obstinately refuse: if you leave him alone he remains obstinately silent, and then complains that you are wasting his time and money. Any sympathy will be repelled; any lack of sympathy will be resented. But though the patient may for a time refuse to continue treatment, he almost always returns, realizing the irrationality of his resentment, and the hopelessness of his case without treatment.

Another difficulty in analysis by means of the transference is that whereas

The essential difference between the technique of psychoanalysis and that of direct reductive analysis is that the former liberates the emotion by means of the transference to the physician, whereas in direct reductive analysis we liberate it by going back to the original experiences which gave rise to it, and in which it was originally repressed, and release it towards the person or experiences to whom it properly belongs. In other words we attach the fear, depression, anger or love craving to *their proper objects.* This has the added advantage that the emotion is released with much greater intensity than by its vicarious expression towards the analyst, and a readjustment to the situation is more effective.

Transference is the displacement of affect to a person *to whom it does not properly belong*: then why not relate it directly to the person *to whom it properly belongs?* It is, as Freud has said, a morbid condition, a form of neurosis; then why not avoid it, and

transference is a personal relationship, many of the experiences of early childhood which produce psychoneurotic symptoms are not of a personal kind, but related to situations other than persons, experiences like terror from falling, starvation, suffocation, or again feelings of depression which arise from digestive troubles, a very common source of psychoneurotic depression. Reductive analysis deals directly with these. To those who find the cause of every psychoneurosis in the Oedipus complex, the treatment by means of the transference is a logical and convincing method: but to those of us who do not see in this complex the universal source of all the psychoneuroses, such a method neglects many important issues. This difference in technique represents a different point of view. The significant fact for us is the emotion itself which the patient is experiencing, whether fear, anger, love or self-pity, not the person towards whom the emotion is directed which is of secondary importance. We prefer, for instance, to speak of what the child is experiencing of love or hate, rather than say that it may be a mother complex.

A further difficulty is that transference may be used by the patient as a means of evading the unpleasant experiences of the past by attaching the emotion to the analyst, and in analysing by means of the transference we are often playing into the hands of the patient.

It is at the stage of negative transference that the analyst is most likely to reveal his own complexes and become impatient, irritable, and cast the blame on the patient for the obstruction in treatment, as though it is something for which the patient is responsible and as though he were being deliberately obstinate. For the analyst to be severe or annoyed with so recalcitrant a patient (as he may well be since the patient has a shrewd intuition into the weak points of the analyst's character) is to mishandle the situation, for it simply reproduces the situation of lack of love which in childhood first made the patient aggressive and obstinate: it also satisfies the patient's sense of power that he has succeeded in rattling the doctor.

It is not surprising then, as has been suggested by Freud, that the handling of the transference is the most difficult part of analysis and may actually prevent the complexes from emerging. Suttie (*The Origins of Love and Hate,* p. 221) has pointed out that patients are hindered from getting down to the deeper layers of experience in relations with the mother because they have clung to the father attachment in him, which is the very objection which Freud raised to the treatment under hypnosis. The transference has made the deeper layers of the individual's experience inaccessible even to the psychoanalysts.

with it avoid the complications and difficulties incidental to the attachment of these morbid emotions to the physician.

We do not of course deny that transference is an effective method of releasing repressed emotions or else it would not have been successfully used all these years by the psychoanalysts; although in our experience it both complicates and prolongs the treatment. Nor do we deny that transference occurs even in direct reductive analysis. But it is one thing to recognize it as a phenomenon, and another to employ it as a technique for the release of repressed emotions. Freud himself did not use it in his original work which was undoubtedly successful. In the majority of our cases the analysis has been conducted through from the beginning to end without any reference to the transference relationships since we keep the emotions related to the proper objects to which they originally belonged.

Transitory transferences commonly occur from the simple fact that in analysis we are releasing emotions and cravings, and these naturally fix themselves on the nearest person, namely the analyst, especially as it is he who has aroused them. But when such transference occurs, we immediately take the patient back to the experience in early childhood which gave rise to the hate, jealousy, sex or love, and encourage him to let off his feelings towards the person to whom they really belong. This as a rule is not difficult, because the specific emotion almost invariably arises from the nuclear incident we are at the time analysing.

In some cases we do not succeed in doing this and the tranference has become more "fixed" on to the analyst. A review of these cases, however, shows that such transference is particularly liable to happen under certain circumstances; namely where the analyst has any kind of personal, social or business relationship with the patient, such as by the acceptance of gifts, or the giving of hospitality; or if the patient is an acquaintance or friend; but especially in the "training analysis" of a fellow physician or colleague with whom the analyst has other day-to-day and perhaps professional contacts.

Where such transference occurs, as it occasionally does for these reasons, we regard it as a failure in technique; and it is then necessary to analyse out the transference itself as a symptom, as in the psychoanalytic mode.

We therefore regard the transference not merely as a neurosis but as a mistake; and agree with Jung that transference is "neither necessary nor desirable."

The fact that we do not analyse by means of the transference does not mean that personality does not count in analysis, for this must occur in any clinical work; but the more perfect the technique the less do personal factors come into the situation. Direct reductive analysis is a technique which reduces the personal factor to a minimum since it deals with objective experiences of the past from which the present-day problems arise. Therefore, although analysts necessarily differ in the skill with which they carry out the technique (as is true of any medical work) reductive analysis is one which anyone can carry out by himself without any special gifts; as any doctor can be trained in the technique of doing an appendicitis operation, although they may differ in the individual skill with which they carry it out.

In all analysis the personal factor is still further excluded by the analyst himself being analysed, which helps him to rid himself of prejudice and preconceived ideas, whether of a moral, intellectual or emotional type, due to his own complexes, and enables him to regard the patient's emotional attitudes in an objective way.

A healthy rapport between patient and physician is desirable if the treatment is to be successful. Such a feeling of confidence is not "transference," nor, like transference, is it a neurosis. It is a natural and biologically valuable relationship, similar to the confidence of the patient in the surgeon who operates on him: it is directed to the physician, not so much as a person, but as skilled in his work and willing to help him. To keep it on that plane is part of the technique of the analyst.

The term transference should not therefore be used, as it frequently is, of *any* affective relationship of the patient to the physician, such as gratitude to him, or even a dislike of him, which may be quite normal, but only of the transference to him of emotions which do not properly belong to him, as Freud says.

The personal relation of analyst and patient. What then is to be this attitude of the analyst to the patient? Is he to be entirely detached? Is the motive of the psycho-physician, as some say, to be nothing but scientific interest? Every analyst must take up the attitude that is natural to him, and it is useless to assume an attitude that is not sincere; for the psychoneurotic, because of his tendency to introspection, usually has a shrewd insight into the psychology of the physician and it is useless to try to bluff him. The analyst must be natural if he expects the patient to be forthcoming.

The physician must also believe in his patient who has usually ceased to believe in himself: he must see his potentialities. The physician who despises his patient as a "neurotic" or "weakling" will not help him much. We must see the patient not as he is but as he is capable of being: we must believe in him if we are to lead him to believe in himself. *The patient is cured by the faith of the physician in him.* Otherwise he would never persevere in his analysis.

The attitude we find most conducive to efficiency in treatment is one of *understanding sympathy.* This is demanded of the physician not only on humanitarian grounds because the patient is sick and in need of help, but because a completely disinterested or still more an impatient attitude will discourage the patient, and produce poor results. *The patient,* as has been said, *is cured by the love of the physician.* The detached attitude necessarily adopted by the physician who spends years in attending incurable psychotics in a mental hospital is therefore not the best approach to the treatment of the psychoneuroses, for the treatment of the psychoneuroses requires that the physician enters into the feelings of his patient. Indeed, it is more necessary for the physician to be *en rapport* with his patient, than that the patient should have a transference to the physician.

But there are other and more technical grounds for such sympathetic understanding, for it is in such an atmosphere that the patient will most easily bring out his complexes and give expression to his feelings. All neurotics, according to our view, are fundamentally suffering from a feeling of deprivation of love: only in an atmosphere of sympathy therefore can such feelings be released. The patient is reluctant to wear his heart on his sleeve for the unsympathetic analyst to peck at.

But whilst the physician requires to have sympathetic understanding, it is important that such sympathy should not be too active or too personal; for that is the most direct road to a positive transference. What is required is rather an *atmosphere* of sympathy. If the sympathy is too active the patient's attention is directed towards the person of the analyst rather than to the causes of the disorder, which is precisely what we wish to avoid. He prefers to remain in the oasis of sympathy instead of progressing to a life of self-dependence.

Whilst analysis should therefore be conducted in an atmosphere of sympathy, it is also true, as someone has said, that analysis must be conducted in an atmosphere of deprivation. Both are necessary to bring out complexes.

When the near relations of a person suffering from neurosis ask, as they frequently do, what attitude they should adopt, one can only comfort them by telling them what they have already discovered, that whatever they do is wrong! This is because owing to the duality in his personality, whichever part of his nature they try to satisfy, it is bound to be opposed by the other part of his personality. In the case of an hysteric whose pain is due to a repressed craving for sympathy: if we give him plenty of sympathy it encourages his self-pity: if we are severe with him and tell him to pull himself together, we are reproducing the very conditions which produced the original repression, and he gets worse. Only analysis can solve this problem by resolving the duality. But the relative, like the physician, should err on the side of sympathy, for it is fundamentally on account of the feeling of lack of affection that the patients are what they are, and to deny them further affection is to drive them back into their neurosis. But all the sympathy in the world will not cure their neurosis.

The analysis of the super-ego. Commonly, with the release of the repressed emotions, the super-ego is swept away: the war-shocked man who relives his terror when blown up can no longer maintain his phantasy that he knows no fear; the obsessional girl whose hate is released can no longer maintain the attitude of the sweet martyr. But sometimes in spite of this the super-ego does not go, but may persist side by side with the released emotions, so that not only does this lead to greater distress of mind temporarily, but as long as the super-ego persists in regarding these tendencies as wrong or shameful, there is little chance of their being properly freed and sublimated to the use of the personality. The patient holds on to the super-ego as the one thing necessary: yet it is the one thing most necessary to modify, if the repressed tendencies which cause the symptoms are to be released. In the psycho-neuroses it is not only the symptom but the super-ego which is abnormal.

It is often necessary, therefore, in the treatment of psycho-neurotic conditions that the false super-ego should itself be shaken out of its complacency, and this means that the analysis has to be definitely directed towards it, instead of, as previously, towards releasing the repressed emotions. The girl who has been jilted assumes the attitude of haughty pride, and represses her resentment and need of affection which therefore manifest themselves as headaches. She cannot be cured as long as she persists in this attitude of disdain. In hysteria it may be just as important to get the patient to realize that his pose of independence and self-sufficiency is abnormal since it is keeping his craving for love repressed, as it is to show him that he is full of self-pity which is being repressed by his independence. The obsessional needs to have his sense of guilt revealed; but it may be as necessary to realize his morbid self-righteousness, which perpetuates his guilt.

But this analysis of the super-ego, when necessary, is often a most difficult phase in the analysis, because whereas the repressed emotions themselves assist the analysis in that they have in themselves a dynamic urge towards expression, there is no such urge in the super-ego which is a much more static attitude and concerned with the maintenance of the *status quo*. Therefore, the analyst does not get the same help from the super-ego as he does from the repressed impulses. That is why the analysis of the propitiatory obsessions, in which the super-ego is dominant, is so difficult. The difficulty in analysing the super-ego is still further complicated when it is projected on to other people. The patient feels that other people are preventing her doing what she wants, that they expect this or that of her, when in fact nobody is stopping her or expecting things of her except her own super-ego. She says she cannot bear to let other people down, when she really means that she cannot let herself down, her standards of rectitude. When the patient realizes that she can do as she likes and that no one is forbidding her doing these things except herself, then for the first time she has the power of choice, whether she chooses rightly or wrongly, and becomes for the first time a moral being instead of acting under compulsion.

A patient complained that he got tired after business, and instead of reading would go to sleep, a fact of which he was very ashamed. When he was encouraged to allow himself to go to sleep if he wanted to, he found he no longer wanted to and was no longer sleepy. His trouble was discovered to be a tough super-ego phantasy of "never being tired," and when he gave this up his repressed ego ceased to make its demands since it was now conciliated, and he therefore ceased to protest against his tyrannical super-ego by being tired.

One can best get rid of the super-ego by revealing the morbid reasons for its formation. The most direct approach to this analysis is by carrying through the nuclear incident till we discover the *resulting attitude of mind* adopted as a result of the conflict, for this often constitutes the super-ego. That is why in analysing the nuclear incident, it is most necessary to see not only what was repressed, why it was repressed, and by what it was repressed, but also to discover *in favour of what* attitude it was repressed. One of the commonest causes of disappointment in analysis is the failure to carry it through to this point and explain the falsity of the super-ego which was adopted as a result of the mental conflict. The patient will then be led to recognize the false motives which were behind them; he will see that his ingratiation was not real sociability but a selfish desire to curry favour; that his courage was bravado to cover fear; that his moral punctiliousness was for fear of punishment. He will then realize for himself that his super-ego is false, and itself his worse symptom.

Certain short cuts in treatment have been attempted. Since the super-ego is the stumbling block why can we not go straight to it and analyse it out by direct assault, instead of going round about by the symptom? For if the super-ego were got rid of, all the repressed tendencies would be released. In mild cases this is possible and when the patient can be shown that his standards are wrong and too rigorous he may be induced to abandon them and accept more natural and healthy ones, which is what the normal adolescent does. A case was given of this under Persuasion.[1]

But in most cases to attack the super-ego directly is an impossibility for the following reasons:

(a) The patient does not regard his ideals as false and cannot be persuaded that they are, and is therefore unwilling that his super-ego should be analysed and treated as if it were a symptom. To him, the super-ego is the one thing that is right, and he will refuse to co-operate in a treatment which he regards as an assault upon his personality.

Incidentally that is also why we cannot analyse ourselves completely. *Self-analysis* can proceed quite satisfactorily as long as it is a process of introspection; we can analyse out our own complexes by tracing back our symptom, by applying the principle of projection, over-compensation, and the rest, as a clue to the abnormality. But when the time comes for the analyst to put *himself* in the melting-pot, to analyse out his own super-ego, it is tantamount to committing psychological suicide! We cannot pursue an analysis and at the same time maintain a balanced judgment with a mind, the reliability of whose standards of judgment is being called in question!

(b) A second reason why the patient refuses to let go his super-ego is that it was originally formed to deliver him from a most distressing conflict: and to abandon it would be to fall back into these dreaded fears, that deep depression, that awful rage. Even when in analysis he sees the abnormality of his super-ego it often requires a considerable act of faith to let it go; but when in fact he does let go he experiences a great sense of relief, since the conflict is thereby resolved.

Bringing the analysis up-to-date. Having now discovered the root cause of the trouble, we bring the analysis up-to-date. A neurosis though originating in the past is due to residues left in

[1] P. 392.

the patient's present personality and problems: our object in treatment is to go into the past to discover the origins and there find the key to the present trouble; and having discovered it open the door to the problems of our present-day pains, fears and obsessions. A patient having discovered that in early childhood he deliberately made use of a pain to get the sympathy he wanted from his mother is brought to see that unconsciously he is doing the same thing now with his wife, and that each time he gets the hysteric pain it is because this same motive is at work. Having once seen it in the past he cannot very well deny it in the present, however distasteful: indeed, one of the advantages of going into the past is that a patient is more willing to admit these things in his childhood, but having done so is compelled to admit that it is still true.

Similarly with the release of emotion: when we release the emotional responses repressed in childhood, we are of course really releasing them at the present day. The patient who feels angry with the nurse in a childhood experience, is releasing these feelings, whereby the repression is removed which has in the past, as in the present, been keeping him from normal expression of assertiveness in life. When therefore we speak of going into past experiences, it is not really the past, but the dispositions and complexes left behind by those past experiences, which persist and affect the mind at the present. It is in the depths of the present psychology of the individual where lie the morbid springs of action. But these are derived from the past and can best be elucidated by going to their origins in the past.

It is important therefore that the patient should come to realize that *the dynamic process which perpetuates the neurosis always belongs to the present*, however much it may be caused by experiences of the past. It is because we *still* have these morbid feelings within us that the neurosis is perpetuated. We then realize that they are no longer applicable; but if they are we deal with the present-day causes.

Analysis, therefore, makes us face up to our moral responsibilities and forces us to make moral decisions. Analysis does not absolve us from the difficulties of life nor from the exercise of our will, but by getting rid of our complexes it makes us capable of making these moral decisions and accepting our responsibilities.

THE RATIONALE OF CURE

It is curious that so few of those who actually treat and cure these disorders stop to consider *what it is that cures*. Various theories and various objections to analysis have been raised. How can knowing the cause cure? What is the use of raking up the past? it will only make the patient worse. Why make the patient more introspective? he is already introspective enough! These and such objections are natural enough and indeed partially justified.

Indeed so obvious are these objections that there must be some reason why analysts persist in what appears to be so irrational a method of treatment. That reason is the incontestible fact that by the reliving of the experiences of the past which caused the neurosis, the patient gets well, as is dramatically illustrated in traumatic cases like "shell-shock." But how and why does he get well?

Temporarily it is true that analysis makes a person more introspective: indeed analysis is a process of introspection. But *introspection is nature's method of compelling us to face our inner problems;* its true function is to solve them. Introspection and self-consciousness are not in themselves morbid processes: they raise man above the lower animals in enabling him to observe, judge and therefore alter his behaviour. *Morbid introspection* occurs when it fails to solve the problem. The psychoneurotic has a problem which he cannot solve because he does not know what it is and therefore suffers from morbid introspection. Analysis is a method of *effective introspection*, by means of which the patient discovers the causes, solves his problem and thereafter ceases to be introspective.

(i) *The discovery of the cause of the neurosis* is the first step in radical treatment. But the objection is immediately raised. "Does knowing the cause cure?" Sometimes in fact it does, but usually it does not. Suppose a patient could be told exactly in detail all that happened to him when he was blown up, it would not cure his war neurosis. A patient may accept the fact that he has an "Oedipus" complex, a sexual fixation to his mother, but still retains his headache, phobia or obsession. That is the weakness of interpreting the cause to the patient. It is like seeing a joke; it always seems a poor one if it has to be explained. The pleasure is in seeing it for oneself. The mere discovery of the cause may simply stir up a patient's complexes and make him worse, as we have seen.

(ii) *Release of emotion.* According to the original Freudian *theory of catharsis* the mere letting off of the repressed emotion itself produced the cure, just as purging the body got rid of the toxins, and opening up the abscess let out the pus.

There is much to support this idea, for anyone who has seen a shell-shocked soldier go through the throes of being blown up, experience all the fear and then emerge with a sense of relief and his symptom gone, would naturally come to the conclusion that it was this release of bottled-up emotion alone which produced the cure.

But the objection is often raised "What is the use of raking up the past?—it will only make the patient worse. Why not let sleeping dogs lie?" There is in fact plenty of evidence that "raking up the past" may *temporarily* make the patient worse as we should expect. But if experience goes for anything there is one incontestable fact, already mentioned, and proved by innumerable cases treated by analysts all over the world, that when the experiences which originally produced the complexes are completely revived, and the emotions contained in them released, it is sometimes *immediately* followed by the disappearance of the symptom, proving that the cure was the direct result of the treatment. The explanation may be in doubt, the fact is incontestable. We also should have expected with the critics that raking up the past would only make the patient worse; in fact it often has the opposite effect; it makes him well.

This is confirmed by cures which sometimes take place spontaneously without treatment.

A soldier who lost his memory suffered from anxiety and headache. One day he wandered in London and saw a huge crane overhead and thought of its falling on him. That night he dreamt of an experience, which he had forgotten, of having been buried in a trench and next morning he wakened with his headache gone. In spite of this hint from nature as to cure, the neurologist continued to give him bromides, until he was removed to another hospital where further forgotten experiences of the war were recovered by analysis with the result that his anxiety also disappeared.

Analysis is therefore in line with nature's method.

But it is not the release of emotions alone, any more than knowing the cause, which itself cures, but the readjustment of the personality to the experience, as we may prove experimentally.

We had the case of the soldier with a shaking head, who under hypnosis had relived the whole terrifying experience of being blown up, and when wakened from his hypnosis had forgotten the incident, and so was little or no better. We have then, under hypnosis, and without further abreaction, told him he will remember what he has come through on waking, and this readjustment to conscious memory has immediately brought about a cure. Something more than the release of emotion was obviously necessary; it required to be linked up to the present mind. Freud himself recognized this when he insisted that the patient should "talk it out." This proves the inadequacy of the theory of catharsis as such.

Further, if merely letting off the repressed emotion was sufficient to produce cure, surely the patient suffering from anxiety states would be cured by the constant expression of his fear, the sex pervert by his indulgence and the man with bad temper by his constant outbursts! That is far from being the case.

The cathartic theory is partly responsible for the popular idea that analysis releases all that is undesirable in human nature, disagreeable traits that are best left alone. A humorist has remarked that the difference between Freudian analysis and others is that you go down deeper, stay down longer and come up dirtier. The humour may be appreciated without its being accepted as a just criticism either of psychoanalysis or of any other form of analysis.

The truth is that though complexes are morbid reactions, they are formed of natural impulses necessary to a healthy life and may be so used when they are released. It is unfortunate that even some psychotherapists unknowingly regard these repressed tendencies in a sorry light, and their attitude towards the patient who discovers these things is, "You now see what sort of a person you are, full of self-pity, mean, cowardly, bad-tempered," as though exposing unpleasant characteristics. That censorious attitude is bad psychotherapy in that it encourages the original repression which made these impulses express themselves only in morbid ways, and perpetuates the self-righteousness both of the patient and the physician.

Our aim in treatment is not to humiliate our patients but to give them confidence by the release and full development of all their powers. Symptoms are merely perverted potentialities. The mind of the neurotic is a veritable Pandora's box, which when opened releases all the Evils, but also Hope, the very release of these "evils" in analysis bringing with it the hope of the restoration of the personality to completeness and fulfilment.

The theory of abreaction is an advance on the theory of catharsis, although they are often identified. Catharsis is a purging; abreaction means an emotional reaction to the original situation which was then not properly reacted to: the patient now reacts to the situation as he *should* have reacted. Fear of a cruel nurse, and therefore of all in authority, is first felt, the fear being directed to its proper object, and then gives place to a reaction of resentment against her cruelty, which the patient could not give vent to as a child. The anger abolishes the fear, and the patient having thus reacted to the nurse obliterates all thought of her and relegates her to the limbo of the past. The theory of catharsis regards these emotions as something noxious to be got rid of; abreaction regards the process as a natural response of the personality to an abnormal situation.

A clergyman whose cringing attitude made him acceptable to authority but whose resentment came out as a psychoneurotic delinquency, pictured his jealous father scolding him and when the patient looked sulky shouting, "Don't look at me like that!" His first reaction to this experience in analysis was fear, weeping and depression. But going through this nuclear incident a second time his reaction is different; he sat up on the couch, his eyes still closed, and shaking his fist shouted, "I'll bl . . . dy well look at you as I like!" and thereupon lost his fear, and his personality was liberated. The principle of the "expulsive power of a new emotion" was long ago enunciated by the great Scottish preacher, though he might not have used this illustration!

This abreaction of the repressed emotion means the abolition of a morbid emotion by the release of an opposite emotion. As timidity may be swept away by the anger and resentment, so morbid resentment may be swept away by the arousal of pity or affection.

But reaction to an experience is of two kinds; reaction to the situation as we should have reacted at the time if it had been possible—that is *abreaction*; secondly, reaction to the situation as we now see it—which we may call *reassociation*.

(iii) *Reassociation and reconditioning*. This means a readjustment to the whole experience as far as it affects our *present* life. The discovery of the cause and the release of emotion is often followed by a spontaneous readjustment to the situation. The patient with bad obsessional propitiations and depressions sees himself as the pious little prig in childhood and says, "What a nauseating picture! I'd like to kick his backside!" Then realizing that he is *still* self-righteous he is disgusted with it, gets rid of it, and so loses his obsession.

But even such readjustment involves various processes of cure.

(a) In the first place, the morbid emotion is *attached to its rightful object*. In neuroses the emotion has been detached from its original object and attached to other objects and situations, the moral fear to open spaces, the sex feelings to a fetichistic object, the moral compulsions to ritual acts and the guilt to irrelevant sins. In analysis the emotion is attached to its original and proper object which is most effectively done in reductive analysis.

(b) The original cause of the emotion is then *seen to be no longer justified* however justified it may have been at the time. What terrified us in childhood and made us repress our assertiveness or sexual feelings, terrifies us no longer; what seemed most shameful under the threat of mother's disapproval is seen to be no longer so: or if it is regarded still as shameful as in the case of the prig, then we may abandon it, now that we know what it is. A woman who has the unconscious habit of scowling at everyone, although she did not know why and could not help it, attaches this to the nurse who was cruel to her. She realizes that people are not now unkind to her, so her scowl is unnecessary and is dispelled in an atmosphere of good humour.

(c) These processes of readjustment may also be put in terms of *reconditioning*. Analysis is a process of reconditioning in which all the main factors in the production of the morbid reactions are discovered and revived, and then reconditioned with healthier ideas and emotions. Thus an experience of which we were originally terribly ashamed is now seen in the light of a sense of humour. But we must realize that *we cannot adequately recondition an emotional experience without reviving it*, any more than we could condition the dog to the sound of the bell without at first putting the meat on its tongue. That is why the release of the emotion itself is necessary before reconditioning can be effective. That also is why it is not enough merely to *know* that we were badly treated, had a mother fixation, hated our father, or were made to feel shame and that these were unjustified. Explanation alone is useless unless we experience the fear, feel the shame as we originally felt it, and then reassociate them with healthier reactions of confidence, indifference or good humour.

(d) *Spontaneous development*. But what are we to do with these emotions when they are aroused? If we arouse the old feelings of hate or fear, will these feelings not get the better of us? We have difficulty enough in controlling them as it is. Analysis is often criticized on the ground that it is a breaking-up process, a pulling down; analysis, we are told, is all very well, but what about synthesis? The analyst pulls you to pieces, what about building you up again? The criticism is based on a false psychological conception, the old notion of the mind as static, built up of a number of units, which may be broken down and built up again. The modern view of the mind sees the personality as dynamic, as functions and potentialities working towards a common end. If we regard the mind statically we must follow our analysis by a building-up synthetic process. If we regard the mind dynamically, analysis is a process of release, of the liberation of repressed tendencies, which are then utilized and directed to higher forms: it is not a process of synthesis but a process of development. This is not mere theory, because one of the strangest facts in analysis is that when the causes are discovered in the original complex, and these emotions liberated, the repressed emotional tendencies *develop as they would have developed if they had never been repressed.* So there is a spontaneous development of self-pity into love, assertiveness into confidence and will-power, sex perversion into adult forms of love and sex.

The patient who had the hate of her own baby discovers that it was *originally* hate of her baby sister. "But what is the use of expressing my hate for my sister when I know she has done nothing to deserve it?" First because she transfers it back to its proper original object of hate and therefore no longer to her baby; secondly, because she realizes it was not her sister's fault, but her own need of security, which no longer applies; thirdly, because the emotion of hate being now released is tranformed into assertiveness and ultimately into will power. The woman who suffered from an exorbitant fatigue whenever she took her children out in the perambulator demonstrated by this symptom a strong repressed craving for sympathy. In the analysis she gave vent to her sobbing as she revived the sadness of her experience as a child, but instead of this increasing her self-pity, her need for love immediately and spontaneously developed into maternal love for her children, which would have happened if it had never been repressed in childhood.

The cure therefore comes about not merely as the result of the release, but of the spontaneous development of dynamic tendencies which have been arrested in development because of repression. In analysis, therefore, there is no need to synthetize: the wise physician is careful not to interfere with the developmental process. We must avoid "meddlesome analysis" as we are told to avoid "meddlesome surgery."

When therefore the question is raised, what is the use of releasing these morbid emotions, our reply is that they are only morbid because they are repressed, and if they are released they develop naturally as they should have developed, and can be used as all natural tendencies were meant to be used for the functions of the personality as a whole.

Patients often express the fear that if they release their emotional impulses, these will overmaster them. The reverse is usually the case: *properly liberated emotions can be controlled more easily than those which are repressed*: for as long as they are dissociated they are not really under control, but when they have been completely released they can be brought under the dominance of the will.

A serious difficulty of many patients is "What use is it to liberate tendencies if there is no opportunity of giving expression to them or of having them satisfied?" an objection particularly urgent in the case of the sexual instinct of the unmarried woman. The reply is first that the repression of sexuality implies discord and unhappiness in the personality, the removal of the repression brings the relief of this tension. Secondly, because only when they are released can they be adequately controlled; and thirdly, only when they are released can they be properly sublimated. But for this release it is only necessary to give *psychological* expression to these feelings of rage or sex, and not necessarily expression of them in objective life. Indeed to give such outward expression to these emotions in their primitive form may not only lead to objective complications, but to further anxiety in the personality itself. The patient deals with the released emotions in a common sense way like anyone without such repressions.[1]

It may further be asked what guarantee have we that these released emotions will be redirected to useful ends. Why should the analysed person with his unrestrained aggressions or sexual excesses released not become a delinquent? The reason is that the patient already has standards of moral conduct in his super-ego: indeed it is these which have kept repressed his primitive emotions and causes the neurosis. When therefore these emotions are liberated there are these controlling forces all ready waiting for them: and although the super-ego has to be greatly modified as a result of treatment, it is not altogether destroyed. Indeed its modification into healthy forms means that it can now accept and utilize these forces which it previously condemned: it adopts a change of

[1] The analyst cannot claim that "What the patient does outside is no concern of his," for the analyst has brought about the release of these impulses, and it is his responsibility to ensure that the patient reserves the expression of these emotions to the analysis until a readjustment is made, and does not do things which he may later regret, like having a row with his boss and losing his job, when he is releasing his anger against his father. It is therefore a rule to make that the patient should not do anything irrevocable, like getting married, whilst undergoing analysis. What he does after analysis is then truly his own responsibility, and one he willingly assumes.

attitude towards them, because it has itself changed, and directs them instead of repressing them. The psychotic, on the other hand, is constitutionally incapable of control: therefore to release these tendencies may precipitate him into a worse psychosis. That is why analysis is dangerous in the treatment of psychotics.

(e) *Sublimation* differs from development. Development is a natural spontaneous process in which primitive impulses like sex naturally pass through various phases from infancy to adult life, changing their form from time to time not primarily as a result of environmental conditions but as a result of maturation. This is most clearly seen in sexual development. But many of our natural propensities are frustrated by our environment, by social taboos, by psychological repression, and by our super-ego. Our daily work may give no outlet to our natural assertiveness or creative abilities: some women cannot marry and under present social custom have no opportunity of either married love or children although there may be no repression. Are they doomed to frustration or neurosis?

McDougall[1] and Freud have pointed out that the primitive potentialities or "instincts" can be diverted from their original ends and redirected towards social ends. This is fortunate considering that the individual has to live in a community in which his natural impulses too often conflict with the demands of society, which constitutes one of the fundamental problems of civilization, sociology, ethics and psychopathology.

Sublimation differs from natural development in that it is the redirection of our energies, conscious and unconscious, in conformity with social demands. In its simplest form, sublimation means the automatic and often unconscious expression of frustrated energy in ways not incompatible with the super-ego, thus avoiding the conflict: instead of murdering we may fell a tree. It may also occur when an impulse is aroused but, frustrated by social taboos, finds automatic outlet in ways not tabooed. So a person may tease another either from love or hate. In its highest form sublimation means that the native and even acquired dispositions are directed towards ends both satisfying to the individual and serviceable to the community.

But this lays an obligation upon society not to make too severe demands upon the individual for this must inevitably result in either repression or rebellion. It also places the community under an obligation to provide *opportunities* for the expression and sublimation of all these tendencies in human nature, if mental health and happiness are to be attained.

[1] *Social Psychology.*

More than all it lays upon the parent the delightful task of providing for the child that atmosphere of protective love in which it will find confidence to face life, free to develop, free to love, free to live without fear, and accepting frustration with good grace.

It is also the gratifying task of the psycho-physician to free the individual whose early conditions have put him under the bondage of fear and release his personality so that it may fulfil its true purpose and functions in life.

Radical analysis is a long and arduous process and every analyst can treat but a few score patients during his lifetime. But if these investigations into the deep-seated causes of behaviour disorders help to solve the problems of human life, these labours will not have been in vain, nor the time ill spent.

*

INDEX

THE END